FIBRINOLYSIS AND THROMBOLYSIS

Edited by **Krasimir Kolev**

Fibrinolysis and Thrombolysis
http://dx.doi.org/10.5772/57039
Edited by Krasimir Kolev

Contributors

Alexi Surette, David Waisman, Giuseppe Filiberto Serraino, Debasish Bhattacharyya, Payel Bhattacharjee, Imre Varju, Krasimir Kolev, Emma Beatriz Casanave, Juan Tentoni, Toshio Saito, Dominic Pepperell, Marie-Christine Morel-Kopp, Christopher Ward, Yutaka Inaba, Yohei Yukizawa, Tomoyuki Saito, Eduardo Fuentes, Luis Guzman, Marcelo Alarcón, Rodrigo Moore-Carrasco, Ivan Palomo

Published by InTech

Janeza Trdine 9, 51000 Rijeka, Croatia

Publishing Process Manager Iva Lipovic

Technical Editor InTech DTP team

Cover InTech Design team

First published May, 2014

Printed in Croatia

Additional hard copies can be obtained from orders@intechopen.com

Fibrinolysis and Thrombolysis, Edited by Krasimir Kolev

p. cm.

ISBN 978-953-51-1265-5

Meet the editor

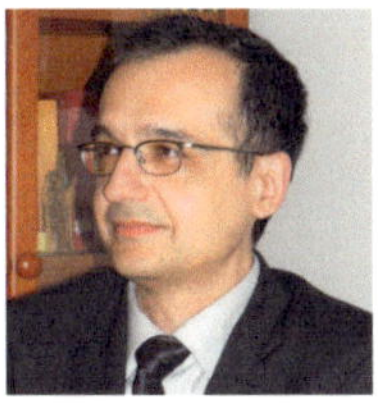

Krasimir Kolev is the head of the Hemostasis Division in the Department of Medical Biochemistry at Semmelweis University, Budapest and president of the Hungarian Society on Thrombosis and Hemostasis. He has published more than 50 original papers and 10 book chapters in the field of fibrinolysis. His early interest was in the enzymology of fibrin resolution focusing on mathematical modelling of the process. Recently his team has described the contribution of red blood cells, shear forces, cellular constituents (DNA, histones, myosin, phospholipids) to the modification of fibrin structure and its mechanical and lytic stability. His work has contributed to the current understanding of the impaired fibrinolysis in antiphospholipid syndrome and the role of various proteases in the pathomechanism of stroke.

Contents

Preface

Can the 21st century bring any news in fibrinolysis?

In the first decades of the 21st century cardio- and cerebrovascular diseases continue to be the leading mortality cause worldwide, being responsible for 23.6 % of the total deaths in the world (WHO statistics, Mortality database. http://apps.who.int/gho/data/node.main.887?lang=en). Thrombolysis targets blood clots, the immediate cause of acute ischemic damage in stroke or myocardial infarction and at present it is based on the administration of plasminogen activators (urokinase, streptokinase, tissue-type plasminogen activator, tPA and its recombinant variants), which convert plasminogen to plasmin, which in turn dissolves fibrin (fibrinolysis), the solid matrix of thrombi. However, thrombolysis often fails and effective doses of plasminogen activators are associated with significant bleeding side effects, often fatal. Furthermore, only a fraction of eligible stroke patients receive treatment (Adams HP Jr, del Zoppo G, Alberts MJ, Bhatt DL, Brass L, Furlan A, Grubb RL, Higashida RT, Jauch EC, Kidwell C, Lyden PD, Morgenstern LB, Qureshi AI, Rosenwasser RH, Scott PA, Wijdicks EF; American Heart Association/American Stroke Association Stroke Council; American Heart Association/American Stroke Association Clinical Cardiology Council; American Heart Association/American Stroke Association Cardiovascular Radiology and Intervention Council; Atherosclerotic Peripheral Vascular Disease Working Group; Quality of Care Outcomes in Research Interdisciplinary Working Group. Guidelines for the early management of adults with ischemic stroke: a guideline from the American Heart Association/American Stroke Association Stroke Council, Clinical Cardiology Council, Cardiovascular Radiology and Intervention Council, and the Atherosclerotic Peripheral Vascular Disease and Quality of Care Outcomes in Research Interdisciplinary Working Groups: The American Academy of Neurology affirms the value of this guideline as an educational tool for neurologists. Circulation. 2007;115(20):e478-534.), due to dangers of bleeding in elderly patients especially. Mechanical percutaneous coronary intervention is the favored treatment for myocardial infarction (Armstrong PW, Gershlick AH, Goldstein P, Wilcox R, Danays T, Lambert Y, Sulimov V, Rosell Ortiz F, Ostojic M, Welsh RC, Carvalho AC, Nanas J, Arntz HR, Halvorsen S, Huber K, Grajek S, Fresco C, Bluhmki E, Regelin A, Vandenberghe K, Bogaerts K, Van de Werf F; STREAM Investigative Team. Fibrinolysis or primary PCI in ST-segment elevation myocardial infarction. N Engl J Med. 2013;368(15):1379-87.), but demands rapid treatment in local specialist centers, otherwise enzymatic thrombolysis remains the recommended reperfusion strategy and thrombolysis is the first-line treatment in ischemic stroke. Hence, there is still a persevering need for improved understanding of the factors that affect fibrinolysis in vivo and novel tools for plasminogen activation and fibrinolysis in coronary and brain arteries. The present book delineates several promising trends in the field that could bring about substantial developments in the theory of thrombolysis and their translational application in the therapeutic practice.

In the introductory chapter Bhattacharjee and Bhattacharyya describe the process of fibrin formation and a variety of factors that modulate fibrin structure (Bhattacharjee P, Bhattacharyya D. An insight into the abnormal fibrin clots: its pathophysiological roles. This book). The authors have selected several pathological conditions to illustrate how abnormal clot structure would affect the stability of fibrin, its susceptibility to lysis. A logical conclusion emerging from the current knowledge about the impact of fibrin structure on the process of clot resolution is that, in addition to the classic plasminogen-dependent fibrinolytic system, novel enzymatic tools (potentially derived from natural sources) may be necessary to overcome the lytic resistance of thrombi in different disease states. A special case of abnormal thrombus structure is discussed by Varjú and Kolev in relation to inflammation (Varjú I, Kolev K. Fibrinolysis at the Interface of Thrombosis and Inflammation: The Role of Neutrophil Extracellular Traps. This book). This chapter summarizes the current state of the role of neutrophil extracellular traps in the modulation of fibrin assembly and the consequences regarding plasminogen activation and plasmin action. Because inflammatory cells infiltrate thrombi, the current data clearly indicate that thrombolysis would greatly benefit from enzymes that target the destruction of the major neutrophil extracellular trap components (DNA, histones).

Surette and Waisman summarize a novel aspect of the pericellular regulation of fibrinolysis through the S100A10, a cell surface protein that co-localizes plasminogen with its activators (Surette AP, Waisman DM. S100A10: A Key Regulator of Fibrinolysis. This book). The endothelial S100A10 participates in intravascular fibrinolysis and thus its modification in hyperhomocysteinemia appears to be a potential mechanism for impaired fibrinolysis in this disease state. In addition, S100A10 represents a new link between fibrinolysis and oncogenesis. It has been identified as a tumor biomarker in human malignancies. Tumor progression and metastasis are probably facilitated through S100A10 dependent plasmin generation.

Animal models are a widely applied tool to study human disease and many important insights into the function of different fibrinolytic proteins have been gained from work with knock-out mice. However, results from such investigations should be treated with due caution in view of essential differences between the human and the animal fibrinolytic systems. The chapter of Casanave and Tentoni provides helpful information in this respect through the discussion of the comparative aspects of the fibrinolytic pathways in vertebrates (Casanave EB, Tentoni J. Comparative vertebrate Fibrinolysis. This book). Alternative natural fibrinolytic products that could expand the repertoire of fibrinolytic agents are discussed by Fuentes and co-workers (Fuentes E, Guzmán L, Alarcón M, Moore R, Palomo I. Thrombolytic/Fibrinolytic Mechanism of Natural Products. This book).

The translational section of the book summarizes several clinical aspects of fibrinolysis. Although routine diagnostic fibrinolytic assays (except for D-dimer) are not widely applied at present, global information on the fibrinolytic state of the patients could have crucial therapeutic and prognostic significance. The chapter of Pepperell, Morel-Kopp and Ward presents a comprehensive overview of the association of the plasma levels of separate fibrinolytic factors and disease states with thrombotic or bleeding trends (Pepperell D, Morel-Kopp MC, Ward C. Clinical Application of Fibrinolytic Assays. This book). The authors focus on the interpretation of two global hemostatic assays (thromboelastography and overall hemostatic potential) in terms of fibrinolysis and highlight their diagnostic value in arterial and venous thrombosis for prediction of recurrent thrombotic events. Inaba, Yukizawa and Saito specify the role of soluble fibrin and plasminogen activator inhibitor-1 determination as a tool for assessment of the individual thrombotic risk in patients undergoing major orthopedic surgery (Inaba Y, Yukizawa Y, Saito T. Coagulation and fibrinolysis markers and their use for the prediction of high risk patients with venous thromboembolism following total hip arthroplasty. This book). In their chapter Serraino and Renzulli call the attention to the significance of correct diagnosis for the success of thrombolytic therapy with the example of primary thrombosis versus fibrous tissue overgrowth in prosthetic valve complications (Serraino GF, Renzulli T. Thrombolysis or Operation: that is the question in prosthetic valve thrombosis. This book). A non-conventional aspect of fibrinolysis is addressed in the chapter of Saito, which summarizes several interesting facts about coagulation and fibrinolysis abnormalities in muscular dystrophy and their involvement in the microcirculation disorder accompanying this disease (Saito T. Coagulation and fibrinolysis abnormalities in patients with muscular dystrophy. This book).

In summary, the present book familiarizes the reader with some recent trends in the theory and practice of thrombolysis. Hopefully, both basic researchers and clinicians will benefit from its content as a source of inspiring ideas for their future work.

Krasimir Kolev
Department of Medical Biochemistry, Semmelweis University,
Budapest, Hungary

Section 1

Thrombolysis: Basic Science

Chapter 1

An Insight into the Abnormal Fibrin Clots — Its Pathophysiological Roles

Payel Bhattacharjee and Debasish Bhattacharyya

Additional information is available at the end of the chapter

http://dx.doi.org/10.5772/57335

1. Introduction

Blood coagulation and its dissolution (thrombolysis) are integrated and highly regulated process to maintain the homeostasis. The mechanism of blood clotting and declotting and the equilibrium between them exclusively depends on an intricate interplay between series of elements – the coagulation factors (mostly proteolytic enzymes), platelet and endothelium [1]. Under normal conditions, tissue factor (TF) is not expressed by cells that are in direct contact with blood. However, TF is exposed to blood following the damage to the endothelial cell wall, where it is free to bind plasma factor VII and initiate the clotting cascade consisting of two separate pathways – 'intrinsic' and 'extrinsic' that ultimately converge on the 'common' pathway and serve to activate prothrombin, the precursor of the enzyme thrombin (factor IIa) by factor Xa [2]. The intrinsic pathway is initiated by the Hageman factor (factor XII) once it binds to the anionic surfaces *e.g.* polyphosphates from platelets or RNA in inflammatory loci [3,4]. A complex of prekallikrein and High Molecular Weight Kininogen (HMWK) also interacts with the exposed surface in close proximity to the bound factor XII and activates it. During activation, the single chain protein of the native factor XII is cleaved into two chains of 50 and 28 kDa that remain linked by a disulphide bond. The light chain of 28 kDa contains the active site and the molecule is referred to as activated factor XIIa, which in turn activates prekallikrein to form kallikrein. The kallikrein thus produced can then also cleave factor XII and a further amplification mechanism is triggered. The factor XIIa remains in close contact with the activating surface and activate factor XI. This step requires Ca^{2+}. At this stage, HMWK, binds to factor XI and facilitates the activation of factor X to form factor Xa [5,6]. The extrinsic system, in contrast to the intrinsic pathway, involves both blood and vascular elements and provides rapid response to tissue injury by generating activated factor X. TF and factor VII are the unique proteins present in this pathway. Once exposed to blood plasma, TF binds rapidly to factor VII which becomes activated to form factor VIIa. Factor VIIa along with Ca^{2+} and a phospholipid rapidly activates factor X forming factor Xa (Figure 1). Factors II, VII, IX, and X are the zymogen forms of vitamin K-dependent serine proteases. Vitamin K is an essential cofactor for post-translational modification of these proteins, in the course of which a carboxyl group is added to the 10 to 12 Glu residues in the amino terminal portion of these proteins. Without this modification, the cell-based coagulation complexes remain unassembled that leads to ineffective clot formation [7].

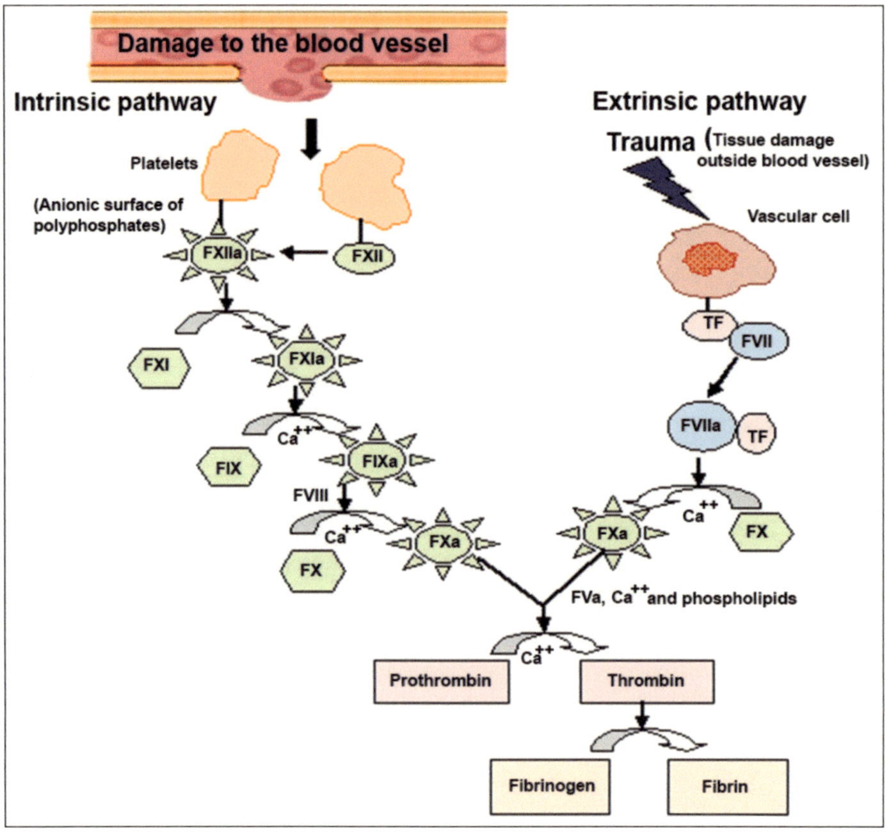

Figure 1. The classical blood coagulation cascade.

2. Formation of fibrin clot

Fibrinogen, a 340 kDa plasma protein, is present at a concentration of 2–4 mg/ml in blood under normal conditions [8]. Composition of fibrinogen, its cleavage by thrombin and subsequent polymerization reactions leading to blood clot are as described in Scheme 1.

http://dx.doi.org/10.5772/57335

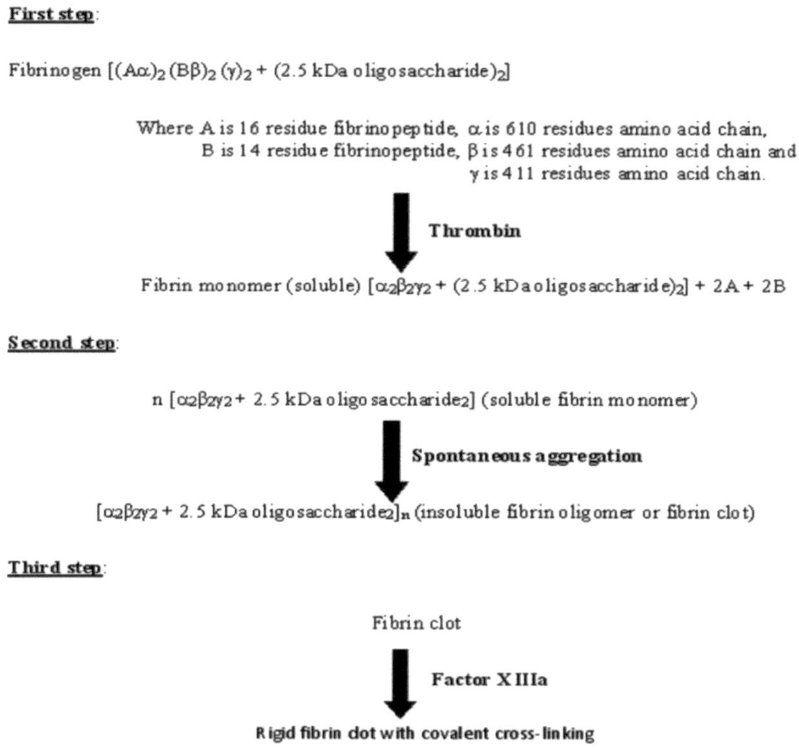

Scheme 1. Steps of fibrin clot formation.

It is noteworthy that unlike an organic chemistry reaction of the type A+B →C, where the structures of A, B and C are defined, Scheme I does not imply that the products of the reactions are chemically and physically homogeneous. The extent of cross-linking, elongation and branching of the fibrils, incorporation of other proteins present in blood plasma *etc* affect the molecular weight, conformation, size and shape, stability and rigidity of the fibril structure. Thus the subsequent steps associated with such reactions may be represented as A+B →C →C_1 → C_2 →C_3 … *etc* together with the simultaneous reactions A+B →C →C_1; C → C_2; C→C_3 …. *etc* or a combination thereof. Further, in case of A+B →C, the rate of formation of C is proportional to the concentrations of A and B. However, with variation of fibrinogen and thrombin concentrations in the presence of other interfering blood components, the rate of formation of different conformers of fibrin also varies. Overall, due to so many variable parameters, the process is rather complex and the products formed are still difficult to predict qualitatively and quantitatively.

For a healthy person, when a clot is formed under normal physiological conditions following the above mentioned steps, it may be considered as normal. However, from a chemical point of view, when any one of the reaction conditions is altered, an abnormal clot is likely to be formed. The interferences may originate from alteration of the concentration of the substrate or corresponding enzyme. In addition, the composition of the reaction medium during the course of the reactions, particularly presence of other biomolecules that interfere, may vary. In either situation, the structure and composition of the products formed may differ significantly. In a diseased condition, the concentration of fibrinogen or thrombin may increase leading to greater accumulation of soluble monomeric form of fibrin [9]. Since the monomeric form of fibrin leads to physically heterogeneous aggregates and the reaction involves bulky macromolecules like proteins, the structure of the product *i.e.* fibrin clot is dependent on the rate of the reaction as well. In other words, unlike the reactions of small organic molecules where the structures of the products are defined and not flexible, structure of fibrin is dependent on the rate of its formation. Further, the process of fibrin aggregation being occurred in a biological environment may recruit other adhering proteins too leading to co-aggregate formation. Thus, whenever the composition of blood differs from normal, the nature and composition of the co-aggregate also differ. The altered structure of fibrin is stabilized in the third step where factor XIIIa enters to form covalent cross links within fibrin clots. If this factor acts favorably, the clot formed will be more stable and hard. The extent of deformation, intramolecular cross linking and incorporation of other proteins in the fibrin structure affect its susceptibility to lysis by plasmin (discussed elaborately later). Usually deformed clots which are resistant to lysis cause medical complications. For a patient, this complication is in addition to those for which normal blood composition is not maintained.

Upon injury, thrombin cleaves off two short peptides from the N-termini of the Aα- and Bβ-chains of fibrinogen, releasing fibrinopeptides A and B, respectively from the center of the fibrinogen molecule, converting it to fibrin monomer, which polymerizes into half-staggered oligomers that lengthen to form ~10 nm wide protofibrils. These protofibrils aggregate laterally to make ~ 100 nm thick fibers. Branching along with lateral and longitudinal growth of fibers leads to the formation of three-dimensional network or gel, which tends to remain localized to the phospholipid-rich sites, *e.g.*, on the surface of activated platelets [10]. Blood clotting factor XIIIa, a plasma transglutaminase specifically cross-links glutamine and lysine residues of adjacent γ- and α-chains of fibrin molecules. These cross-links are formed within and between the protofibrils to stabilize the fibrin gel [11]. The activity of factor XIIIa plays a crucial role at this stage because it determines the stiffness of the clot. In case the clot is too soft, normal pressure of blood flow may break it leading to continuation of bleeding. Alternately, if the clot is too hard, it inhibits the pathway for normal healing of the wound. A serious concern is that the clots may be degraded to clot-lets by the hydrolyzing enzymes and these microemboli[1] enter into the circulation leading to heart attacks and strokes [12]. An optimum degree of cross-linking does not make the fibrin network mechanically very stable rather it can bend where its elasticity is apparent. In a dynamic system, the elasticity offers access of hydrolytic enzymes to the cleavable polypeptide chain of fibrin network [13]. Activation of the clotting cascade subsequently initiates the fibrinolytic cascade that regulates the size of the ultimate clot. Perturbation in this equilibrium due to excess or abnormal thrombus formation may lead to serious pathological problems.

1 When a thrombus detaches from the vessel wall and circulates in the blood.

http://dx.doi.org/10.5772/57335

Based on above discussions, varieties of fibrin clot may be viewed as described in Figure 2. The differences between the clots appear to be the thickness of the fibers and the porosity of the mesh structure that are primary determinants of the action of plasmin. What is hidden is the extent of branching of the chains. All these factors contribute to the elasticity of individual fiber and finally elasticity of the fibrin clot. The elasticity of the clots is an important physical parameter that determines the stability of the clots against the pressure of blood flow. In case the clots are sufficiently elastic, they may get enough time to be degraded by lytic enzymes. Otherwise, clot-lets may form and carried downstream in the blood circulatory system [14].

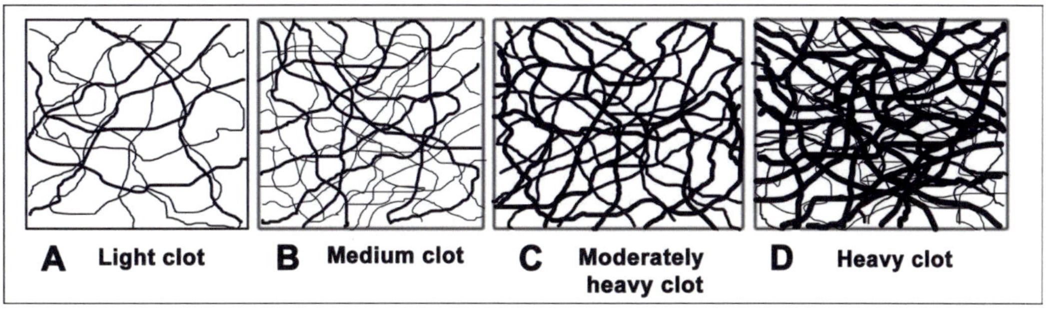

Figure 2. Hypothetical structures of fibrin clot of variable fiber thickness and porosity.

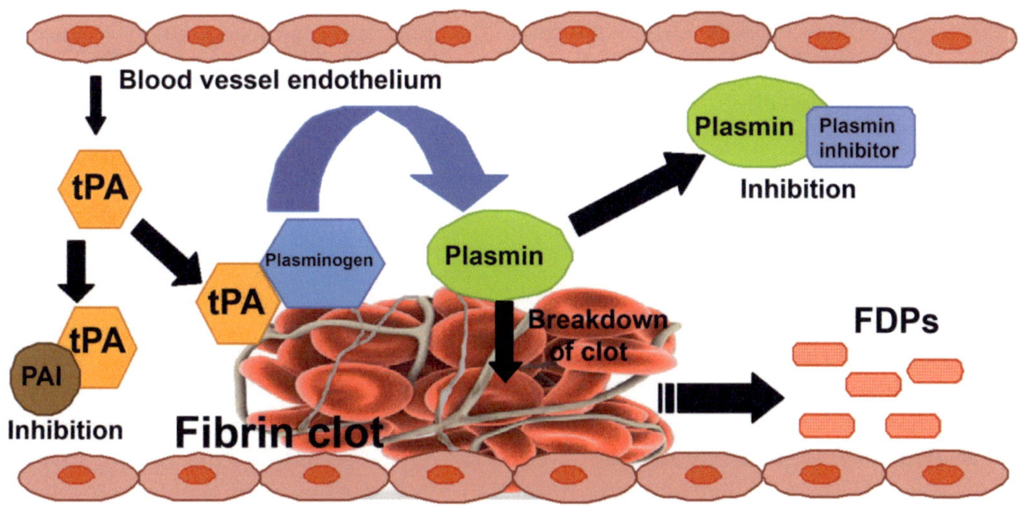

Figure 3. Interplay of enzymes in the process of fibrinolysis. Abbreviations used are FDPs, fibrin degradation products; PAI, plasminogen activator inhibitors; tPA, tissue plasminogen activator.

3. Mechanism of fibrinolysis

When a clot is formed, some mechanism is necessary to limit the clot at the site of injury and ultimately to remove the clot during healing of the injury. Platelet-poor areas of the clot are more prone to fibrinolysis than platelet-rich areas [15]. Fibrin actively regulates its self-dissolution through numerous interactions with fibrinolytic and anti-fibrinolytic components. This pathway consists of plasminogen, a variety of activators and several inhibitors (Figure 3). The 148-160 stretch of residues of the Aα-chain of fibrin becomes exposed and available for plasminogen binding after the conversion of fibrinogen to fibrin. Activation of plasminogen to form plasmin is accomplished either by factor XII-dependent pathway or by plasminogen activators like tissue plasminogen activator (tPA) and urokinase-like plasminogen activator (uPA) [16]. The tPA, which is synthesized primarily by microvascular endothelial cells is most active when attached to fibrin. The affinity for fibrin makes tPA a useful therapeutic agent, since its activity is largely confined to the sites of recent thrombosis [17]. uPA lacks fibrin binding activity, circulates in an inactive single chain form (scu-PA) in plasma and can activate plasmin in the circulation [18]. Plasmin interferes with the fibrin polymerization and initiates cleavage of fibrinogen or soluble fibrin from the C-terminal end of its α-polypeptide chain and gradually forms smaller fragments leading to formation of fibrin degradation products (FDPs) fragments X, Y, D and E in plasma. Cleavage of cross-linked fibrin by plasmin produces degraded products of variable lengths known as X-oligomers, that subsequently degrade into Y, D and E fragments [19]. Elevated levels of FDPs are clinically significant in diagnosing abnormal thrombotic states including Disseminated Intra-Vascular Coagulation (DIC), deep venous thrombosis or pulmonary thromboembolism (described in detail later). The activity of plasmin is tightly regulated to prevent excessive fibrinolysis, which is manifested by a bleeding tendency. Free plasmin rapidly forms a complex with circulating α_2-plasmin inhibitor and is inactivated. Endothelial cells further modulate the coagulation/anticoagulation balance by releasing plasminogen activator inhibitors (PAIs), which block fibrinolysis and confer an overall procoagulation effect. Thrombin also upregulates the expression of uPA and tPA and their inhibitor PAI-1 and regulates fibrinolysis [20].

4. Abnormal fibrin clot

Alteration in fibrin polymerization, heterogeneous fibrillization or unusual structural conformation may lead to the formation of an unstable thrombus. Abnormal fibrin network can make thrombi excessively resistant to degradation or too fragile [21]. Binding of plasminogen to fibrin during fibrinolysis has been reported to be dependent on the fibrin network conformation and fiber diameters. Fibrin fibers are generally intersected laterally rather than by progressive uniform cleavage around the fiber [22]. Clots with a fine fibrin (tight) conformation display a slower lysis than those with a coarse fibrin (loose) conformation, whereas, clots made of thin fibers may be lysed faster than clots having thick fiber. Fibrin network architecture rather than fibrin fiber diameter regulates the distribution or accessibility of fibrinolytic components during the course of fibrinolysis [23]. Longstaff *et al*, (2011) recently showed that accessibility of the clot to fibrinolytic proteins and alterations in binding of tPA and plasminogen were both regulated by fibrin structure [24].

5. Factors affecting formation of abnormal clots

The structure and functions of fibrin clot are determined by genetic and acquired factors. Other parameters such as microgravity, pH, temperature, reducing agents and concentration of chloride and calcium ions may also affect the conversion of fibrinogen to fibrin; *e.g.* calcium stabilizes the structure of fibrinogen, accelerates fibrin formation and can partially protect fibrinogen from degradation. With advancement of space research substantial rise in quantity and quality of manned space flights has provided opportunity for the eventual long-term inhabitation of space, either on stations or other planets. Within space, a variety of altered circumstances including changes in gravitational status, neuro-immunoendocrine modulations, radiation affect the dynamic equilibrium of human body. Traumatic injuries often occur to the astronaut during space travel for which efficient healing is required. Microgravity plays an important role during wound healing. It has been found that fibrin gels formed in such microgravitational condition are more homogeneous than those formed at normal gravity, although the fibre diameter and matrix porosity remain unaltered. Changes in temperature and concentration of proteins like, fibrinogen and thrombin substantially affect fiber diameters and porosity of fibrin clot [9,25,26].

5.1. Genetic factors

Genetic abnormalities in the fibrinogen genes (4q28.1, 4q28.2, and 4q28.3) may cause low levels of fibrinogen in blood, even fibrinogen production may be stopped. It leads to bleeding problems in patients [27]. On the other hand, other genetic abnormalities may lead to the production of fibrinogen molecules with abnormal structure and function which affect the binding of fibrinogen with thrombin, resulting in the defective polymerization of fibrin molecules or fibrinolytic inactivation by plasmin. This condition, known as 'dysfibrinogenaemia', has an autosomal dominant or recessive mode of inheritance [28]. Changes in chromosomes 5, 6, 9, 16 and 17 in which the quantitative trait loci for fibrin structure are located lead to formation of abnormal architechture of clot [29]. A Common fibrinogen Bβ-chain polymorphism, BβArg448Lys, has been shown to affect fibrin structure in plasma clots. Fibrinogen β-chain plays a crucial role in conformational changes in Cα- region and lateral aggregation of fibrin protofibrils. This determines fiber thickness and final ultrastructure of the clot. The location of the BβArg448Lys polymorphism is relatively close to three important areas, the proposed β-chain polymerization site; a β-chain interaction site for the Cα-region and a β-chain calcium-binding site. Thus this polymorphism affects the fibrin structure and rigidity. Recombinant Lys 448 and wild type fibrinogens also showed differences in fibrin structure, both in purified systems and in plasma [30]. The α-chain Thr312Ala polymorphism is associated with formation of thick fibrin fiber with increased cross-linkage, because, this polymorphism lies close to the factor XIIIa cross-linking site at position Aα 328 [31]. Clots produced with a splice variant of γ fibrinogen (γ′ fibrinogen) have thinner fibers, more branching which are more resistant to lysis [32]. Fibrinogen Naples I, is an abnormal fibrinogen with a single base substitution (G to A) in the Bβ-chain gene (Ala68Thr). This polymorphism results in inefficient binding between fibrin and thrombin causing decreased release of fibrinopeptide A and B in both homozygous and heterozygous abnormal fibrinogens. Individuals homozygous for this defect had a severe history of both arterial and venous thrombosis [33]. Most of the plasma glycoproteins have N-linked oligosaccharides attached to the appropriate Asn moieties of the peptide core; for example, fibrinogen contains sialic acid, galactose, mannose, and N-Acetylglucosamine which occurs as a biantennary complex, N-linked to Asn364 of each Bβ and to Asn52 of each γ chain [34]. Six hereditary dysfibrinogens have been reported to have an amino acid substitution that generates an Asn-X-Ser/Thr type sequence containing extra oligosaccharide at an Asn residue with the same biantennary structures found in normal fibrinogen. These are, fibrinogen Pontoise at BβAsn333, Asahi at γAsn308, Lima at AαAsn139, Caracas II at AαAsn434, Niigata at BβAsn158 and Kaiserslautern at γAsn380. Carbohydrate moieties in fibrinogen have been proposed to be involved in the regulation of fibrin assembly and form stable fibrin networks. However the extra-glycosylated dysfibrinogens cause altered fibrin assembly at various stages of fibrin network formation [35].

Factor XIII polymorphisms, *i.e.* G to T transition in codon 34, with subsequent replacement of valine with leucine (factor XIII Val34Leu) is associated with altered fibrin structure [36]. Thrombin activates factor XIII Leu34 more efficiently as compared to Val34. Early activation of factor XIII and presence of high concentrations of fibrinogen result in the formation of less permeable clots with smaller pores, thinner fibers and ineffective cross-linking [37]. 'Dusart syndrome' is a congenital dysfibrinogenemia characterized by reduced plasminogen binding, impaired fibrin-dependent plasminogen activation by tPA and abnormal fibrin polymerization and clot structure. 'Dusart' fibrinogen molecules contain disulfide-linked albumin molecules, most of which are bound in the carboxy-terminal region of the Aα554 [38, 39]. The Factor V Leiden is a single point mutation at position 1691 in exon 10 that cause G to A transition resulting in Glu506Arg substitution. G to A transition at position 20210 of the prothrombin gene results in G20210A prothrombin mutations that elevates the plasma concentration of prothrombin and in turn increases thrombin generation. These two mutations affect clot structure resulting in Venous Thrombo-Embolism (VTE) [40].

5.2. Acquired factors

The acquired risk factors include abnormal concentration of thrombin and factor XIII in plasma, blood flow, platelet activation, oxidative stress, hyperglycemia, hyperhomocysteinemia, medications, cigarette smoking, particulate matters in environment and interaction of fibrin with other proteins, the role of which are discussed in details.

Notably prothrombin concentration plays a major role in regulating fibrin structure as the fiber diameter of fibrin decreases with increasing prothrombin levels [41]. In both purified fibrinogen and plasma-based systems, clots produced with high thrombin concentrations (0.25 U/mL) are characterized by thin fibers that form a network with small pores [9]. Whereas in hemophilia B, reduced thrombin generation is associated with the formation of lysis susceptible to loosely packed fibrin with thick fiber. Recombinant factor VIIa increases the rate of thrombin generation and clot stability [42].

There are controversies regarding the effect of blood flow on the structure and physical properties of blood clot. One study found no effect of flow on fiber diameter, whereas another group reported formation of thick and stiff fibers in the direction of flow, with thinner fibers interconnecting these larger fibers perpendicularly [43-45]. Blood flow also causes location-dependent changes in fibrin structure due to mechanical forces (radial, axial and circumferential) acting on the vessel wall. Thinner fibers with smaller pores that are formed on the surface of thrombi are resistant to lysis with plasmin [46].

Fibrinogen is 20 times more susceptible to oxidation than albumin and may therefore scavenge oxidants and protect other proteins from oxidation [47]. Oxidation of fibrinogen following exposure to oxygen, metals and myeloperoxidase-derived oxidants decreases the rate of clot formation, whereas, exposure of fibrinogen to Fe^{3+} ascorbate promotes clot formation and enhances platelet aggregation [47,48]. Fibrin structure and its lysability are also affected by nitration of two β-chain tyrosines in the fibrinogen molecule [49]. F2-isoprostanes, a marker of oxidative stress, shown to be associated with reduced clot permeability and fibrinolysis in cardiovascular patients [50].

Platelets release proteins at the sites of platelet aggregation that alters the properties of fibrin clot. Increased amounts of platelet factor 4 and PAI-1 contributes to the formation of compact clot structures and impaired fibrin degradation [51]. Polyphosphate, a polymer of 60-100 phosphate residues is a platelet-derived proinflammatory and procoagulant mediator that directly bind and activate factor XII. It affects intrinsic pathway by modulating the fibrinolytic system, factor V activation and fibrin structure. Polyphosphates lead to the formation of tight and thick fibrin aggregates having 3-fold higher turbidity [52]. It also impairs binding of plasminogen and tPA to partially lysed fibrin causing prolonged clot lysis. This process is Ca^{2+} dependent and independent of factor XIII activation [4,53].

Altered fibrin structure in hyperglycemia is attributed to fibrinogen glycation, which interferes with fibrin polymerization, cross-linking by factor XIIIa, tPA and plasminogen binding and production of plasmin. Fibrinogen purified from hyperglycemic patients produces denser and lysis-resistant clots. Treatment with insulin makes this fibrin more permeable as it decreases fibrinogen glycation [54].

Homocysteine (Hcy), a product of methionine metabolism, increases the risk for Coronary Artery Disease (CAD) and thrombosis. The ε-amino group of fibrinogen lysines can be modified by a highly reactive thioester, Hcy thiolactone, which is present in small amounts (0.2 nM) in plasma. Elevated level of Hcy thiolactone introduces free sulfhydryl groups to ten lysine residues in the D- and Cα-regions of fibrinogen that increases the size of the modified amino acid. This modification decreases the ability of fibrin to support tPA-induced plasminogen activation. This results in the formation of fibrin with thinner and more tightly packed fibers leading to increased resistance to fibrinolysis [55,56].

The smoking-related fibrin abnormalities appear to be determined largely by elevated fibrinogen and enhanced oxidative stress. It has been reported that following acute exposure to cigarette smoke, fibrin clots have dense and compact fibers compared to nonsmoking samples [57]. Particulate matter which contained soluble components such as metal ions as well as ultra-fine particles (< 0.22 μm in diameter) has been reported to be capable of causing alterations to fibrin structure and clot permeability in an oxidation-dependent manner [58].

Aspirin (75 mg/day) reversibly increases clot permeability and fiber mass-length ratio up to 65%. *In vitro* model of acetylation of fibrinogen by aspirin showed that acetylation reduced rigidity of clots and enhanced lysis of clot. Aspirin inhibits factor XIII activation and fibrinogen oxidation. Ingestion of 300 mg aspirin increase clot permeability in subjects possessing the Leu34 allele of factor XIII [59,60]. S-nitrosoglutathione (GSNO), a low Mw member of S-nitrosothiols, is an important biological signaling molecule and has been used clinically as an antithrombotic agent. It has been reported to bind to Cα-region of fibrinogen and alters its secondary structure and the kinetics of fibrin polymerization. It also inhibits factor XIIIa activity and fiber cross-linking in a dose-dependent manner. GSNO at higher dose induces abnormal fibrin structures and fibrin agglomerates producing coarse clot networks with decreased fibrin density and increased fiber diameter which are more susceptible to lysis [61]. Fenfluramine (3-trifluoromethyl-*N*-ethylamphetamine), a drug used as a regulator of serotonin has been reported to cause clotting abnormalities [62]. Apart from cholesterol-lowering effects, statins reduce cardiovascular morbidity and mortality by increasing fibrin permeability and shorter lysis time. Quinapril, an angiotensin-converting enzyme inhibitor at 10 mg/day for 1 month can increase clot permeability by decreasing formation of thrombin in CAD patients [63]. Metformin, an oral antidiabetic drug affects the fibrin structure by interfering with fibrin polymerization and reduction of factor XIII-mediated cross-linking that leads to increased lysability [64]. Anticoagulant treatment with vitamin K antagonists, heparins, direct thrombin inhibitors, indirect thrombin inhibitors and direct activated factor X inhibitors affects fibrin structure and physical properties through reduced thrombin generation. This accounts for the formation of less compact and more lysable fibrin [65].

Vascular wall components like proteins (decorin or collagen fragments *etc.*) and glycosaminoglycans (chondroitin sulfate and dermatan sulfate *etc*) entrapped in the fibrin network affect mechanical and chemical stability of fibrin clot. The architecture of the fibrin network is not significantly influenced by the negatively charged glycosmanoglycans, but fully glycosylated decorin, containing the same sugar subunits, modify the fibrin structure. Protein modulators cause faster lysis of the clot, whereas glycosaminoglycans enhance plasmin mediated clot lysis [66].

Several plasma proteins are known to bind to fibrin and change the properties and function of the clot; *e.g.* lipoprotein(a) (Lp(a)) which is structurally similar to plasminogen, can compete with plasminogen for the binding of fibrin and thereby inhibit the formation of plasmin and eventually fibrinolysis. Lp[a] comprises of a heterogenous class of lipoprotein particles having a core of neutral lipids and a protein moiety containing one mole of apoB-100 covalently linked by a di-sulfide bond to one mole of apo[a]. The C-terminal domain of apo[a] containing the catalytic triad, His4350-Asp4393-Ser4481 exhibits a high degree of homology with the serine protease domain of human plasminogen. Apo[a] contains up to 54 kringles, among which, kringles IV and V (KIV and KV) are homologous to plasminogen. Kringles are involved in interactions with small molecules, for example, KIV-5, KIV-8 and KIV-10 have a high binding affinity for lysine, lysine analogs, and fibrin(ogen) [67]. Elevated Lp(a) levels cause formation of thin fibrin fibers with less permeability and reduced susceptibility to fibrinolysis [68]. The fibrin clot is stabilized against tPA-induced fibrinolysis in the presence of 0.6 to 1.0 μM myosin. In the bound form the tPA-cofactor property of myosin is masked and the fibrin-myosin clot starts disassembling at a slower rate through plasmin degradation than the pure fibrin clot. Myosin weakens the interactions of FDPs leading to its polymerization that increased solubility of the partially degraded fibrin-myosin clot [69].

Binding of fibronectin to a fibrin clot is a two step process; non-covalent and reversible binding of fibronectin to fibrin is preceeded by covalent cross-linking by factor XIIIa. Fibronectin contains three domains with fibrin binding affinity. Low-affinity fibrin-binding sites are contained within the C-terminal region and the high-affinity fibrin binding site resides within the NH_2- terminus of the fibronectin molecule. Covalent cross linking between glutamine in fibronectin and the ε-amino group of a lysine residue in the α-chain of fibrin is mediated by factor XIIIa [70] Binding of fibronectin to fibrin upon injury is important for wound healing and tissue repair [71]. Increased concentration of fibronectin in blood causes the fibrin network to have thicker fibers and larger pores and is associated with arterial thrombosis [72]. Other proteins that bind to fibrin includes α_2-plasmin inhibitor, plasminogen activator inhibitor-2 (PAI-2), hepatocyte-derived fibrinogen-related protein-1 (HFREP-1), albumin, fibroblast growth factor-2, vascular endothelial growth factor, interleukin-1b, factor Xa, tissue factor pathway inhibitor, thrombin-activatable fibrinolysis inhibitor (TAFI), von Willebrand factor, thrombospondin, actin, factor V and factor XIII. α_2-plasmin inhibitor, PAI-2, TAFI, von Willebrand factor, thrombospondin, actin and factor V have been reported to cross-link with fibrin via factor XIIIa. Howes *et al*, described the total protein composition of the whole clot and identified proteins that are cross-linked via factor XIIIa [73]; whereas Talens et al, identified eighteen different fibrin clot-bound proteins, which are not cross-linked to fibrin via factor XIIIa [74]. These authors classified eleven out of the eighteen fibrin clot-bound proteins has been classified into three groups related to their function: blood coagulation, protease inhibition and high density lipoprotein (HDL) metabolism. Plasminogen, factor XIII and thrombin are involved in blood coagulation while α_2-macroglobulin and α_1-antitrypsin are protease inhibitors and haptoglobin, serum amyloid P and apolipoproteins A-I, A-IV, J and E are involved in HDL metabolism [74]. β-amyloid 1-42 (Aβ42) peptide may bind to each identical ends of fibrinogen and specifically interacts near the C-terminus of the fibrinogen β-chain and induces oligomerization. Fibrin clots formed in the presence of Aβ42 have abnormal structure and are resistant to degradation by plasmin. This abnormal fibrin co-deposit with Aβ42 and increase neurovascular damage in blood vessels [75]. Figure 4 shows co-aggregation of different plasma proteins with fibrin. When fibrinogen (1.5 μM) was incubated with thrombin (100 μU/ml), it forms a thread like fibrin fibers. Upon incubation with 1 μM of the plasma proteins, the fibrin forms unusually dense network with less porous structure. Fibrin and α-synuclein co-aggregate forms thread-like structure interspersed with dense network. These SEM images of co-aggregates support the previous finding that binding of plasma proteins with fibrin alters its fiber diameter, porosity. The dense clumps of aggregates might show poor lysability.

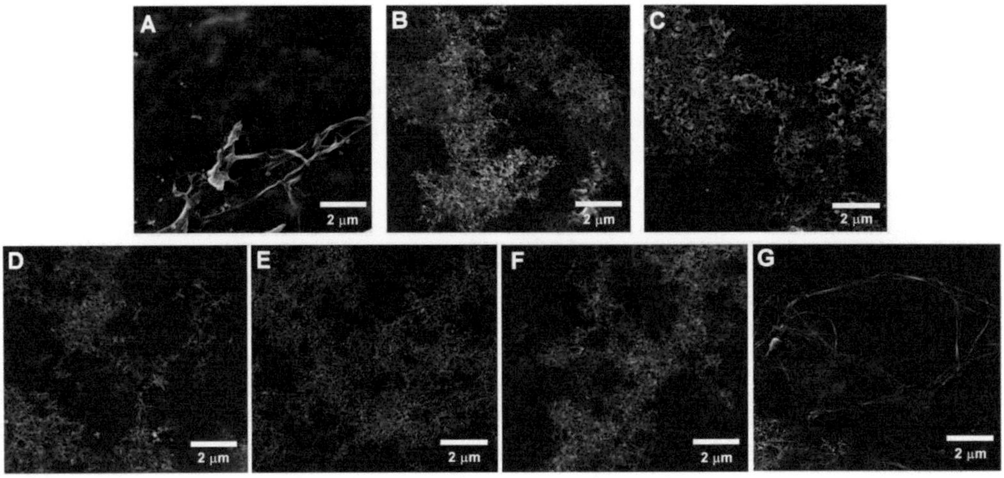

Figure 4. Morphology of abnormal fibrin co-aggregate. A. Normal fibrin network; B. Fibrinogen - fibronectin co-aggregate; C. Fibrinogen- Aβ42 co-aggregate; D. Fibrinogen - transthyretin co-aggregate; E. Fibrinogen - human serum albumin co-aggregate; F. Fibrinogen - lysozyme co-aggregate and G. Fibrinogen-A53T α-synuclein co-aggregate. In these experiments, 1.5 μM fibrinogen was incubated with 100 μU/ml of thrombin (after dilution from bovine thrombin, 1000 NIH Units, Sigma Aldrich, USA) at 37°C for 24 hr to form fibrin clot. The co-aggregate was prepared under identical conditions with 1 μM of the plasma proteins as stated above. Morphological analysis of protein aggregates was done using scanning electron microscope (Model: Vega II LSU, Tescan Digital Microscopy Imaging, Czechoslovakia). The sample (10 μl) was placed on a carbon coated 300-mesh grid for 5 min at 25°C and the unbound substrate was removed by blotting paper. To stain the adhered particles, the grid was treated with 2% uranyl acetate for 20 sec and the excess reagent was removed as stated. The grid was dried under vacuum, sputter coated with gold-palladium alloy and viewed under SEM at 10.0 kV voltages and 20,000 x magnification.

6. Pathophysiological role of abnormal clots

Abnormally structured clots may also generate emboli that can lodge in critical organs, disrupting the blood flow with potentially fatal consequences like liver diseases, ischemic stroke, myocardial infarction, venous thromboembolism, atherothrombotic vascular disease, peripheral artery disease, coronary artery disease, adult respiratory distress syndrome, retinal vein occlusion, end-stage renal disease, acute pancreatitis, rheumatoid arthritis, type 1 and type 2 diabetes and Alzheimer disease.

6.1. Liver diseases

The increased sialic acid content in the oligosaccharide of the abnormal fibrinogen impairs polymerization of fibrin monomers leading to severe dysfibrinogenemia in patients with End Stage Liver Disease (ESLD) [76,77]. Accelerated fibrinolysis is attributed by the impaired clearance of tPA and other fibrinolytic enzymes by the diseased liver, without an appropriate increase in plasminogen activator inhibitors [78]. Impaired hepatic synthesis of fibrinolytic inhibitors like, α_2-plasmin inhibitor and TAFI contributes to increased levels of plasmin. The hemostatic imbalance in ESLD occasionally favors hypercoagulability, predisposing to thrombosis [79].

6.2. Ischemic stroke

Four types of inherited abnormalities of fibrinolysis (plasminogen deficiency, plasminogen activator deficiency, dysfibrinogenemia and factor XII/prekallikrein deficiencies) are related to thrombosis. Fibrin clots were formed more rapidly and had a compact structure composed of thicker fibers and reduced permeability compared to those made from plasma obtained from healthy controls [80].

6.3. Myocardial infarction (MI)

The term myocardial infarction pathologically denotes the death of cardiac myocytes due to extended ischemia. Rupture of the atherosclerotic plaque[2] in an epicardial coronary artery contributes to the activation, adhesion and aggregation of platelets and the production of thrombin, causing subsequent thrombus formation which occludes the vessels and impedes blood flow [81]. Acute MI patients show the tendency to form less permeable and lysable fibrin clots that are composed of thicker fibers [82].

6.4. Venous thromboembolism (VTE)

Forming thrombus inside the vessel (intravascular thrombosis) of the lower extremities and to a lesser extent in the upper extremities may lead to partial or complete blockage of blood flow through this vessel causing a serious pathological problem known as deep vein thrombosis (DVT). When an embolus goes up through the circulation settling in an arterial branch in the lungs, it cause pulmonary embolism (PE). DVT and PE together are called venous thromboembolic disorders (VTE). In addition to abnormalities in the blood coagulation system due to increased thrombin generation, it can be caused by defective plasminogen, tPA deficiency and higher level of TAFI. These indicate enhanced fibrin formation and degradation [83]. Curnow *et al*, 2007 showed that patients with arterial thrombosis, VTE, pregnancy complications or autoimmune diseases have increased fibrin generation and reduced fibrinolysis [84].

6.5. Peripheral arterial disease (PAD)

It results from progressive narrowing of the peripheral arteries, most commonly in the pelvis and legs. In middle-aged and elderly PAD patients, it has been shown that plasma fibrin clots contain thicker fibers and smaller pores, which form more rapidly, but are lysed at a reduced rate, compared with those made from plasma obtained from healthy individuals [16].

---

2 Deposition of a solid substance in the lining of the artery wall leading to hardening of the arteries. The core of the plaque is made of fatty substances, cholesterol, waste products from the cells, calcium, and fibrin, which is separated from arterial bloodstream only by a slender and fragile layer of tissue, the fibrous cap.

6.6. Coronary artery disease (CAD)

It is caused by the narrowing and hardening (atherosclerosis) of arteries which supply blood to the cardiac muscles. In CAD patients, plasma fibrin clots are denser and less permeable than healthy individuals. The fibrin clots with tightly packed, thin fibers and small pores are associated with the number and severity of coronary artery stenoses (diseased arterial tissue) documented by angiography. C reactive protein (CRP) binds to fibrin(ogen) and may alter fibrin network formation, clot permeability and susceptibility to lysis both in healthy and CAD patients [85].

6.7. Adult respiratory distress syndrome (ARDS)

Alveolar fibrin deposition is one of the hallmarks of this syndrome. In ARDS the increased PAI and α_2-plasmin inhibitor levels lead to decreased fibrinolytic activity and increased alveolar fibrin deposition [86]. It appears to contribute to the magnitude of the inflammatory response by virtue of their ability to cleave and degrade products to promote chemotaxis, increase vascular permeability and exert modulatory effects on various immune cells. It also causes lung fibrosis by providing a matrix for macrophage migration and by promoting angiogenesis and collagen deposition [87].

6.8. Rheumatoid arthritis (RA)

During inflammation, the exudation of plasma into joints results in accumulation of high concentration of coagulation factors at the synovial fluid and often accompanied by fibrin deposits. Patients with RA have faster clot formation, higher clot absorbance at 405 nm, indicating presence of thicker fibrin fibers than healthy individuals. Moreover, the clot is less permeable and lysis time is longer. Fibrin deposition is correlated with fibrinogen, tPA, PAI-1, PAI-2, CRP, platelet count and 8-iso-prostaglandin F_2 alpha, an inducer of oxidative stress [88]. Local activation of complement system helps to stabilize fibrin clots thereby decreasing the fibrinolytic potential at the joint. Local production of the regulatory factor C4B-binding protein (C4BP) by rheumatoid synovial fibroblasts as well as its co-localization with fibrin-rich areas at the synovial tissue contributes to fibrin deposition at synovial joints. Fibrin is one of the major substrate for peptidyl deiminases that transform Arg residues into Cit (citrulline)of fibrin and subsequently change its physical properties inside inflamed joints. This modification makes the clot resistant to proteolytic degradation by altering the binding sites for plasmin. Further, the deformity turns the molecule antigenic [89].

6.9. Type 1 and type 2 diabetes

Diabetic patients suffer from persistent hyperglycaemia, which cause protein glycation. Protein glycation generates glycoaldehyde that induces post-translational modification in fibrinogen, which impairs the fibrinolytic process. Decreased binding of tPA and plasminogen to fibrin, reduced plasmin generation on the clot surface and increased cross-linking cause formation of dense, less porous fiber with reduced lysability in diabetic patients as compared to healthy non-diabetic persons [90].

6.10. Retinal vein occlusion (RVO)

Abnormal fibrin clot with poor lysability contribute to the hyperviscosity reported in this disease. Elevated level of CRP, which binds to fibrinogen might be responsible for this abnormality [91].

6.11. End-stage renal disease (ESRD)

In ESRD patients, plasma fibrin clots have reduced permeability, faster protofibril formation, increased fiber size and mass, decreased susceptibility to fibrinolysis, compared with healthy individuals. The plasma concentration of the acute phase protein fibrinogen plays major role in regulating fibrin structure properties. Besides the levels of other acute phase proteins such as orosomucoid, CRP and interleukin 6 (IL-6) have also been reported to affect the tightness and density of plasma clots [50,92,93].

6.12. Alzheimer disease (AD)

Fibrinogen circulates through the brain and spinal cord vasculature without entering the central nervous system (CNS) due to blood brain barrier (BBB) [94,95]. However, in pathological conditions like injury or diseases associated with vascular disruption, infection or inflammation, the concentration of fibrinogen increases beyond its normal limit (2-4 mg/ml) and enters into CNS through disrupted BBB [96]. The synergistic effect of higher fibrinogen level and presence of Aβ peptide produce lysis resistant clots in neurovascular diseases, which contributes to vascular deficiencies, decreased blood flow, increased inflammation and neuronal death leading to higher severity of AD [75]. Aβ can alter fibrinolysis by three independent mechanisms; Aβ intercalates into fibers during formation of fibrin network promoting generation of clots with an abnormally dense fiber network, blocks binding of plasminogen to fibrin and therefore blocks generation of plasmin and finally as a result, alters the rate of plasmin-mediated fibrinolysis [97,98].

7. Role of plasmin

The suitability of a protein as a substrate of a proteolytic enzyme primarily depends on two factors; specificity of the enzyme *i.e.* the peptide bond of the amino acids that the enzyme targets to hydrolyze and accessibility of the hydrolysable bond to the catalytic site of the protease. Thus, mere existence of a proteolytically cleavable bond in the primary amino acid sequence of a protein does not ensure it to be hydrolyzed by a protease until the bond is physically accessed by the catalytic site of the enzyme. Because of this stringency, many proteins can survive proteolysis while maintaining compact configuration of the native state in an environment of proteases whereas the partially or fully denatured state of the same protein is easily degraded by the proteases. Sometimes it also happens that a proteolytically sensitive region of a protein is first cleaved off by a protease followed by complete unraveling of the molecule in a cooperative manner leading to its fragmentation. For large multi-domain proteins, usually the domains are connected by proteolytically sensitive hinge regions. Once the domains are cleaved off, structural integrity of each domain is lost facilitating digestion by the proteases. Therefore, if the peptide bonds of fibrin polymer (clot) that are otherwise hydrolysable by plasmin are no more accessible to the enzyme due to alteration of the structure of the clots, fibrin in its modified form may be partly or completely resistant to plasmin. For example, tighter fibrin networks composed of thin fibers are degraded less efficiently by plasmin than those composed of thick fibers due to two reasons; first, an increased number of fibers to be cleaved and second, decreased porosity of tighter fibrin networks make the fibrinolytic enzymes inaccessible to the hydrolysable bonds [99]. In case the fibrin clot is not constituted of pure fibrinogen rather a copolymer with other protein/s or ligand, the situation becomes even more complicated. The added molecules may sterically protect the hydrolysable bonds of fibrin from the action of plasmin. Taken together, the fibrin clot may be completely resistant to plasmin, *e.g.* Aβ binds to the fibrinogen β-chain near the β-hole, which is in close proximity to residues 148-160 of the Aα-chain and modifies the structure in such a way that it inhibits plasmin to bind the copolymer [98].

In the dissolution of the clots, the substrate (fibrin) is virtually static. It is only the enzyme plasmin that is free in the solution and is capable of searching and recognizing the hydrolysable bonds. From an enzymologist's point of view, these reactions are difficult to take place, slow and are not supposed to follow normal Michaelis-Menten relation of enzyme kinetics. From the above discussion, it is apparent that when dealing with abnormal clots, presence of plasmin may not be limiting. It is the deformation of the structure of the fibrin clot that prevents it from being degraded by plasmin.

8. Prevention and treatment

At present, there are three major classes of medicines to treat patients with a thrombophilic disorders: antiplatelet, anticoagulant and thrombolytic agents. There are several medications that are used to inhibit platelet aggregation through the process by which platelets clump together to plug the injured surface. Among them aspirin, dypyridamole, ticlopidine and clopidogrel are orally administered, glycoprotein IIb/IIIa (GP IIB/IIIA) inhibitors are intravenous (IV) forms, whereas, non-steroidal anti-inflammatory drugs (NSAIDs) are available in either of the forms stated. The anticoagulants, which act through inhibiting or altering steps in the coagulation cascade, include warfarin (Coumadin), heparin *etc*. Thrombolytic medications serve to break up the fibrin clot. This includes streptokinase, uPA, tPA and their recombinant variants. Streptokinase binds with plasminogen and ultimately forms streptokinase and plasmin complexes. These complexes are more efficient than plasmin alone at breaking down a clot. Excessive bleeding is a serious consequence of using these medications [100]. The specific impact of the abnormal fibrin structure on the efficiency of each of these therapeutic agents has not been comprehensively characterized to date.

The activity of fibrinolytic enzymes isolated from natural sources often resembles the activity of plasmin and plasminogen activators [101]. Earthworms have been used in East-Asian traditional folk medicine for thousand years for the antithrombotic effect. Later, Mihara *et al*, 1983 first isolated lumbrokinase (LK), a fibrinolytic enzyme from the *Lumbricus rubellus* (earthworm) [102]. Few fibrinolytic enzymes have been isolated from earthworm *Perionyx excavates*, which show rapid hydrolysis on both coagulated fibrous fibrin and soluble fibrinogen monomers in absence of activators such as tPA or urokinase [103]. Snake venom proteases possess coagulatory and fibrinolytic activities. Fibrino(geno)lytic enzymes have been isolated from the venoms of *Agkistrodon acutus, A. contortrix, A. rhodostoma, A. halys brevicaudus, A. piscivorus piscivorus, A. piscivorus conami* and *Crotalus atrox etc* [104]. Russell's viper (*Daboia russelli russelli*) venom contains a fibrinolytic enzyme that also shows hemorrhagic activity. Exposure to 90°C irreversibly destroys the hemorrhagic activity of this enzyme while its fibrinolytic activity could be restored on cooling [105]. Caffeic acid phenethyl ester (CAPE), a phenolic compound found in honey bee product has been reported to have fibrinolytic activity [106].

Microbial fibrinolytic enzymes have been isolated from bacteria (*e.g. Streptomyces sp, Actinomyce sp etc*), fungi, and algae. Streptokinase and staphylokinase are two well-known plasminogen activators from *Streptococcus hemolyticus* and *Streptococcus aureus*, which have been found to be effective in thrombolytic therapy. Fibrinolytic enzymes have also been purified from fermented products like Japanese natto, Korean Chungkook-Jang soy sauce, dochi, fermented shrimp paste, salt-fermented fish, fermented vegetables, *e.g.* Kimchi and Indonesia soy products, *e.g.* Tempeh [107]. The first commercial fibrinolytic enzyme, nattokinase was purified and characterized from natto, a popular soybean food in Japan, which is fermented by *Bacillus subtilis natto* [108]. Fibrin(ogen)olytic enzymes have been identified from mushrooms like *Pleurotus ostreatus, Armillaria mellea, Tricholoma saponaceum, Cordyceps militaris, Ganoderma lucidum, Fomitella fraxinea, Cordyceps sinensis, Flammulina velutipes, Fusarium sp.* and *Schizophyllum commune* [107].

Antioxidant therapy using vitamin C showed satisfactory result in patients having type 2 diabetes with CAD by regulating the fibrinolytic system [109]. High dosages of vitamin C and vitamin E in combination have been reported to improve endothelial function and decrease plasma levels of PAI-1, von Willebrand factor and PAI-1/tPA ratio in chronic smokers, thereby keeping under control the excessive thrombotic trend in these patients [110]. Astaxanthin, a red pigment carotenoid found in salmons and crustacean species, protects experimental animal models from vascular oxidative damage, hypertension and cerebral thrombosis [111]. It has been found that folic acid, vitamin B6 and vitamin B12 are very effective at lowering homocysteine and thereby prevent thrombosis [112]. Therapeutic approaches using these natural product-derived fibrin(ogen)olytic enzymes and antioxidants showed promising results in both experimental and clinical settings. However, there are no reports regarding the application of these molecules for prevention of abnormal fibrin clot formation.

9. Conclusion

Abnormal blood clots are formed by a variety of reasons leading to variable structures of the clots. Therefore, it is difficult to conceive that they could be treated by a general protocol. Information on this part is scanty. Our ongoing investigations indicate that there are fibrinolytic enzymes from plant and mammalian sources that are capable of efficient degradation of the fibrin-plasma protein co-aggregates (P. Bhattacharjee and D. Bhattacharyya, manuscript to be communicated elsewhere). Whether these enzymes may be upgraded to drugs remains speculative at this stage. We have a feeling that remedies for combating abnormal clots will be available from natural sources in due course.

Acknowledgements

P.B. is a University Grants Commission – National Eligibility Test senior research fellow. Mr T. Muruganandan of this institute assisted in scanning electron microscopy. The publication was supported by CSIR- Network Project (miND BSC 0115).

Author details

Payel Bhattacharjee and Debasish Bhattacharyya*

*Address all correspondence to: debasish@iicb.res.in

Division of Structural Biology and Bioinformatics, CSIR-Indian Institute of Chemical Biology, Kolkata, India

References

[1] Lefkowitz JB. Coagulation Pathway and Physiology. In: Hemostasis Physiology. JB Lippincott Co, Philadelphia, PA. 2006. p3-12.

[2] Butenas S., Mann KG. Active tissue factor in blood. Nature Medicine 2004; 10(11) 1155-1156.

[3] Kannemeier C., Shibamiya A., Nakazawa F., Trusheim H., Ruppert C., Markart P., Song Y., Tzima E., Kennerknecht E., Niepmann M., von Bruehl M-L., Sedding D., Massberg S., Gu°nther A., Engelmann B., Preissner KT. Extracellular RNA constitutes a natural procoagulant cofactor in blood coagulation. Proceedings of the National Academy of Sciences USA 2007; 104(15) 6388–6393.

[4] Müller F., Mutch NJ., Schenk WA., Smith SA., Esterl L., Spronk HM., Schmidbauer S., Gahl WA., Morrissey JH., Renné T. Platelet polyphosphates are proinflammatory and procoagulant mediators in vivo. Cell 2009; 139(6) 1143–1156.

[5] Colman RW., Clowes AW., George JN., Goldhaber SZ., Marder VJ. Overview of hemostasis. In: Hemostasis and Thrombosis: Basic Principles and Clinical Practice. 5th ed. JB Lippincott Co, Philadelphia, PA. 2006. p3-16.

[6] Hoffman M. Remodeling the blood coagulation cascade. Journal of Thrombosis and Thrombolysis 2003; 16, 17-20.

[7] Butenas S., Orfeo T., Brummel-Ziedins KE., Mann KG. Tissue factor in thrombosis and hemorrhage. Surgery 2007; 142, 2-14.

[8] Weigandt KM., White N., Chung D., Ellingson E., Wang Y., Fu X., Pozzo DC. Fibrin Clot Structure and Mechanics Associated with Specific Oxidation of Methionine Residues in Fibrinogen. Biophysical Journal 2012; 103(11) 2399–2407.

[9] Wolberg AS., Campbell RA. Thrombin generation, fibrin clot formation and hemostasis. Transfusion and Apheresis Science 2008; 38(1) 15–23.

[10] Ferry JD., Morrison PR. Preparation and properties of serum and plasma proteins. VIII. The conversion of human fibrinogen to fibrin under various conditions. Journal of American Chemical Society 1947; 69(2) 388–400.

[11] Ariëns RAS., Lai TS., Weisel JW., Greenberg CS., Grant PJ. Role of factor XIII in fibrin clot formation and effects of genetic polymorphisms. Blood 2002; 100(3) 743-754.

[12] Collet J-P., Lesty C., Montalescot G., Weisel JW. Dynamic Changes of fibrin architecture during fibrin formation and intrinsic fibrinolysis of fibrin-rich clots. Journal of Biological Chemistry 2003; 278(24) 21331-21335.

[13] Collet J-P., Shuman H., Ledger RE., Lee S., Weisel JW. The elasticity of an individual fibrin fiber in a clot. Proceedings of the National Academy of Sciences USA 2005; 102(26) 9133-9137.

[14] Weisel JW. Structure of fibrin: impact on clot stability. Journal of Thrombosis and Haemostasis 2007; 5, 116–124.

[15] Collet J-P., Montalescot G., Lesty C., Weisel JW. A structural and dynamic investigation of the facilitating effect of glycoprotein IIb/IIIa inhibitors in dissolving platelet-rich clots. Circulation Research 2002; 90(4) 428-434.

[16] Undas A., Nowakowski T., Cieœla-Dul M., Sadowski J. Abnormal plasma fibrin clot characteristics are associated with worse clinical outcome in patients with peripheral arterial disease and thrombangiitis obliterans. Atherosclerosis 2011; 215(2) 481–486.

[17] Kooistra T., Schrauwen Y., Arts J., Emeis JJ. Regulation of endothelial cell tPA synthesis and release. International Journal of Hematology 1994; 59(4) 233-255.

[18] Wojta J., Hoover RL., Daniel TO. Vascular origin determines plasminogen activator expression in human endothelial cells. Renal endothelial cells produce large amounts of single chain urokinase type plasminogen activator. Journal of Biological Chemistry 1989; 264(5) 2846-2852.

[19] Gaffney PJ. Breakdown products of fibrin and fibrinogen: molecular mechanisms and clinical implications. Journal of Clinical Pathology 1980; 33, 10-17.

[20] Carpenter SL., Mathew P. Alpha2-antiplasmin and its deficiency: fibrinolysis out of balance. Haemophilia 2008; 14(6) 1250-1254.

[21] Kim E., Kim OV., Machlus KR., Liu X., Kupaev T., Lioi J., Wolberg AS., Chen DZ., Rosen ED., Xua Z., Alber M. Correlation between fibrin network structure and mechanical properties: an experimental and computational analysis. Soft Matter 2011; 7, 4983-4992.

[22] Diamond SL. Engineering design of optimal strategies for blood clot dissolution. Annual Review of Biomedical Engineering 1999; 1, 427-462.

[23] Collet J-P., Park D., Lesty C., Soria J., Soria C., Montalescot G., Weisel JW. Influence of fibrin network conformation and fibrin fiber diameter on fibrinolysis speed: dynamic and structural approaches by confocal microscopy. Arterial thrombosis and vascular biology 2000; 20(5) 1354-1361.

[24] Longstaff C., Thelwell C., Williams SC., Silva MM., Szabó L., Kolev K. The interplay between tissue plasminogen activator domains and fibrin structures in the regulation of fibrinolysis: kinetic and microscopic studies. Blood 2011; 117(2) 661-668.

[25] Farahani RM., DiPietro LA. Microgravity and the implications for wound healing. International Wound Journal 2008; 5(4) 552–561.

[26] Nunes CR., Roedersheimer MT., Simske SJ., Luttges MW. Effect of microgravity, temperature, and concentration on fibrin and collagen assembly. Microgravity Science and Technology 1995; 8(2) 125-130.

[27] Kant JA., Fornace AJ., Saxe D., Simon MI., McBride OW., Crabtree GR. Evolution and organization of the fibrinogen locus on chromosome 4: gene duplication accompanied by transposition and inversion. Proceedings of the National Academy of Sciences USA 1985; 82(8) 2344-2348.

[28] Acharya SS., Dimichele DM. Rare inherited disorders of fibrinogen. Haemophilia 2008; 14(6) 1151-1158.

[29] Williams FM., Carter AM., Kato B., Falchi M., Bathum L., Surdulescu G., Kyvik KO., Palotie A., Spector TD., Grant PJ. Identification of quantitative trait loci for fibrin clot phenotypes: the EuroCLOT study. Arteriosclerosis, Thrombosis, and Vascular Biology 2009; 29(4) 600–605.

[30] Ajjan R., Lim BCB., Standeven KF., Harrand R., Dolling S., Phoenix F., Greaves R., Abou-Saleh RH., Connell S., Smith DAM., Weisel JW., Grant PJ., Ariens RAS. Com-

mon variation in the C-terminal region of the fibrinogen β-chain: effects on fibrin structure, fibrinolysis and clot rigidity. Blood 2008; 111(2) 643-650.

[31] Carter AM., Catto AJ., Grant PJ. Association of the α-fibrinogen Thr312Ala polymorphism with poststroke mortality in subjects with arterial fibrillation. Circulation 1999; 99(18) 2423-2426.

[32] Pieters M., Kotze RC., Jerling JC., Kruger A., Ariëns RAS. Evidence that fibrinogen γ′ regulates plasma clot structure and lysis and relationship to cardiovascular risk factors in black Africans. Blood 2013; 121(16) 3254-3260.

[33] Koopman J., Haverkate F., Lord ST., Grimbergen J., Mannucci PM. Molecular basis of fibrinogen Naples associated with defective thrombin binding and thrombophilia. Homozygous substitution of B beta 68 Ala----Thr. Journal of Clinical Investigation 1992; 90(1) 238-244.

[34] Langer BG., Weisel JW., Dinauer PA., Nagaswarni C., Bell WR. Deglycosylation of fibrinogen accelerates polymerization and increases lateral aggregation of fibrin fiber. Journal of Biological Chemistry 1988; 263(29) 15056-15063.

[35] Sugo T., Nakamikawa C., Takano H., Mimuro J., Yamaguchi S., Mosesson MW., Meh DA., DiOrio JP., Takahashi N., Takahashi H., Nagai K., Matsuda M. Fibrinogen Niigata with impaired fibrin assembly: an inherited dysfibrinogen with a Bβ Asn-160 to Ser substitution associated with extra glycosylation at Bβ Asn-158. Blood 1999; 94(11) 3806-3813.

[36] Hancer VS., Diz-Kucukkaya R., Bilge AK., Ozben B., Oncul A., Ergen G., Nalcaci M. The association between factor XIII Val34Leu polymorphism and early myocardial infarction. Circulation Journal 2006; 70(3) 239-242.

[37] Ariëns RAS., Philippou H., Chandrasekaran N., Weisel JW., Lane DA., Grant PJ. The factor XIII V34L polymorphism accelerates thrombin activation of factor XIII and affects cross-linked fibrin structure. Blood 2000; 96(3) 988-995.

[38] Collet J-P., Soria J., Mirshahi M., Hirsch M., Dagonnet FB., Caen J., Soria C. Dusart syndrome: a new concept of the relationship between fibrin clot architecture and fibrin clot degradability: hypofibrinolysis related to an abnormal clot structure. Blood 1993; 82(8) 2462-2469.

[39] Mosesson MW., Siebenlist KR., Hainfeld JF., Wall JS., Soria J., Soria C., Caen JP. The relationship between the fibrinogen D domain self-association/cross-linking site (gammaXL) and the fibrinogen Dusart abnormality (Aα R554C-Albumin) clues to thrombophilia in the "Dusart Syndrome". Journal of Clinical Investigation 1996; 97(10) 2342–2350.

[40] Abdullah WZ., Kumaraguru S., Ghazali S., Yusoff NM. Factor V Leiden and prothrombin G20210A mutations among healthy Indians in Malaysia. Lab Medicine 2010; 41, 284-287.

[41] Wolberg AS. Thrombin generation and fibrin clot structure. Blood Review 2007; 21(3) 131–142.

[42] Wolberg AS., Allen GA., Monroe DM., Hedner U., Roberts HR., Hoffman M. High dose factor VIIa enhances clot stability in a model of hemophilia B. British Journal of Haematology 2005; 131(5) 645–55.

[43] Gersh KC., Edmondson KE., Weisel JW. Flow rate and fibrin fiber alignment. Journal of Thrombosis and Haemostasis 2010; 8(12) 2826–2828.

[44] Neeves KB., Illing DA., Diamond SL. Thrombin flux and wall shear rate regulate fibrin fiber deposition state during polymerization under flow. Biophysical Journal 2010; 98(7) 1344-1352.

[45] Weisel JW., Litvinov RI. Mechanisms of fibrin polymerization and clinical implications. Blood 2013; 121(10) 1712-1719.

[46] Varju′ I., So′ tonyi P., Machovich R., Szabo′ L., Tenekedjiev K., Silva MMCG., Longstaff C., Kolev K. Hindered dissolution of fibrin formed under mechanical stress. Journal of Thrombosis and Haemostasis 2011; 9(5) 979–986.

[47] Olinescu R., Kummerow F. Fibrinogen as an efficient antioxidant. Journal of Nutritional Biochemistry 2001; 12(3) 162–169.

[48] Feng YH., Hart G. In vitro oxidative damage to tissue-type plasminogen activator: a selective modification of the biological functions. Cardiovascular Research 1995; 30(2) 255–261.

[49] Parastatidis I., Thomson L., Burke A., Chernysh I., Nagaswami C., Visser J., Stamer S., Liebler DC., Koliakos G., Heijnen HF., Fitzgerald GA., Weisel JW., Ischiropoulos H. Fibrinogen β-chain tyrosine nitration is a prothrombotic risk factor. Journal of Biological Chemistry 2008; 283(49) 33846–33853.

[50] Undas A., Kolarz M., Kopec G., Tracz W. Altered fibrin clot properties in patients on long-term haemodialysis: relation to cardiovascular mortality. Nephrology Dialysis Transplantation 2008; 23(6) 2010–2015.

[51] Undas A., Ariëns RAS. Fibrin clot structure and function: a role in the pathophysiology of arterial and venous thromboembolic diseases. Arteriosclerosis, Thrombosis and Vascular Biology 2011; 31(12) e88-e99.

[52] Smith SA., Morrissey JH. Polyphosphate enhances fibrin clot structure. Blood 2008; 112(7) 2810–2816.

[53] Smith SA., Mutch NJ., Baskar D., Rohloff P., Docampo R., Morrissey JH. Polyphosphate modulates blood coagulation and fibrinolysis. Proceedings of the National Academy of Sciences USA 2006; 103(4) 903–908.

[54] Pieters M., Covic N., van der Westhuizen FH., Nagaswami C., Baras Y., Toit Loots D., Jerling JC., Elgar D., Edmondson KS., van Zyl DG., Rheeder P., Weisel JW. Glycaemic

control improves fibrin network characteristics in type 2 diabetes - a purified fibrinogen model. Thrombosis and Haemostasis 2008; 99(4) 691-700.

[55] Sauls DL., Wolberg AS., Hoffman M. Elevated plasma homocysteine leads to alteration in fibrin clot structure and stability: implications for the mechanism of thrombosis in hyperhomocysteinemia. Journal of Thrombosis and Haemostasis 2003; 1(2) 300–306.

[56] Sauls DL., Lockhart E., Warren ME., Lenkowski A., Wilhelm SE., Hoffman M. Modification of fibrinogen by homocysteine thiolactone increases resistance to fibrinolysis: a potential mechanism of the thrombotic tendency in hyperhomocysteinemia. Biochemistry 2006; 45(8) 2480–2487.

[57] Barua RS., Sy F., Srikanth S., Huang G., Javed U., Buhari C., Margosan D., Ambrose JA. Effects of cigarette smoke exposure on clot dynamics and fibrin structure: an ex vivo investigation. Arteriosclerosis, Thrombosis, and Vascular Biology 2010; 30(1) 75–79.

[58] Metassan S., Ariëns RAS., Scott DJ., Routledge MN. Changes to the structure of blood clots formed in the presence of fine particulate matter. Journal of Physics 2009; 151, 1-7.

[59] Williams S., Fatah K., Hjemdahl P., Blombäck M. Better increase in fibrin gel porosity by low dose than intermediate dose acetylsalicylic acid. European Heart Journal 1998; 19(11) 1666–1672.

[60] Undas A., Brummel-Ziedins KE., Mann KG. Antithrombotic properties of aspirin and resistance to aspirin: beyond strictly antiplatelet actions. Blood 2007; 109(6) 2285-2292.

[61] Bateman RM. Ellis CG., Suematsu M., Walley KR. S-Nitrosoglutathione Acts as a Small Molecule Modulator of Human Fibrin Clot Architecture. PloS One 2012; 7(8) e43660.

[62] Carr ME., Carr SL., Martin EJ., Johnson BA. Rapid clot formation and abnormal fibrin structure in a symptomatic patient taking fenfluramine--a case report. Angiology 2001; 52(5) 361-366.

[63] Undas A., Celinska-Lowenhoff M., Lowenhoff T., Szczeklik A. Statins, fenofibrate, and quinapril increase clot permeability and enhance fibrinolysis in patients with coronary artery disease. Journal of Thrombosis and Haemostasis 2006; 4(5) 1029–1036.

[64] Standeven KF., Ariëns RAS., Whitaker P., Ashcroft AE., Weisel JW., Grant PJ. The effect of dimethylbiguanide on thrombin activity, FXIII activation, fibrin polymerization, and fibrin clot formation. Diabetes 2002; 51(1) 189–197.

[65] Blombäck M., He S., Bark N., Wallen HN., Elg M. Effects on fibrin network porosity of anticoagulants with different modes of action and reversal by activated coagulation factor concentrate. British Journal of Haematology 2011; 152(6) 758–765.

[66] Rottenberger Z., Komorowicz E., Szab o L., B ota A., Varga Z., Machovich R., Longstaff C., Kolev K. Lytic and mechanical stability of clots composed of fibrin and blood vessel wall components. Journal of Thrombosis and Haemostasis 2013; 11(3) 529–538.

[67] Scanu AM., Edelstein C. Learning about the structure and biology of human lipoprotein [a] through dissection by enzymes of the elastase family: facts and speculations. Journal of Lipid Research 1997; 38(11) 2193-2206.

[68] Undas A., Stepien E., Tracz W., Szczeklik A. Lipoprotein(a) as a modifier of fibrin clot permeability and susceptibility to lysis. Journal of Thrombosis and Haemostasis 2006; 4(5) 973–975.

[69] Kolev K., Tenekedjiev K., Ajtai K., Kovalszky I., Gombás J., Váradi B., Machovich R. Myosin: a noncovalent stabilizer of fibrin in the process of clot dissolution. Blood 2003; 101(11) 4380-4386.

[70] Corbett SA., Lee L., Wilson CL., Schwarzbauer JE. Covalent Cross-linking of Fibronectin to Fibrin Is Required for Maximal Cell Adhesion to a Fibronectin-Fibrin Matrix. Journal of Biological Chemistry 1997; 272(40) 24999-25005.

[71] Makogonenko E., Tsurupa G., Ingham K., Medved L. Interaction of fibrin(ogen) with fibronectin: further characterization and localization of the fibronectin-binding site. Biochemistry 2002; 41(25) 7907-7913.

[72] Weisel JW. Fibrinogen and fibrin. In: Fibrous Proteins: Coiled-coils, collagen and elastomers. Advances in Protein Chemistry 2005; 70, 248-285.

[73] Howes J-M., Keen JN., Findlay JB., Carter AM. The application of proteomics technology to thrombosis research: the identification of potential therapeutic targets in cardiovascular disease. Diabetes and Vascular Disease Research 2008; 5(3) 205–212.

[74] Talens S., Leebeek FWG., Demmers JAA., Rijken DC. Identification of fibrin clot-bound plasma proteins. PloS One 2012; 7(8) e41966.

[75] Ahn HJ., Zamolodchikov D., Cortes-Canteli M., Norris Sidney EH., Glickman JF., Strickland S. Alzheimer's disease peptide β-amyloid interacts with fibrinogen and induces its oligomerization. Proceedings of the National Academy of Sciences USA 2010; 107(50) 21812–21817.

[76] Roberts HR., Stinchcombe TE., Gabriel DA. The dysfibrinogenaemias. British Journal of Haematology 2001; 114(2) 249–257.

[77] Kujovich JL. Hemostatic defects in end stage liver disease. Critical Care Clinics 2005; 21(3) 563–587.

[78] Fletcher AP., Biederman O., Moore D., Alkjaersig N., Sherry S. Abnormal plasminogen-plasmin system activity (fibrinolysis) in patients with hepatic cirrhosis: its cause and consequences. Journal of Clinical Investigation 1964; 43(4) 681–695.

[79] Lisman T., Leebeek FW., Mosnier LO., Bouma BN., Meijers JC., Janssen HL., Nieuwenhuis HK., De Groot PG. Thrombin-activatable fibrinolysis inhibitor deficiency in cirrhosis is not associated with increased plasma fibrinolysis. Gastroenterology 2001; 121(1) 131–139.

[80] Undas A., Podolec P., Zawilska K., Pieculewicz M., Jedliński I., Stępień E., Konarska-Kuszewska E., Węglarz P., Duszyńska M., Hanschke E., Przewłocki T., Tracz W. Altered fibrin clot structure/function as a novel risk factor for cryptogenic ischemic stroke. Stroke 2009; 40, 1499-1501.

[81] Gutstein DE., Fuster V. Pathophysiology and clinical significance of atherosclerotic plaque rupture. Cardiovascular Research 1999; 41(2) 323-333.

[82] Undas A., Szuldrzynski K., Stepien E., Zalewski J., Godlewski J., Tracz W., Pasowicz M., Zmudka K. Reduced clot permeability and susceptibility to lysis in patients with acute coronary syndrome: effects of inflammation and oxidative stress. Atherosclerosis 2007; 196(2) 551-558.

[83] Undas A., Zawilska K., Ciesla-Dul M., Lehmann-Kopydłowska A., Skubiszak A., Ciepłuch K., Tracz W. Altered fibrin clot structure/function in patients with idiopathic venous thromboembolism and in their relatives. Blood 2009; 114(19) 4272-4278.

[84] Curnow JL., Morel-Kopp MC., Roddie C., Aboud M., Ward CM. Reduced fibrinolysis and increased fibrin generation can be detected in hypercoagulable patients using the overall hemostatic potential assay. Journal of Thrombosis and Haemostasis 2007; 5(3) 528-534.

[85] Undas A., Plicner D., Stepien E., Drwila R., Sadowski J. Altered fibrin clot structure in patients with advanced coronary artery disease: a role of C-reactive protein, lipoprotein(a), and homocysteine. Journal of Thrombosis and Haemostasis 2007; 5(9) 1988–1990.

[86] Idell S., Peters J., James KK., Fair DS., Coalson JJ. Local abnormalities of coagulation and fibrinolytic pathways that promote alveolar fibrin deposition in the lungs of baboons with diffuse alveolar damage. Journal of Clinical Investigation 1989; 84(1) 181-193.

[87] Fan J., Kapus A., Li YH., Rizoli S., Marshall JC., Rotstein OD. Priming for enhanced alveolar fibrin deposition after hemorrhagic shock. American Journal of Respiratory Cell and Molecular Biology 2000; 22(4) 412-421.

[88] Kwasny-Krochin B., Gluszko P., Undas A. Unfavorably altered fibrin clot properties in patients with active rheumatoid arthritis. Thrombosis Research 2010; 126(1) e11-16.

[89] Sanchez-Pernaute O., Filkova M., Gabucio A., Klein M., Maciejewska-Rodrigues H., Ospelt C., Brentano F., Michel BA., Gay RE., Herrero-Beaumont G., Gay S., Neidhart M., Juengel A. Citrullination enhances the pro-inflammatory response to fibrin in rheumatoid arthritis synovial fibroblasts. Annals of the Rheumatic Diseases 2013; 72(8) 1400-1406.

[90] Alzahrani SH., Ajjan RA. Coagulation and fibrinolysis in diabetes. Diabetes and Vascular Disease Research 2010; 7(4) 260-273.

[91] Karska-Basta I., Kubicka-Trza̧ska A., Romanowska-Dixon B., Undas A. Altered fibrin clot properties in patients with retinal vein occlusion. Journal of Thrombosis and Haemostasis 2011; 9(12) 2513–2515.

[92] Fatah K., Hamsten A., Blombäck B., Blombäck M. Fibrin gel network characteristics and coronary heart disease: relations to plasma fibrinogen concentration, acute phase protein, serum lipoproteins and coronary atherosclerosis. Thrombosis Haemostasis 1992; 68(2) 130-135.

[93] Stenvinkel P., Alvestrand A. Inflammation in end-stage renal disease: sources, consequences and therapy. Seminars in Dialysis 2002; 15(5) 329-337.

[94] Davalos D., Akassoglou K. Fibrinogen as a key regulator of inflammation in disease. Seminars in Immunopathology 2012; 34(1) 43-62.

[95] Tennent GA., Brennan SO., Stangou AJ., O'Grady J., Hawkins PN., Pepys MB. Human plasma fibrinogen is synthesized in the liver. Blood 2007; 109(5) 1971–1974.

[96] Adams RA., Passino M., Sachs BD., Nuriel T., Akassoglou K. Fibrin mechanisms and functions in nervous system pathology. Molecular Interventions 2004; 4(3) 163–176.

[97] Cortes-Canteli M., Zamolodchikov D., Ahn HJ., Strickland S., Norris EH. Fibrinogen and altered hemostasis in Alzheimer's disease. Journal of Alzheimer's Disease 2012; 32(3) 599–608.

[98] Zamolodchikov D., Strickland S. Aβ delays fibrin clot lysis by altering fibrin structure and attenuating plasminogen binding to fibrin. Blood 2012; 119(14) 3342-3351.

[99] Lord, ST. Molecular mechanisms affecting fibrin structure and stability. Arteriosclerosis, Thrombosis, and Vascular Biology 2011; 31(3) 494-499.

[100] Fedan JS. Anticoagulant, antiplatelet, and fibrinolytic (thrombolytic) drugs. In: Modern pharmacology with clinical applications, 6th ed. Craig CR, Stitzel RE (Eds.), Lippincott Williams & Wilkins, Philadelphia, USA; 2003. p269-278.

[101] Kotb E. Fibrinolytic bacterial enzymes with thrombolytic activity, Springer Briefs in Microbiology, NY, U.S.A; 2012. p1-74.

[102] Mihara H., Sumi H., Akazawa K. Fibrinolytic enzyme extracted from the earthworm. Thrombosis and Haemostasis 1983; 50, 258-263.

[103] Phan TTB., Ta TD., Nguyen DTX., Van Den Broek LAM., Duong GTH. Purification and characterization of novel fibrinolytic proteases as potential antithrombotic agents from earthworm Perionyx excavates. AMB Express 2011; 1(1) 1-11.

[104] Lu C-L., Chen S-N. Fibrinolytic enzymes from medicinal mushrooms. In Protein Structure, Eshel Faraggi (Ed.), Rijeka, InTech, Croatia; 2012. p 978-953.

[105] Maity G., Mandal S., Bhattacharjee P., Bhattacharyya D. Thermal detoxification of the venom from Daboia russelli russelli of Eastern India with restoration of fibrinolytic activity. Toxicon 2011; 57(5) 747-754.

[106] Abuzar ME., Rosline H., Zamzuri I., Zulkifli MM., Wan-Arfah N., Zaidah AN. Fibrinolytic activity of caffeic acid phenethyl ester (CAPE): in vitro study on whole blood clot. International Journal of Pharmacy and Pharmaceutical Sciences 2013; 5, 459-462.

[107] Peng Y., Yang X., Zhang Y. Microbial fibrinolytic enzymes: an overview of source, production, properties, and thrombolytic activity in vivo. Applied Microbiology and Biotechnology 2005; 69(2) 126-132.

[108] Fujita M., Nomura K., Hong K., Ito Y., Asada A., Nishimuro S. Purification and characterization of a strong fibrinolytic enzyme (nattokinase) in the vegetable cheese natto, a popular soybean fermented food in Japan. Biochemical and Biophysical Research Communications 1993; 197(3) 1340–1347.

[109] Tousoulis D., Antoniades C., Tountas C., Bosinkou E., Kotsopoulou M., Toutouzas P., Stefanadis C. Vitamin C affects thrombosis/fibrinolysis system and reactive hyperemia patients with type 2 diabetes and coronary artery diseases. Diabetes Care 2003; 26(10) 2749-2753.

[110] Antoniades C., Tousoulis D., Tentolouris C., Toutouza M., Marinou K., Goumas G., Tsioufis C., Toutouzas P., Stefanadis C. Effects of antioxidant vitamins C and E on endothelial function and thrombosis/fibrinolysis system in smokers. Thrombosis and Haemostasis 2003; 89(6) 990-995.

[111] Sasakia Y., Kobaraa N., Higashinoa S., Giddingsb JC., Yamamotoa J. Astaxanthin inhibits thrombosis in cerebral vessels of stroke-prone spontaneously hypertensive rats. Nutrition Research 2011; 31(10) 784–789.

[112] de Jong SC., van den Berg M., Rauwerda JA., Stehouwer CD. Hyperhomocysteinemia and atherothrombotic disease. Seminars in Thrombosis and Hemostasis 1998; 24(4) 381-385.

Chapter 2

Fibrinolysis at the Interface of Thrombosis and Inflammation — The Role of Neutrophil Extracellular Traps

Imre Varjú and Krasimir Kolev

Additional information is available at the end of the chapter

http://dx.doi.org/10.5772/57259

1. Introduction

As a response to inflammatory stimuli, polymorphonuclear (PMN, neutrophil) cells are able to expel a mixture of their nuclear and granular elements. These web-like substances are called neutrophil extracellular traps (NETs), structures that are able to entrap invading pathogens. NETs are composed of DNA, histones, granular enzymes and proteins (such as cathepsin G or elastase), and seem to be a universal tool of defense: humans, animals and even plants [1] are capable of extracellular trap formation, indicating that these webs provide an evolutionarily conserved protective mechanism.

Besides their protective function, a role for NETs is emerging in the pathogenesis of many diseases [2,3], and may be of interest regarding the pathogenesis of thrombosis. Stimulation of coagulation by NETs can result in unwanted thrombosis [4] and infection is a common event in the development of deep vein thrombosis [5,6]. Targeting the release of nucleosomes, development of NETs and the availability of circulating histones could be a strategy for prevention or therapeutic intervention in venous thromboembolism, sepsis and other diseases involving cell death and lysis.

This chapter describes the formation and structure of NETs and discusses the possible connections and interrelations between this newly recognized form of innate immunity and components of the haemostatic system.

2. Triggers of NET formation

NETs can be formed in response to all major types of microbes (bacteria, fungi, protozoa, viruses) and their products, as well as inflammatory mediators, ROS, cell-cell interactions, and certain non-infectious or non-physiological stimuli. Table 1. shows a set of examples for various triggers.

Microbial stimuli	Chemical stimuli
Bacteria	**Microbial toxins and components**
Enterococcus faecalis	*δ-Toxin from Staphylococcus epidermidis*
Escherichia coli	*fMLP (+rapamycin)*
Haemophilus influenzae	*Glucose oxidase*
Helicobacter pylori	*M1 protein-fibrinogen complex*
Klebsiella pneumoniae	*Lipophosphoglycan*
Lactococcus lactis	*Lipopolysaccharide (LPS)*
Listeria monocytogenes	*Panton-Valentin leukocidin*
Mannheimia haemolytica	**Inflammatory mediators and citokines**
Mycobacterium tuberculosis/canettii	*Antibodies*
Serratia marcescens	*Calcium ions*
Shigella flexneri	*GM-CSF + C5a/ LPS*
Staphylococcus aureus	*Hydrogen peroxide*
Streptococcus dysgalactiae/pneumoniae	*Interferon + eotaxin*
Yersinia enterocolitica	*Interferon-α/γ + C5a*
Fungi	*Interleukin 1-β/8/23*
Aspergillus fumigatus	*Nitric oxide*
Candida albicans	*Platelet activating factor*
Cryptococcus gattii/neoformans	*Platelets through TLR-4*
Protozoa	*TNF-α*
Leishmania amazonensis donovani/major/chagasi	**Non-physiological stimuli**
Virus	*Phorbol-12-myristate-13-acetate (PMA)*
Feline Leukemia Virus	*PMA + ionomycin*
HIV-1	*Statins*
Influenza A	

Table 1. Triggers of NET formation. Several microbial and chemical stimuli have been identified. A summary based on [7-10].

http://dx.doi.org/10.5772/57259

3. Formation of NETs

3.1. NET formation as a form of cell death

NETs are the results of a unique cell death program that is different from apoptosis or necrosis [11]. It is characterized by the loss of intracellular membranes before the plasma membrane integrity is compromised (NETosis). To release NETs, activated neutrophils undergo dramatic morphological changes [12]. Minutes after activation by PMA, they flatten and firmly attach to the substratum, while showing a multitude of granules and a lobulated nucleus [13]. During the next hour, the nucleus loses its lobules, the chromatin decondenses and swells, and the inner and outer nuclear membranes progressively detach from each other. Concomitantly, the granules disintegrate. After one hour, the nuclear envelope seems to disaggregate into vesicles and the contents of nucleoplasm, cytoplasm and granules are able to freely mix. After approximately 4 hours, the cells round up and seem to contract until the cell membrane ruptures and the internal components are ejected to the extracellular space [13,14]. It is important to note, that depending on stimuli and donor, only a certain percentage of the activated neutrophils make NETs [13].

Apoptosis, another form of programmed cell death, is characterized by membrane blebbing, phosphatidylserine exposure on the cell surface, nuclear chromatin condensation and DNA fragmentation *without* membrane disintegration [8]. Necrosis is characterized by PS exposure during the early steps, cellular swelling and bursting, and plasma membrane damage/rupture *without* nuclear membrane disintegration. The program of NETosis, on the other hand, shows disintegration of the nuclear envelope *without* DNA fragmentation; loss of internal membranes and organelles, and membrane rupture (and therefore PS exposure) *after* mixing of the nuclear and cytoplasmic elements.

3.2. Alternative ways of extracellular trap formation

Besides the above described, first observed form of NETosis (also called *'suicidal' NETosis*), several other types have been reported [15].

In contrast with the PMA-induced 3-4 hour-long cell death program, a recently described form, *'vital' NETosis*, leads to rapid NET formation without neutrophil cell death [16-18]: Staphylococcus aureus appears to induce NETs in a rapid fashion [16], and LPS-activated platelets are also capable of inducing NETosis within minutes [19]. 'Vital' NETosis does not only spare the neutrophil from 'suicidal' lysis, but transforms them into anuclear cytoplasts capable of chasing and imprisoning live bacteria [18]. The third difference between 'suicidal' and 'vital' forms (besides timing and functional capacity of the involved neutrophils) is the mechanisms employed to create and cast out NETs: in contrast to the above described form, vital NETosis requires budding of the nuclear envelope, and vesicular trafficking of nuclear components to the plasma membrane, thereby delivering the NET out of the cell without requiring membrane perforation [16]. *Mitochondrial ETosis* originally observed in eosinophils, and later in neutrophils could also be considered as a subtype of the 'vital' form [20,21].

4. Structure and composition of NETs

NETs released from neutrophils in the extracellular space consist of nuclear DNA and various histones decorated with granular proteins. NETs are fragile, complex structures composed of smooth 'threads', approximately 15-25 nm in diameter, which are likely to represent a chain of nucleosomes from unfolded chromatin. High-resolution scanning electron microscopy (SEM) revealed that the NET threads are studded to variable extent with globuli of 30-50 nm [14] that contain the multiple cathelicidin antimicrobial peptides which originate from the neutrophil granules (or lysosomes). Several 'threads' can be wound into 'cables' that can be up to 100 nm in diameter (Figure 1.).

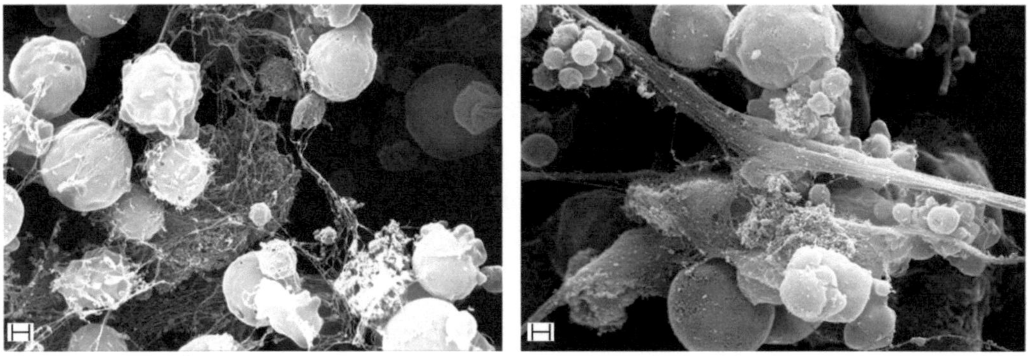

Figure 1. SEM images of NETs produced by PMA-activated neutrophils. Images are taken at 10,000x magnification. Scale bars=1 μm.

These cables then form complex three-dimensional structures that, using SEM, can be hard to distinguish from fibrin networks [22]. Analysis of cross sections of NETs by transmission electron microscopy (TEM) revealed that fibers are not surrounded by membranes [23]. When produced in multiwell plates in vitro, NETs float within the medium, rather like a spider's web does in moving air [24]. The fact that they are 'sticky' as a result of their electrostatic charge and that they extend over areas of several microns makes them very effective at trapping [25], and possibly killing microorganisms [24].

DNA is a major structural component, because several intercalating dyes stain NETs strongly, and deoxyribonuclease (DNAse) treatment results in the disintegration of NETs, whereas protease treatment has no such effect [23]. Accounting for approximately 70%, the most abundant component of NETs are histones [26]. All core histones as well as linker histones can be found in NETs (H1, H2A, H2B, H3, H4), although in an enzymatically processed form (see later). The aforementioned globuli contain proteins and enzymes from the primary (azurophilic) granules (e.g. neutrophil elastase, cathepsin G, myeloperoxidase, bactericidal permeability increasing protein BPI), secondary (specific) granules (e.g. lactoferrin), and tertiary granules (e.g. gelatinase or MMP-9, peptidoglycan recognition proteins PGRPs [27]) of neutrophils [28]. Cytoplasmic components, like calprotectin, a heterodimer of cytosolic S100A8 and S100A9, are rarely found in NETs [26].

These proteins exert various antimicrobial actions [29]: MPO is responsible for microbicidal HOCl generation; serine proteases (neutrophil elastase NE, cathepsin G, proteinase 3, tryptase, neutrophil serine protease 4 NSP4 [30]) are able to inactivate bacteria by cleaving their virulence factors [23]; cathelicidin LL37, BPI, defensins, and histones can disintegrate pathogen cell membranes challenging their viability [31,32]; calprotectin [26,33], calgranulin and lactoferrin chelate ions that are vital for microbial growth, altogether making NETs an effective tool virtually against all types of microbes.

NETs produced from mitochondrial DNA release have a slightly different structure [21]. NE and MPO co-localize with mitochondrial DNA, but certain nuclear (lamin B, nuclear matrix protein-45, poly-ADP-ribose polymerase, histones) and other (cytoplasmic caspase-3, beta-actin, mitochondrial cytochrome c, membrane markers CD15 and 16) elements are absent, which suggests a different type of host-NET interaction in the case of mitochondrion-derived NETs.

5. Intracellular events leading to NET formation

A unifying theory describing the subsequent steps of NET formation is still missing, but many mechanisms have been identified to contribute to NET expulsion.

5.1. Signaling events

The signaling mechanisms leading to the formation of NETs are poorly understood, and it is very likely that different triggers are able to induce NETosis through different pathways (Figure 2. [34]).

The protein kinase C (*PKC*) enzyme family is comprised of conventional, novel and atypical isoforms [35]. There are at least four conventional isoenzymes: PKCα, PKCβI, PKCβII and PKCγ. The novel isoenzyme group has four subtypes: PKCδ, PKCε, PKCη and PKCθ. The third group, atypical isoenzymes, consists of PKCζ and PKCι [35]. PMA (phorbol-12-myristate-13-acetate), a widely used inducer of NETs, stimulates conventional (α, βI, βII, γ) and novel (δ, ε, η, θ) PKC by mimicking the activating ligand diacylglycerol (DAG) [35]. PKC isoforms of all classes have been reported in neutrophils from healthy donors [36], and activation of PKC is critical in the generation of NETs [37]. Nevertheless, an intricate antagonism is present between PKC isoforms in the regulation of a crucial element of NETosis, histone deimination: PKCα has a dominant role in the repression of histone deimination, whereas PKCζ is essential in the activation of peptydil arginine deiminase 4 (PAD4, see later) and the execution of NETosis. The precise balance between opposing PKC isoforms in the regulation of NETosis affirms the idea that NET release underlies specific and vitally important evolutionary selection pressures [38].

PK-C activation (e.g. by PMA) is upstream of the *Raf-MEK-ERK* pathway [39] leading to phosphorylation of gp91phox [40] and p47phox [41] which initiates the assembly of the cellular or phagosomal membrane-bound and the cytosolic subunits of another key player of NET formation, NADPH oxidase (see below). An alternative route for activation of ERK is also suggested through generation of reactive oxygen species (ROS) [42]. The Raf-MEK-ERK pathway also upregulates the expression of antiapoptotic protein Mcl-1, which contributes to the inhibition of apoptosis and redirects the death program to NETosis [39].

The monomeric G-protein (rho small GTPase) *Rac2* is also activated upstream of NADPH oxidase activation [43].

The role of *PI3K-Akt-mTOR* pathway is contradictory. Inhibition of mTOR leads to enhancement of fMLP-induced NETosis, because the pathway inhibits autophagy, a process that seems to enhance NET formation (e.g. by blocking apoptosis) [10]. If a different trigger, lipopolysaccharide (LPS) is used, however, mTOR seems to support NETosis by exerting translational enhancement of HIF1α [44].

Certain triggers of NETosis act through a PKC/ROS-independent pathway, possibly mediated by *Src* kinase [45], which may be able to directly activate PAD4.

Cytoskeletal elements may also play a role in transmitting signals from the cell surface to the nucleus, e.g. inhibition of the cell surface receptor integrin *Mac1-cytohesin1* (a guanine exchange factor)-*actin* cytoskeleton pathway results in inhibition of PAD4 activation and NET formation [46].

5.2. NADPH oxidase and ROS formation

Most pathways converge to activate *NADPH oxidase* as a key enzyme of the process [47]. Neutrophils isolated from patients with chronic granulomatous disease (CGD) caused by mutations in NADPH oxidase fail to produce NETs upon PMA-stimulation [13]. Inhibition of the oxidase with diphenyleneiodonium DPI also prevents NETosis in response to several factors [48]. Assembly of the NADPH oxidase responsible for the generation of ROS during the respiratory burst requires phosphorylation of the four cytosolic subunits (p47-phox, p40-phox, p67-phox and Rac) to enable their association with the membrane bound gp91phox-p22phox (cytochrome b558) complex. Once being in the active form, the enzyme generates ROS, out of which the most important seem to be the superoxide ions (O_2^-). O_2^- dismutates (either spontaneously, or by superoxide dismutase [SOD] catalysis) to form H_2O_2. Further metabolization of H_2O_2 can lead to a variety of toxic oxygen derivatives, like the primary mediator of oxidative killing in the phagosome, HOCl, formed by *myeloperoxidase* (MPO) action. The importance of the latter enzyme is underlined by studies in patients suffering from MPO deficiency: the level of NETs they produced correlated with the degree of the enzyme deficiency [49]. How ROS generated during an oxidative burst contribute to NETosis is controversial. One possibility is that they contribute directly to the observed morphological changes by causing direct membrane destruction [50]. A proposed alternative is that ROS directly and indirectly (through activation of NF-κB) inactivate caspases [51-54], while exerting a possible autophagy-enhancing effect [34]. Both mechanisms lead to an inhibition of apopto-

http://dx.doi.org/10.5772/57259

sis, ensuring that the already ongoing cell death program does not take an apoptotic route. ROS also play a crucial role in initializing the events that lead to chromatin decondensation, another key component of this type of cell death (Figure 2.).

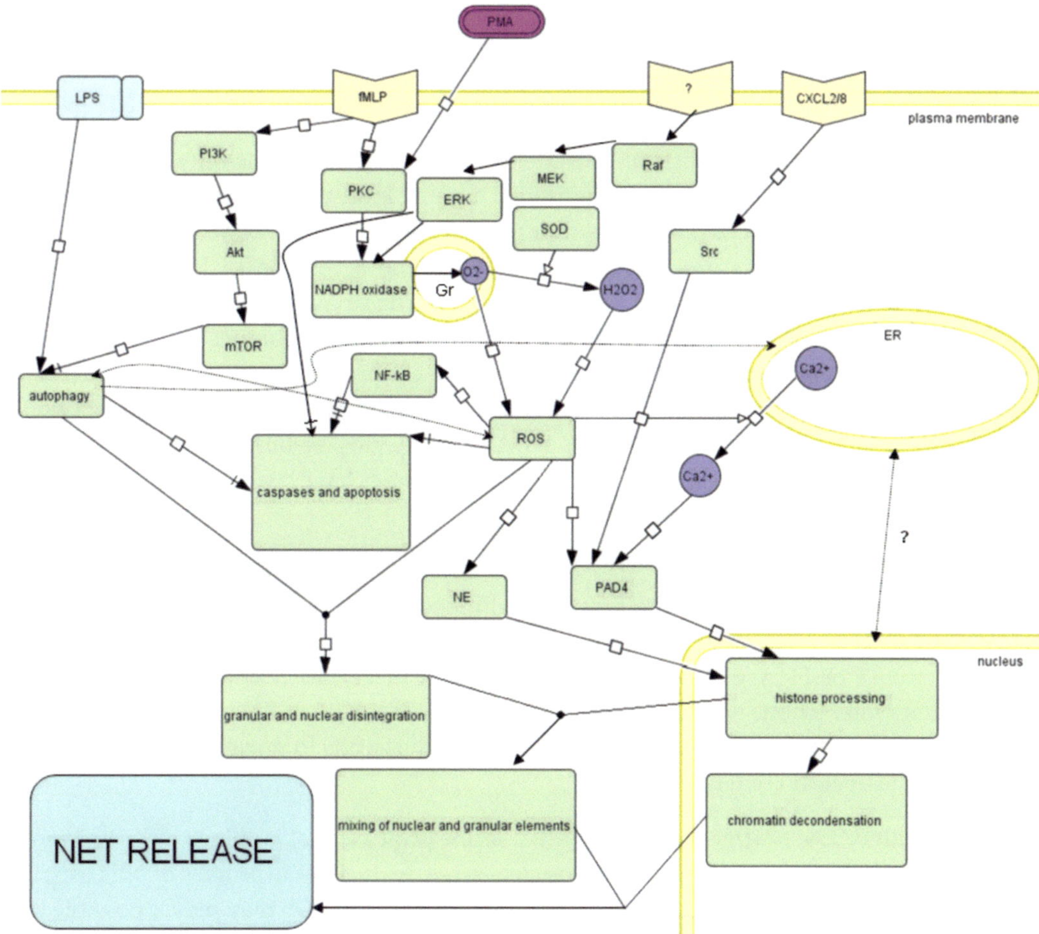

Figure 2. Intracellular steps leading to NET formation. Several signaling pathways can lead to NADPH oxidase activation and ROS formation, which triggers NE and PAD4 action on nuclear histones. Nuclear disintegration and decondensation leads to mixing of the granular and nuclear components, which are later expelled from the cell in the form of NETs. Dashed-end arrows represent inhibition, arrows pointing to the middle of another arrow represent activation of a step. Arrows with dotted lines stand for ambiguous relations. Gr: granule. For other abbreviations and explanation: see text. Modified from [34].

5.3. Chromatin decondensation

One option to weaken the interaction between DNA and highly positively charged histones is the enzymatic processing. At this moment, two enzymes seem to be of greatest importance: PAD4 (peptydilarginine deiminase 4) and NE (neutrophil elastase).

Peptydilarginine deiminases are enzymes catalyzing citrullination (deimination), a posttranslational modification of arginine to citrulline. The process results in the loss of positive charge and hydrogen bond acceptors, therefore leading to weakened protein-protein, RNA-protein, and DNA-protein interactions. Out of the five PAD enzymes expressed in humans and mice (PAD1-4 and 6) [55], PAD2 and 4 are the most abundant in neutrophil granulocytes, and the latter seems to be critical in NET formation: PAD4-deficient mice are unable to decondense chromatin or form NETs [56], whereas overexpression of PAD4 is sufficient to drive chromatin decondensation to form NET-like structures in cells that normally do not form NETs [57].

PAD4, a 74 kDa protein that exists as a head-to-tail dimer [58,59] is the only member of the peptydilarginine deiminase family containing a nuclear localization signal that ensures its trafficking to the nucleus [58,60,61] (although not the only one to be found inside, e.g. PAD2 is also reported to be localized intranuclearly [62]). The activation of PAD4 is calcium-dependent: binding of calcium to the C-terminal catalytic domain induces conformational changes that lead to the adequate positioning of critical active site residues [58]. The calcium-dependency of the enzyme also serves as a possible connection between ROS generation (possibly leading to calcium release from the endoplasmic reticulum) and PAD4 activation. In addition, ROS are possible direct regulators of PAD4 [63]. Cytoskeletal activity and autophagy may also be involved in PAD4 activation, since both processes have been shown to be required for chromatin decondensation during NET generation.

The main nuclear substrates of PAD4 are arginyl residues of PRMT1 (protein arginine methyltransferase 1) [61], PAD4 itself (autocitrullination downregulating the activity of the enzyme [64,65]), and, most importantly regarding the process of NETosis, histones (H2A, H3Arg-8 and-17 or H4Arg3) [66]. Hypercitrullination of arginil residues in histones [67] weakens their interactions with DNA resulting in the dissociation of heterochromatin protein 1-β [57], and the extensive chromatin decondensation that leads to nuclear delobulation and swelling of the nuclear content [66,68].

In concert with PAD4, *neutrophil elastase* (NE), a serine protease that is able to cleave histones, also promotes nuclear decondensation. H1 is cleaved early during the process of NETosis, but nuclear decondensation coincides with degradation of H4 [50]. ROS may play a possible role in the translocation of NE from the azurophilic granules into the nucleus by disrupting the association of NE with the proteoglycan (e.g. serglycin) matrix that is thought to down-regulate protease activity in resting cells [69-71]. The similar, but later occurring translocation route of myeloperoxidase MPO supports the process, which seems to be independent of its enzymatic activity [50]. Once in the nucleus, NE activity is reduced by DNA, which could help in protecting certain NET-components from losing their antimicrobial activity by proteolytic digestion [50]. Interestingly, serpinb1, an inhibitor of neutrophil proteases is also being transported to the nucleus during NETosis, possibly setting a brake of NE action [72]. While NE knockout mice fail to form NETs in a pulmonary model of Klebsiella Pneumoniae infection [50], serpinb1-deficient neutrophils produce overt NETosis in vivo during Pseudomonas aeruginosa lung infection [72], which points to the importance of the fine regulation of NE activity during the process of NET formation.

5.4. Reorganization of membrane structures-the role of autophagy in NETosis

While the decondensated nuclear content expands, the space between the two membranes of the delobulated nuclear envelope starts growing, this which eventually leads to formation of vesicles and disintegration of nuclear membranes. During the final stage, nuclear and granular integrity is completely lost, which allows mixing of the chromatin and the granular components, and a rupture in the plasma membrane causes the release of extracellular chromatin traps.

However, vesicle formation is also seen in neutrophils isolated from CGD patients, which are unable to produce NETs [73]. This observation suggests that vesicles do not necessarily originate from the nuclear envelope, but ER membranes are likely to be assembled as a source of autophagic vesicles [34], in addition to possible *de novo* vesicle formation. A decrease in perinuclear ER membranes may result in lower morphological constraints on nuclear collapse, and calcium leaking form the ER may activate PAD4. Taken together, these events could partially explain that autophagy is needed for nuclear decondensation and NET formation [73]. These speculations are supported by the finding that inhibition of mTOR, a suppressor of autophagy, also leads to enhanced NET production (see before [10]).

6. NETs and haemostasis

NETs are a newly recognized scaffold of venous [74] and arterial [75,76] (Figure 3.) thrombi (besides fibrin and von Willebrand Factor [vWF]) that allows cell localization (neutrophils, red blood cells), platelet activation and aggregation, and promotion of both (extrinsic and intrinsic) pathways of coagulation. Thus, NETs are a focus of cross-talk between immunity, inflammation and haemostasis. Here we discuss the interaction among the various players of the haemostatic system and NET components.

6.1. NETs and the vessel wall

The classic view of the intact endothelial surface emphasizes its anticoagulant role. While endothelial damage is a common initiator of arterial thrombosis, in the case of deep vein thrombosis (DVT), activation of endothelium and Weibel-Palade Body (WPB) release play a crucial role. NETs induce endothelial cell damage and death [17,77-79], an effect that is likely to be assigned to NET-associated proteases, defensins and, most importantly, histones [78,80]. Binding of histones to membrane phospholipids results in pore formation and influx of ions [81-83], this may lead to elevated endothelial calcium levels, vWF release from WPB [84], activation of endothelium, or even endothelial cell death. Endothelial ROS formed under these circumstances may, in turn, trigger NET formation by neutrophils [77]. Perfusion of iliac artery cross sections with NE results in increased thrombogenicity of the arterial wall [85], although it is not clear if NET-bound NE is able to reproduce this effect at the site of vascular damage.

NETs also contribute to the progression of atherosclerotic plaque formation in the subendothelial layer of arteries: neutrophils infiltrate arteries during early stages of atherosclerosis [86], and NETs can be detected in murine and human atherosclerotic lesions [87].

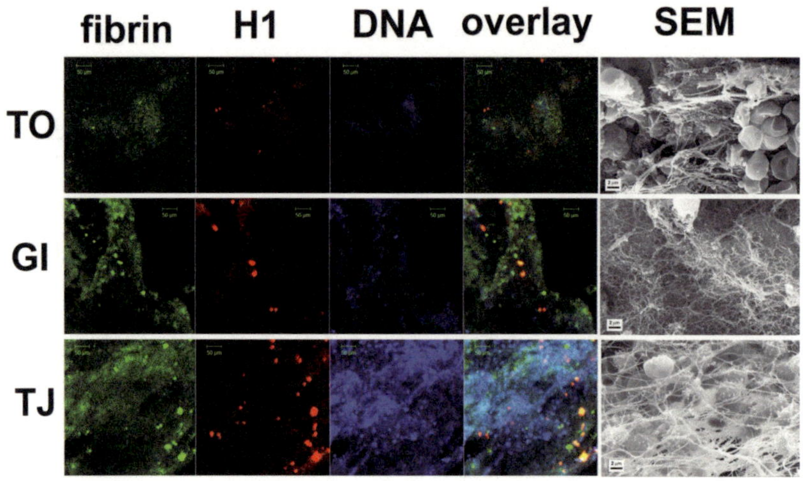

Figure 3. Presence of NET components in arterial thrombi. Following thrombectomy thrombus samples were either frozen for immunostaining or washed, fixed and dehydrated for SEM processing. Sections of frozen samples were double-immunostained for fibrin (green) and histone 1 (red) as well as with a DNA-dye, TOTO-3 (blue). Images were taken at original magnification of ×20 with confocal laser microscope. SEM images were taken from the fixed samples of the same thrombi. There was variable but widespread staining for DNA. Histones were also present though were not so widely dispersed and in some cases were coincident with fibrin aggregates. The size of the thrombus-section area staining for DNA and histone correlated with the leukocyte content of the respective thrombus observed in the SEM images. The red blood cell-rich (TO) and the fibrin-rich (GI) thrombi showed limited DNA-and histone-positive regions in contrast to the extensively stained areas in the leukocyte-rich (TJ) thrombus. TO: a thrombus from popliteal artery, GI: a thrombus from infrarenal aorta aneurysm, TJ: a thrombus from femoro-popliteal graft. Figure from [76].

6.2. NETs and platelets

NET fibres bind platelets directly and/or indirectly, and support their aggregation [88]. When perfused with blood, NETs bind platelets serving as an alternative scaffold for platelet adhesion and activation [89].

The first step of platelet binding involves either electrostatic interactions between NET histones and platelet surface phospholipids [81]/carbohydrates [90], or histone binding to Toll-like receptors 2 and 4 [91]. Platelets also bind double and single stranded DNA in vitro [92,93]. Adhesion molecules may also play a role in thrombocyte-NET interactions, such as vWF (binding histones through its A1 domain) [94], fibronectin or fibrinogen [89,84]. The interaction of histones with platelets results in calcium influx either by pore formation [95] or by opening of existing channels [96], a process, which triggers activation of αIIbβ3 [97]. This chain of events raises the possibility of a sequential histone-induced activation of platelets (first binding to platelet surface, then, following activation, binding to adhesion molecules [88]), which could explain the unsaturable nature of histones binding to platelets [88]. When infused into mice, histones co-localize with platelets and induce thrombocytopenia and thrombosis [83,84,88], possibly partially through potentiation of thrombin-dependent platelet-activation [98].

Serine proteases may also play a role in platelet activation: NETs contain enzymatically active neutrophil elastase NE and cathepsin G [23], and these proteases potentiate platelet aggregation through proteolitically activating platelet receptors [99,100]. Some of these elements, however, play an ambiguous role in the modulation of platelet functions: e.g. NE is also an effective enzyme for the cleavage of vWF under high shear stress [101], helping the detachment of platelets from thrombogenic surfaces.

NETs also seem to bind certain interleukins that may enhance platelet activation and aggregation: the presence of IL17A and-F was shown in NET regions of acute myocardial infarction thrombus specimens [102].

Platelet-NET interaction seems to be bidirectional in many ways. Serotonin released from platelets promotes the recruitment of neutrophils [103]. Activated platelets generate ROS, such as superoxide [104], and secrete human β-defensin 1 [105], both of which can trigger formation of NETs [13,106]. Platelets pre-stimulated with LPS or collagen also induce NETosis in neutrophils [17,108], contributing to the formation of a vicious cycle of NET formation and platelet activation [74].

Interaction between platelets and NETs might also be involved in pathological situations like transfusion-related acute lung injury (TRALI) [108,109], thrombotic microangiopathies [110], or heparin-induced thrombocytopenia (HIT). During HIT, possible binding of NETs to PF4 forming an antigenic complex may offer an explanation for disease progression even after immediate removal of heparin [111].

6.3. NETs and red blood cells

Red blood cells are no longer considered as passively entrapped elements of thrombi, but cells that may promote thrombosis by exposing phosphatydilserine and altering blood viscosity [112]; furthermore, their presence modulates structural parameters of the forming fibrin meshwork through integrin-mediated fibrin(ogen)-red blood cell interactions [113].

Similarly to platelets, RBCs avidly bind to NETs after perfusion of whole blood [89], possibly through direct and indirect mechanisms. RBCs can bind DNA, since it was eluted from the surface of isolated RBCs from cancer patients [114]. Activated neutrophils or platelets (e.g. in NETs) can also recruit RBCs at very low venous shear in vitro [115]. NETs are predominantly found in the red, RBC-rich part of experimental mice DVT thrombus, suggesting that NETs could be important for RBC recruitment to venous thrombi [84].

6.4. NETs and the coagulation system

NETs offer a variety of activators for both the extrinsic and the intrinsic (contact-) pathways of the coagulation cascade [116,107] stimulating fibrin formation and deposition in vitro [89,107,116] (Figure 4.).

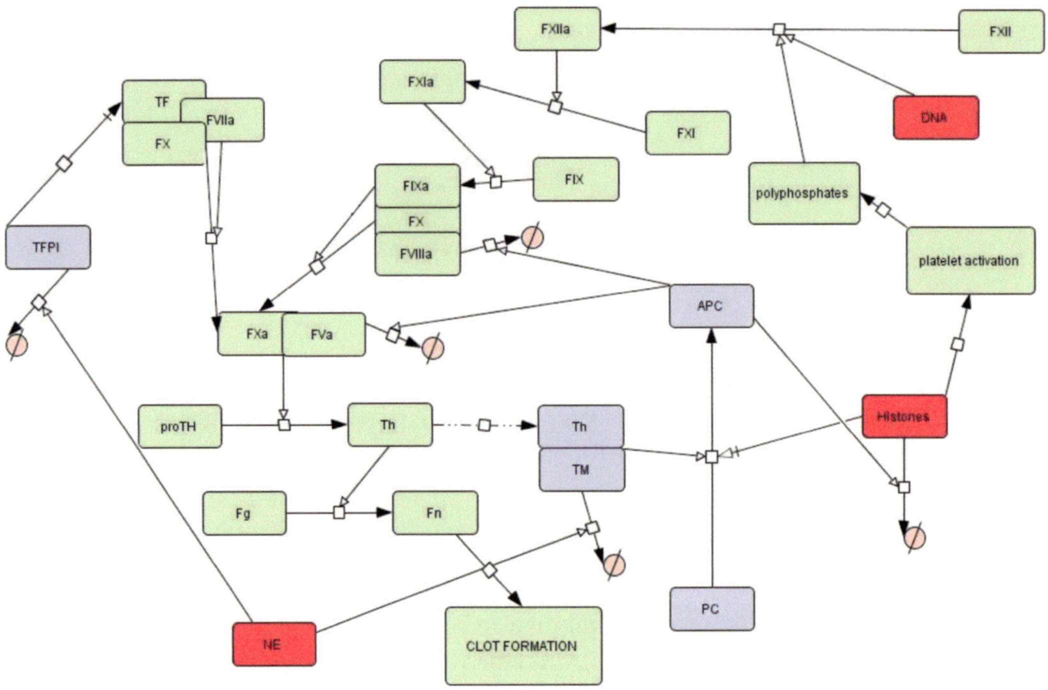

Figure 4. Examples of NET-coagulation interactions. Green boxes indicate prothrombotic elements/steps of the cascade. Blue represents antithrombotic systems. Red boxes stand for NET components. Dashed pink circles symbolize degradation of the respective protein. Dashed arrows represent inhibition, while arrows pointing to the middle of another arrow represent activation of a process. For further explanation, see text.

NE and cathepsin G, two serine proteases that are in the NETs, degrade inhibitors of coagulation [12]. NE is known to cleave tissue factor pathway inhibitor (TFPI) of the *extrinsic pathway*, and enhance factor Xa activity [117]. The cleavage of TFPI by NE is supported by activated platelets that attach to the surface of neutrophils and facilitate NET formation [107]. Neutrophil-expelled nucleosomes also bind TFPI and serve as a platform for the NE-driven degradation of TFPI [107]. NETs do not only release brakes of the extrinsic pathway, but also trigger it: TF was identified as a NET component [116,118]; and disulphide isomerase (PDI) released from damaged or activated endothelial cells and platelets (e.g. in NETs) participates in bringing the inactive (encrypted) TF (e.g. in neutrophils [75,119] and platelets [120,121]) to its active (decrypted) form [122].

NETs also bind factor XII and stimulate fibrin formation via the *intrinsic coagulation pathway* [116]. Faxtor XII can be activated following contact with pathogens (e.g. entrapped in NETs), damaged cells (e.g. endothelial damage by NETs), and negatively charged surfaces (such as the NET component DNA, which also enhances the activity of certain coagulation serine proteases [123]). Polyphosphates released from activated platelets following stimulation by histones may also serve as coagulation-triggering negatively charged molecules [91,124].

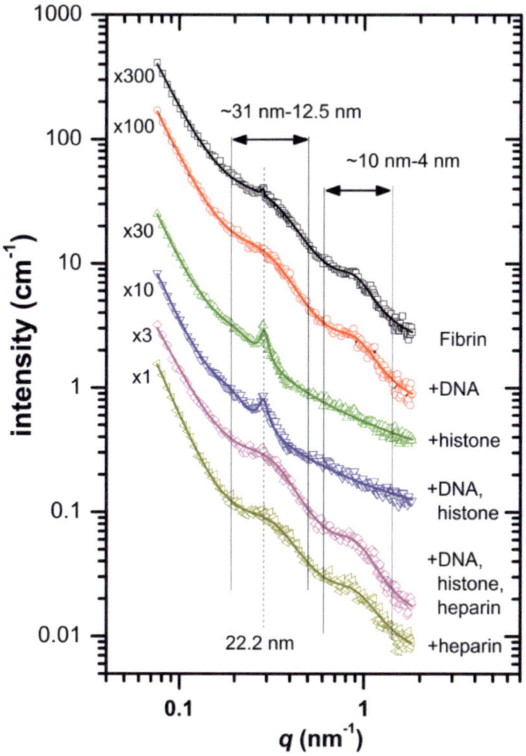

Figure 5. Small-angle X-ray scattering in fibrin clots containing DNA, histone, heparin or their combinations at the same concentrations. The general decay trend of the scattering curves reflects the fractal structure of the fibrin clot and its effect can be modeled as a background signal with empirical power-law equations. The peaks arising above this background reflect the longitudinal and cross-sectional alignment of fibrin monomers. A small, but sharp peak in pure fibrin at q-value of ≈0.285 nm-1 corresponds to the longitudinal periodicity of d=2π/q'=22 nm that is in agreement with earlier SAXS studies [128] and a little bit lower than the values reported for dried samples in transmission electron microscopic investigations [129]. This peak cannot be resolved in fibrin containing DNA or heparin indicating that these additives disrupt the regular longitudinal alignment of the monomeric building blocks. In contrast, the addition of histone does not interfere with the longitudinal periodicity, the related scattering peak is even more pronounced. In pure fibrin two additional broad scattering peaks can be resolved spanning over the q-ranges of ≈0.2 to 0.5 nm-1 and ≈0.6 to 1.5 nm-1. The first peak can be attributed to periodicity of ≈12.5 to 31 nm in cluster units of the fibers, while the second one corresponds to periodicity of ≈4 to 10 nm characteristic for the average protofibril-to-protofibril distance based on the structural models of Yang et al. [130] and Weisel [129]. Both of these broad peaks are most profoundly affected by the presence of histone (a 10-fold decrease in the area of Peak 1 and complete loss of Peak 3) suggesting that this additive interferes with the lateral organization of protofibrils resulting in lower protofibril density. Earlier studies [131] have shown that lower protofibril density can correspond to thicker fiber diameter, which is in qualitative agreement with SEM results [76]. The structure modifying effects of histone are preserved in the presence of DNA, but these effects are completely reversed in the quaternary system of fibrin/DNA/histone/heparin; Curves are shifted vertically by the factors indicated at their origin for better visualization. Symbols represent the measured intensity values, while solid lines show the fitted empirical functions. The dashed vertical line indicates the longitudinal periodicity of fibrin of about 22 nm (representing the approximate half-length of a fibrin monomer), while the solid vertical lines show the boundaries of the broad peaks that characterize the lateral structure of the fibrin fibers. q (momentum transfer)=4π/λ sinθ, where θ is half the scattering angle and λ is the wavelength of the incident X-ray beam. Figure from [76].

Besides its crucial role in NET-driven thrombosis [125], PAD4 has also been shown to citrullinate antithrombin (ATIII) in vitro [126], which weakens its thrombin-inhibiting efficiency and this may be an additional factor contributing to increased thrombin generation associated with NETs. Histones also bind to fibrinogen and prothrombin [127], and can aggregate vWF [94], the significance of which is not clear.

NET components also interfere with the *anticoagulant* systems in plasma. Despite the historically attributed anticoagulant properties of histones [131,132] (prolonging the plasma based standard clotting assays, probably due to their affinity for negatively charged phospholipids, such as phosphatidylserine [81]), nowadays they are viewed as clear procoagulant substances, due to their platelet-activating nature (see before) and their modulatory effects on the thrombin-thrombomodulin(TM)-activated protein C (APC) pathway. Histones interact with *TM* and *protein C* and inhibit TM-mediated protein C activation [134]. Interestingly, in return, APC cleaves histones (H2A, H3, H4) and reduces their cytotoxicity [83], possibly serving as a basis for a counter-regulatory process. Cleavage of histones is relatively slow, but is augmented substantially by membrane surfaces, particularly those that best support APC anticoagulant activity [83], although NET-bound histones may be more difficult to cleave [78]. Thrombomodulin is also cleaved by NE and may also be rendered inactive by neutrophil oxidases (such as MPO) [135,136] present in NETs.

Heparin, a highly sulfated polyanion (GAG) is able to interfere with DNA-histone complexes [76] (Figure 5.). Heparin can remove histones from NET chromatin fibres, leading to their destabilization [89,116]: NETs are dismantled after perfusion with heparinized blood [116]. Heparin also blocks the interaction between the positively charged histones and platelets [74], in this way adding newly recognized elements to its long-known anticoagulant effects.

6.5. NETs, thrombolysis, NET lysis

Whilst there are extensive studies on the interaction between NET components and coagulation, little is known about their effects on fibrinolysis.

Histones and DNA, representing the main mass of NETs, seem to have *antifibrinolytic* properties. Addition of purified histones and DNA to the forming clot in vitro results in altered clot structure seen under SEM, a finding also confirmed by short axis X-ray scattering (SAXS) [76] (Figure 5.). The structural changes are accompanied by increased mechanical (Figure 6.) and enzymatic resistance of the clot, and a change in the microscopic properties of the lysis front (Figure 7.), especially when DNA and histones are used in combination [137,76]. Lysis may be also delayed by NET components resulting from interactions between fibrin degradation products (FDPs) and DNA/histones [76].

Nevertheless, certain NET components may *promote* thrombolysis: in vitro studies have shown that NE and cathepsin G can degrade fibrin [138], and in plasminogen-knockout mice, more neutrophils infiltrate the clot [139], possibly serving as an auxiliary mechanism when plasmin-mediated fibrinolysis is impaired [140]. Histone 2B can serve as a receptor to recruit plasminogen on the surface of human monocytes/macrophages [141], and perhaps in NETs as well, where the co-localization of NE and plasmin(ogen) could result in amplified formation of mini-

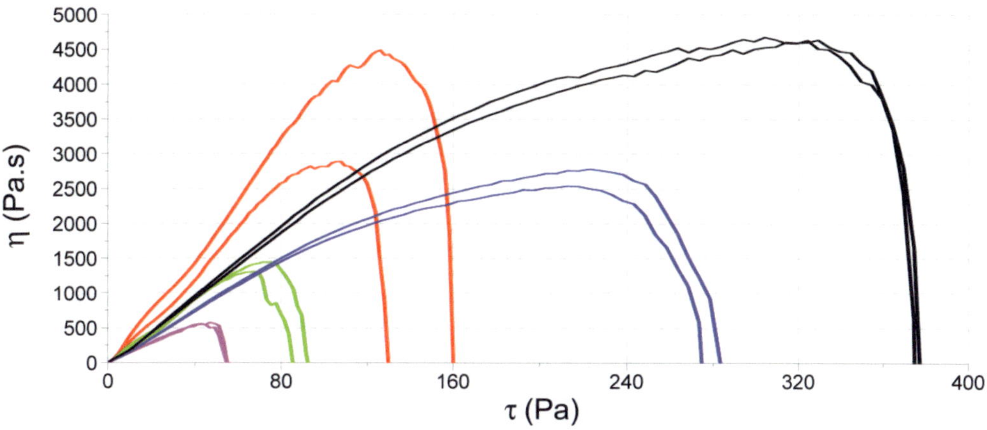

Figure 6. Rheometer studies showing the effect of DNA and histones on the critical shear force needed to disassemble fibrin. Curves are shown for pure fibrin (red), fibrin containing increasing DNA concentrations (green<magenta), histone (blue) and histone+DNA (black). In the presence of DNA alone the curves can be interpreted as increased sensitivity of fibrin to mechanical shear so that the shear force needed to disassemble fibrin (where viscosity approaches zero) is reduced in comparison to the situation without DNA. However, when histones are added to fibrin, and to a greater extent when histones are added to fibrin+DNA, the clots become more stable and resistant to shear forces. τ: shear stress, η: viscosity. Figure from [76].

plasmin, a plasmin-derivative that bears a catalytic efficiency on cross-linked fibrin that exceeds that of plasmin [142]. NE is also able to efficiently disable the major plasmin-inhibitor, α2-antiplasmin, further supporting plasmin action. PAD4 is eventually secreted from neutrophils during NET formation and was shown to citrullinate fibrin in rheumatoid arthritis [144] (although less efficiently than PAD2 [145]), but the significance of this related to thrombolysis is not known.

In vitro and in vivo observations indicate that fibrin, vWF and chromatin form a co-localized network within the thrombus that is similar to extracellular matrix [84,82,116], and it is likely that each of these components should be cleaved by their own appropriate enzyme (plasmin, ADAMTS-13, and DNAses), therefore it is important to assess current knowledge on the possible ways of NET degradation in blood plasma.

NETs can be degraded by *DNases* in vitro. There are two main DNases in human plasma: DNase1 and DNase1-like family, out of which, DNase1-like 3 (DNase1l3) is the most characterized. Both enzymes show calcium/magnesium dependency. DNase1 is secreted into circulation by a variety of exocrine and endocrine organs [146-148], whereas DNase1l3 is released from liver cells, splenocytes, macrophages and kidney cells [149]. DNase1 and DNase1l3 cooperate during in vitro chromatin breakdown (chromatin fragmentation is completely absent if DNase1 and DNase1l3 is inhibited) [150], and preprocessing of NETs by DNAse1 also facilitates their clearance by macrophages [151]. Plasmin is able to cleave histones [152], thus helping DNase action, since DNase1 prefers protein-free DNA. In addition, NE already present in NETs, APC (see before), thrombin [153] and an unidentified protease [154] may also assist in histone degradation. The in vivo relevance of plasmin-DNase cooperation is reflected in the elevated levels of plasma DNA in patients with DVT [74].

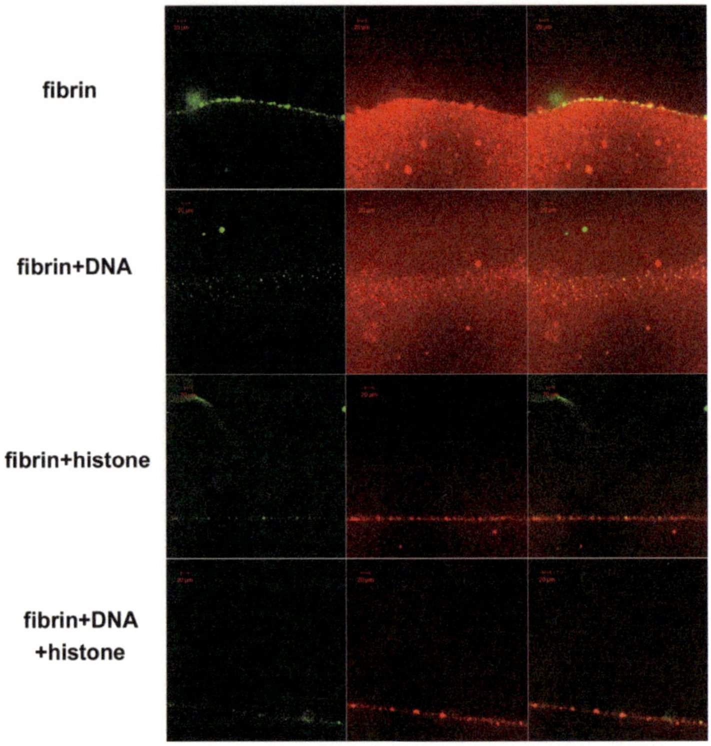

Figure 7. Confocal microscopy studies of lysis front movement using green fluorescent protein-labeled tPA (tPA-GFP) and red fluorescent fibrin after 25 min of fibrinolysis. Each column of micrographs from left to right shows green tPA-GFP fluorescence, red AlexaFluor 546 conjugated fibrin fluorescence and the merged image. The first row shows the accumulation of fibrin aggregates that co-localize with tPA-GFP. The second row, with the addition of DNA, shows less fibrin aggregate formation but a diffuse fibrin clot that remains behind the advancing tPA-GFP front. The lower two rows where clots contain histones and histones+DNA, respectively demonstrate reduced formation of fibrin aggregates within fibrin and less binding of tPA-GFP. Figure from [76].

As a possible counter-regulatory mechanism, NETs seem to protect themselves from bacterial and perhaps human DNases by limiting the availability of divalent cations (see calprotectin) and consequently the activity of these enzymes [155].

7. Conclusion

NETs are 'double-edged swords' of innate immunity. While they seem to be protective against a wide range of pathogens, their contribution to various diseases, and their clear prothrombotic role in the circulation may have dangerous consequences to the host. In terms of thrombosis, they seem to serve as a fundamental scaffold that supports thrombus integrity by providing a surface for activation of procoagulant proteins and platelets, in both venous and arterial thrombi. Further investigation is indispensable to determine their exact role in the process of thrombi dissolution, and to test whether breakdown of NETs (e.g. by DNases) increases the therapeutic efficiency of the current thrombolysis protocols.

Acknowledgements

This work was supported by the Hungarian Scientific Research Fund [OTKA 83023].

Author details

Imre Varjú* and Krasimir Kolev

*Address all correspondence to: varju.imre@med.semmelweis-univ.hu

Department of Medical Biochemistry, Semmelweis University, Budapest, Hungary

References

[1] Hawes MC, Curlango-Rivera G, Wen F, White GJ, Vanetten HD, Xiong Z. Extracellular DNA: the tip of root defenses? Plant Sci. 2011; 180(6):741-5.

[2] Kaplan MJ, Radic M. Neutrophil extracellular traps: double-edged swords of innate immunity. J Immunol. 2012;189(6):2689-95.

[3] Medina E. Neutrophil extracellular traps: a strategic tactic to defeat pathogens with potential consequences for the host. J Innate Immun. 2009;1(3):176-80.

[4] Borissoff JI, ten Cate H. From neutrophil extracellular traps release to thrombosis: an overshooting host-defense mechanism? J Thromb Haemost. 2011;9(9):1791-4.

[5] Esmon CT. Basic mechanisms and pathogenesis of venous thrombosis. Blood Rev. 2009;23(5):225-9.

[6] Smeeth L, Cook C, Thomas S, Hall AJ, Hubbard R, Vallance P. Risk of deep vein thrombosis and pulmonary embolism after acute infection in a community setting. Lancet. 2006;367(9516):1075-9.

[7] Zawrotniak M, Rapala-Kozik M. Neutrophil extracellular traps (NETs)-formation and implications. Acta Biochim Pol. 2013;60(3):277-84.

[8] Goldmann O, Medina E. The expanding world of extracellular traps: not only neutrophils but much more. Front Immunol. 2012;3:420.

[9] Drescher B, Bai F. Neutrophil in viral infections, friend or foe? Virus Res. 2013;171(1): 1-7.

[10] Itakura A, McCarty OJ. Pivotal role for the mTOR pathway in the formation of neutrophil extracellular traps via regulation of autophagy. Am J Physiol Cell Physiol. 2013;305(3):C348-54.

[11] Darrah E, Andrade F. NETs: the missing link between cell death and systemic autoimmune diseases? Front Immunol. 2012;3:428.

[12] Brinkmann V, Zychlinsky A. Neutrophil extracellular traps: is immunity the second function of chromatin? J Cell Biol. 2012;198(5):773-83.

[13] Fuchs TA, Abed U, Goosmann C, Hurwitz R, Schulze I, Wahn V, Weinrauch Y, Brinkmann V, Zychlinsky A. Novel cell death program leads to neutrophil extracellular traps. J Cell Biol. 2007;176(2):231-41.

[14] Brinkmann V, Zychlinsky A. Beneficial suicide: why neutrophils die to make NETs. Nat Rev Microbiol. 2007;5(8):577-82.

[15] Yipp BG, Kubes P. NETosis: how vital is it? Blood. 2013;122(16):2784-94.

[16] Pilsczek FH, Salina D, Poon KK, Fahey C, Yipp BG, Sibley CD, Robbins SM, Green FH, Surette MG, Sugai M, Bowden MG, Hussain M, Zhang K, Kubes P. A novel mechanism of rapid nuclear neutrophil extracellular trap formation in response to Staphylococcus aureus. J Immunol. 2010;185(12):7413-25.

[17] Clark SR, Ma AC, Tavener SA, McDonald B, Goodarzi Z, Kelly MM, Patel KD, Chakrabarti S, McAvoy E, Sinclair GD, Keys EM, Allen-Vercoe E, Devinney R, Doig CJ, Green FH, Kubes P. Platelet TLR4 activates neutrophil extracellular traps to ensnare bacteria in septic blood. Nat Med. 2007;13(4):463-9.

[18] Yipp BG, Petri B, Salina D, Jenne CN, Scott BN, Zbytnuik LD, Pittman K, Asaduzzaman M, Wu K, Meijndert HC, Malawista SE, de Boisfleury Chevance A, Zhang K, Conly J, Kubes P. Infection-induced NETosis is a dynamic process involving neutrophil multitasking in vivo. Nat Med. 2012;18(9):1386-93.

[19] Palmer LJ, Cooper PR, Ling MR, Wright HJ, Huissoon A, Chapple IL. Hypochlorous acid regulates neutrophil extracellular trap release in humans. Clin Exp Immunol. 2012;167(2):261-8.

[20] Yousefi S, Gold JA, Andina N, Lee JJ, Kelly AM, Kozlowski E, Schmid I, Straumann A, Reichenbach J, Gleich GJ, Simon HU. Catapult-like release of mitochondrial DNA by eosinophils contributes to antibacterial defense. Nat Med. 2008;14(9):949-53.

[21] Yousefi S, Mihalache C, Kozlowski E, Schmid I, Simon HU. Viable neutrophils release mitochondrial DNA to form neutrophil extracellular traps. Cell Death Differ. 2009;16(11):1438-44.

[22] Krautgartner WD, Klappacher M, Hannig M, Obermayer A, Hartl D, Marcos V, Vitkov L. Fibrin mimics neutrophil extracellular traps in SEM. Ultrastruct Pathol. 2010;34(4):226-31.

[23] Brinkmann V, Reichard U, Goosmann C, Fauler B, Uhlemann Y, Weiss DS, Weinrauch Y, Zychlinsky A. Neutrophil extracellular traps kill bacteria. Science. 2004;303(5663):1532-5.

[24] Cooper PR, Palmer LJ, Chapple IL. Neutrophil extracellular traps as a new paradigm in innate immunity: friend or foe? Periodontol 2000. 2013;63(1):165-97.

[25] Menegazzi R, Decleva E, Dri P. Killing by neutrophil extracellular traps: fact or folklore? Blood. 2012; 119(5):1214-6.

[26] Urban CF, Ermert D, Schmid M, Abu-Abed U, Goosmann C, Nacken W, Brinkmann V, Jungblut PR, Zychlinsky A. Neutrophil extracellular traps contain calprotectin, a cytosolic protein complex involved in host defense against Candida albicans. PLoS Pathog. 2009;5(10):e1000639.

[27] Cho JH, Fraser IP, Fukase K, Kusumoto S, Fujimoto Y, Stahl GL, Ezekowitz RA. Human peptidoglycan recognition protein S is an effector of neutrophil-mediated innate immunity. Blood. 2005;106(7):2551-8.

[28] Wartha F, Beiter K, Normark S, Henriques-Normark B. Neutrophil extracellular traps: casting the NET over pathogenesis. Curr Opin Microbiol. 2007;10(1):52-6.

[29] Lögters T, Margraf S, Altrichter J, Cinatl J, Mitzner S, Windolf J, Scholz M. The clinical value of neutrophil extracellular traps. Med Microbiol Immunol. 2009;198(4): 211-9.

[30] O'Donoghue AJ, Jin Y, Knudsen GM, Perera NC, Jenne DE, Murphy JE, Craik CS, Hermiston TW. Global substrate profiling of proteases in human neutrophil extracellular traps reveals consensus motif predominantly contributed by elastase. PLoS One. 2013;8(9):e75141.

[31] Cho JH, Sung BH, Kim SC. Buforins: histone H2A-derived antimicrobial peptides from toad stomach. Biochim Biophys Acta. 2009;1788(8):1564-9.

[32] Méndez-Samperio P. The human cathelicidin hCAP18/LL-37: a multifunctional peptide involved in mycobacterial infections. Peptides. 2010;31(9):1791-8.

[33] Bianchi M, Niemiec MJ, Siler U, Urban CF, Reichenbach J. Restoration of anti-Aspergillus defense by neutrophil extracellular traps in human chronic granulomatous disease after gene therapy is calprotectin-dependent. J Allergy Clin Immunol. 2011;127(5):1243-52.e7.

[34] Remijsen Q, Kuijpers TW, Wirawan E, Lippens S, Vandenabeele P, Vanden Berghe T. Dying for a cause: NETosis, mechanisms behind an antimicrobial cell death modality. Cell Death Differ. 2011;18(4):581-8.

[35] Way KJ, Chou E, King GL. Identification of PKC-isoform-specific biological actions using pharmacological approaches. Trends Pharmacol Sci. 2000;21(5):181-7.

[36] Balasubramanian N, Advani SH, Zingde SM. Protein kinase C isoforms in normal and leukemic neutrophils: altered levels in leukemic neutrophils and changes during myeloid maturation in chronic myeloid leukemia. Leuk Res. 2002;26(1):67-81.

[37] Gray RD, Lucas CD, Mackellar A, Li F, Hiersemenzel K, Haslett C, Davidson DJ, Rossi AG. Activation of conventional protein kinase C (PKC) is critical in the generation of human neutrophil extracellular traps. J Inflamm (Lond). 2013;10(1):12.

[38] Neeli I, Radic M. Opposition between PKC isoforms regulates histone deimination and neutrophil extracellular chromatin release. Front Immunol. 2013;4:38.

[39] Hakkim A, Fuchs TA, Martinez NE, Hess S, Prinz H, Zychlinsky A, Waldmann H. Activation of the Raf-MEK-ERK pathway is required for neutrophil extracellular trap formation. Nat Chem Biol. 2011;7(2):75-7.

[40] Raad H, Paclet MH, Boussetta T, Kroviarski Y, Morel F, Quinn MT, Gougerot-Pocidalo MA, Dang PM, El-Benna J. Regulation of the phagocyte NADPH oxidase activity: phosphorylation of gp91phox/NOX2 by protein kinase C enhances its diaphorase activity and binding to Rac2, p67phox, and p47phox. FASEB J. 2009;23(4):1011-22.

[41] El Benna J, Han J, Park JW, Schmid E, Ulevitch RJ, Babior BM. Activation of p38 in stimulated human neutrophils: phosphorylation of the oxidase component p47phox by p38 and ERK but not by JNK. Arch Biochem Biophys. 1996;334(2):395-400.

[42] Keshari RS, Verma A, Barthwal MK, Dikshit M. Reactive oxygen species-induced activation of ERK and p38 MAPK mediates PMA-induced NETs release from human neutrophils. J Cell Biochem. 2013;114(3):532-40.

[43] Lim MB, Kuiper JW, Katchky A, Goldberg H, Glogauer M. Rac2 is required for the formation of neutrophil extracellular traps. J Leukoc Biol. 2011;90(4):771-6.

[44] McInturff AM, Cody MJ, Elliott EA, Glenn JW, Rowley JW, Rondina MT, Yost CC. Mammalian target of rapamycin regulates neutrophil extracellular trap formation via induction of hypoxia-inducible factor 1 α. Blood. 2012;120(15):3118-25.

[45] [45] Marcos V, Zhou Z, Yildirim AO, Bohla A, Hector A, Vitkov L, Wiedenbauer EM, Krautgartner WD, Stoiber W, Belohradsky BH, Rieber N, Kormann M, Koller B, Roscher A, Roos D, Griese M, Eickelberg O, Döring G, Mall MA, Hartl D. CXCR2 mediates NADPH oxidase-independent neutrophil extracellular trap formation in cystic fibrosis airway inflammation. Nat Med. 2010;16(9):1018-23.

[46] Neeli I, Dwivedi N, Khan S, Radic M. Regulation of extracellular chromatin release from neutrophils. J Innate Immun. 2009;1(3):194-201.

[47] Almyroudis NG, Grimm MJ, Davidson BA, Röhm M, Urban CF, Segal BH. NETosis and NADPH oxidase: at the intersection of host defense, inflammation, and injury. Front Immunol. 2013;4:45.

[48] Parker H, Winterbourn CC. Reactive oxidants and myeloperoxidase and their involvement in neutrophil extracellular traps. Front Immunol. 2012;3:424.

[49] Metzler KD, Fuchs TA, Nauseef WM, Reumaux D, Roesler J, Schulze I, Wahn V, Papayannopoulos V, Zychlinsky A. Myeloperoxidase is required for neutrophil extracellular trap formation: implications for innate immunity. Blood. 2011;117(3):953-9.

[50] Papayannopoulos V, Metzler KD, Hakkim A, Zychlinsky A. Neutrophil elastase and myeloperoxidase regulate the formation of neutrophil extracellular traps. J Cell Biol. 2010;191(3):677-91.

[51] Fadeel B, Ahlin A, Henter JI, Orrenius S, Hampton MB. Involvement of caspases in neutrophil apoptosis: regulation by reactive oxygen species. Blood. 1998;92(12): 4808-18.

[52] Hampton MB, Stamenkovic I, Winterbourn CC. Interaction with substrate sensitises caspase-3 to inactivation by hydrogen peroxide. FEBS Lett. 2002;517(1-3):229-32.

[53] Wilkie RP, Vissers MC, Dragunow M, Hampton MB. A functional NADPH oxidase prevents caspase involvement in the clearance of phagocytic neutrophils. Infect Immun. 2007;75(7):3256-63.

[54] Sadikot RT, Zeng H, Yull FE, Li B, Cheng DS, Kernodle DS, Jansen ED, Contag CH, Segal BH, Holland SM, Blackwell TS, Christman JW. p47phox deficiency impairs NF-kappa B activation and host defense in Pseudomonas pneumonia. J Immunol. 2004;172(3):1801-8.

[55] Anzilotti C, Pratesi F, Tommasi C, Migliorini P. Peptidylarginine deiminase 4 and citrullination in health and disease. Autoimmun Rev. 2010;9(3):158-60.

[56] Li P, Li M, Lindberg MR, Kennett MJ, Xiong N, Wang Y. PAD4 is essential for antibacterial innate immunity mediated by neutrophil extracellular traps. J Exp Med. 2010;207(9):1853-62.

[57] Leshner M, Wang S, Lewis C, Zheng H, Chen XA, Santy L, Wang Y. PAD4 mediated histone hypercitrullination induces heterochromatin decondensation and chromatin unfolding to form neutrophil extracellular trap-like structures. Front Immunol. 2012;3:307.

[58] Arita K, Hashimoto H, Shimizu T, Nakashima K, Yamada M, Sato M. Structural basis for Ca(2+)-induced activation of human PAD4. Nat Struct Mol Biol. 2004;11(8):777-83.

[59] Liu YL, Chiang YH, Liu GY, Hung HC. Functional role of dimerization of human peptidylarginine deiminase 4 (PAD4). PLoS One. 2011;6(6):e21314.

[60] Nakashima K, Hagiwara T, Yamada M. Nuclear localization of peptidylarginine deiminase V and histone deimination in granulocytes. J Biol Chem. 2002;277(51):49562-8.

[61] Vossenaar ER, Zendman AJ, van Venrooij WJ, Pruijn GJ. PAD, a growing family of citrullinating enzymes: genes, features and involvement in disease. Bioessays. 2003;25(11):1106-18.

[62] Zhang X, Bolt M, Guertin MJ, Chen W, Zhang S, Cherrington BD, Slade DJ, Dreyton CJ, Subramanian V, Bicker KL, Thompson PR, Mancini MA, Lis JT, Coonrod SA. Peptidylarginine deiminase 2-catalyzed histone H3 arginine 26 citrullination facilitates estrogen receptor α target gene activation. Proc Natl Acad Sci USA. 2012;109(33): 13331-6.

[63] Rohrbach AS, Slade DJ, Thompson PR, Mowen KA. Activation of PAD4 in NET formation. Front Immunol. 2012;3:360.

[64] Andrade F, Darrah E, Gucek M, Cole RN, Rosen A, Zhu X. Autocitrullination of human peptidyl arginine deiminase type 4 regulates protein citrullination during cell activation. Arthritis Rheum. 2010;62(6):1630-40.

[65] Méchin MC, Coudane F, Adoue V, Arnaud J, Duplan H, Charveron M, Schmitt AM, Takahara H, Serre G, Simon M. Deimination is regulated at multiple levels including auto-deimination of peptidylarginine deiminases. Cell Mol Life Sci. 2010;67(9): 1491-503.

[66] Wang Y, Li M, Stadler S, Correll S, Li P, Wang D, Hayama R, Leonelli L, Han H, Grigoryev SA, Allis CD, Coonrod SA. Histone hypercitrullination mediates chromatin decondensation and neutrophil extracellular trap formation. J Cell Biol. 2009;184(2): 205-13.

[67] Neeli I, Khan SN, Radic M. Histone deimination as a response to inflammatory stimuli in neutrophils. J Immunol. 2008;180(3):1895-902.

[68] Wang Y, Wysocka J, Sayegh J, Lee YH, Perlin JR, Leonelli L, Sonbuchner LS, McDonald CH, Cook RG, Dou Y, Roeder RG, Clarke S, Stallcup MR, Allis CD, Coonrod SA. Human PAD4 regulates histone arginine methylation levels via demethylimination. Science. 2004;306(5694):279-83.

[69] Serafin WE, Katz HR, Austen KF, Stevens RL. Complexes of heparin proteoglycans, chondroitin sulfate E proteoglycans, and [3H]diisopropyl fluorophosphate-binding proteins are exocytosed from activated mouse bone marrow-derived mast cells. J Biol Chem. 1986;261(32):15017-21.

[70] Kolset SO, Gallagher JT. Proteoglycans in haemopoietic cells. Biochim Biophys Acta. 1990;1032(2-3):191-211. Review.

[71] Reeves EP, Lu H, Jacobs HL, Messina CG, Bolsover S, Gabella G, Potma EO, Warley A, Roes J, Segal AW. Killing activity of neutrophils is mediated through activation of proteases by K+flux. Nature. 2002;416(6878):291-7.

[72] Farley K, Stolley JM, Zhao P, Cooley J, Remold-O'Donnell E. A serpinB1 regulatory mechanism is essential for restricting neutrophil extracellular trap generation. J Immunol. 2012;189(9):4574-81.

[73] Remijsen Q, Vanden Berghe T, Wirawan E, Asselbergh B, Parthoens E, De Rycke R, Noppen S, Delforge M, Willems J, Vandenabeele P. Neutrophil extracellular trap cell death requires both autophagy and superoxide generation. Cell Res. 2011;21(2): 290-304.

[74] Fuchs TA, Brill A, Wagner DD. Neutrophil extracellular trap (NET) impact on deep vein thrombosis. Arterioscler Thromb Vasc Biol. 2012;32(8):1777-83.

[75] Darbousset R, Thomas GM, Mezouar S, Frère C, Bonier R, Mackman N, Renné T, Dignat-George F, Dubois C, Panicot-Dubois L. Tissue factor-positive neutrophils bind to injured endothelial wall and initiate thrombus formation. Blood. 2012;120(10):2133-43.

[76] Longstaff C, Varjú I, Sótonyi P, Szabó L, Krumrey M, Hoell A, Bóta A, Varga Z, Komorowicz E, Kolev K. Mechanical stability and fibrinolytic resistance of clots containing fibrin, DNA, and histones. J Biol Chem. 2013;288(10):6946-56.

[77] Gupta AK, Joshi MB, Philippova M, Erne P, Hasler P, Hahn S, Resink TJ. Activated endothelial cells induce neutrophil extracellular traps and are susceptible to NETosis-mediated cell death. FEBS Lett. 2010;584(14):3193-7.

[78] Saffarzadeh M, Juenemann C, Queisser MA, Lochnit G, Barreto G, Galuska SP, Lohmeyer J, Preissner KT. Neutrophil extracellular traps directly induce epithelial and endothelial cell death: a predominant role of histones. PLoS One. 2012;7(2):e32366.

[79] Villanueva E, Yalavarthi S, Berthier CC, Hodgin JB, Khandpur R, Lin AM, Rubin CJ, Zhao W, Olsen SH, Klinker M, Shealy D, Denny MF, Plumas J, Chaperot L, Kretzler M, Bruce AT, Kaplan MJ. Netting neutrophils induce endothelial damage, infiltrate tissues, and expose immunostimulatory molecules in systemic lupus erythematosus. J Immunol. 2011;187(1):538-52.

[80] Okrent DG, Lichtenstein AK, Ganz T. Direct cytotoxicity of polymorphonuclear leukocyte granule proteins to human lung-derived cells and endothelial cells. Am Rev Respir Dis. 1990;141(1):179-85.

[81] Pereira LF, Marco FM, Boimorto R, Caturla A, Bustos A, De la Concha EG, Subiza JL. Histones interact with anionic phospholipids with high avidity; its relevance for the binding of histone-antihistone immune complexes. Clin Exp Immunol. 1994;97(2): 175-80.

[82] Kleine TJ, Gladfelter A, Lewis PN, Lewis SA. Histone-induced damage of a mammalian epithelium: the conductive effect. Am J Physiol. 1995;268(5 Pt 1):C1114-25.

[83] Xu J, Zhang X, Pelayo R, Monestier M, Ammollo CT, Semeraro F, Taylor FB, Esmon NL, Lupu F, Esmon CT. Extracellular histones are major mediators of death in sepsis. Nat Med. 2009;15(11):1318-21.

[84] Brill A, Fuchs TA, Savchenko AS, Thomas GM, Martinod K, De Meyer SF, Bhandari AA, Wagner DD. Neutrophil extracellular traps promote deep vein thrombosis in mice. J Thromb Haemost. 2012;10(1):136-44.

[85] Wohner N, Keresztes Z, Sótonyi P, Szabó L, Komorowicz E, Machovich R, Kolev K. Neutrophil granulocyte-dependent proteolysis enhances platelet adhesion to the arterial wall under high-shear flow. J Thromb Haemost. 2010;8(7):1624-31.

[86] Drechsler M, Megens RT, van Zandvoort M, Weber C, Soehnlein O.Hyperlipidemia-triggered neutrophilia promotes early atherosclerosis. Circulation. 2010;122(18): 1837-45.

[87] Megens RT, Vijayan S, Lievens D, Döring Y, van Zandvoort MA, Grommes J, Weber C, Soehnlein O. Presence of luminal neutrophil extracellular traps in atherosclerosis. Thromb Haemost. 2012;107(3):597-8.

[88] Fuchs TA, Bhandari AA, Wagner DD. Histones induce rapid and profound thrombocytopenia in mice. Blood. 2011;118(13):3708-14.

[89] Fuchs TA, Brill A, Duerschmied D, Schatzberg D, Monestier M, Myers DD Jr, Wrobleski SK, Wakefield TW, Hartwig JH, Wagner DD. Extracellular DNA traps promote thrombosis. Proc Natl Acad Sci USA. 2010;107(36):15880-5.

[90] Watson K, Gooderham NJ, Davies DS, Edwards RJ. Nucleosomes bind to cell surface proteoglycans. J Biol Chem. 1999;274(31):21707-13.

[91] Semeraro F, Ammollo CT, Morrissey JH, Dale GL, Friese P, Esmon NL, Esmon CT. Extracellular histones promote thrombin generation through platelet-dependent mechanisms: involvement of platelet TLR2 and TLR4. Blood. 2011;118(7):1952-61.

[92] Clejan L, Menahem H. Binding of deoxyribonucleic acid to the surface of human platelets. Acta Haematol. 1977;58(2):84-8.

[93] Dorsch CA. Binding of single-strand DNA to human platelets. Thromb Res. 1981;24(1-2):119-29.

[94] Ward CM, Tetaz TJ, Andrews RK, Berndt MC. Binding of the von Willebrand factor A1 domain to histone. Thromb Res. 1997;86(6):469-77.

[95] Kleine TJ, Lewis PN, Lewis SA. Histone-induced damage of a mammalian epithelium: the role of protein and membrane structure. Am J Physiol. 1997;273(6 Pt 1):C1925-36.

[96] Gamberucci A, Fulceri R, Marcolongo P, Pralong WF, Benedetti A. Histones and basic polypeptides activate Ca2+/cation influx in various cell types. Biochem J. 1998;331 (Pt 2):623-30.

[97] Crittenden JR, Bergmeier W, Zhang Y, Piffath CL, Liang Y, Wagner DD, Housman DE, Graybiel AM. CalDAG-GEFI integrates signaling for platelet aggregation and thrombus formation. Nat Med. 2004;10(9):982-6.

[98] Carestia A, Rivadeneyra L, Romaniuk MA, Fondevila C, Negrotto S, Schattner M. Functional responses and molecular mechanisms involved in histone-mediated platelet activation. Thromb Haemost. 2013;110(5):1035-45.

[99] Renesto P, Chignard M. Enhancement of cathepsin G-induced platelet activation by leukocyte elastase: consequence for the neutrophil-mediated platelet activation. Blood. 1993;82(1):139-44.

[100] Si-Tahar M, Pidard D, Balloy V, Moniatte M, Kieffer N, Van Dorsselaer A, Chignard M. Human neutrophil elastase proteolytically activates the platelet integrin alphaIIbbeta3 through cleavage of the carboxyl terminus of the alphaIIb subunit heavy chain. Involvement in the potentiation of platelet aggregation. J Biol Chem. 1997;272(17): 11636-47.

[101] Wohner N, Kovács A, Machovich R, Kolev K. Modulation of the von Willebrand factor-dependent platelet adhesion through alternative proteolytic pathways. Thromb Res. 2012;129(4):e41-6.

[102] de Boer OJ, Li X, Teeling P, Mackaay C, Ploegmakers HJ, van der Loos CM, Daemen MJ, de Winter RJ, van der Wal AC. Neutrophils, neutrophil extracellular traps and interleukin-17 associate with the organisation of thrombi in acute myocardial infarction. Thromb Haemost. 2013;109(2):290-7.

[103] Duerschmied D, Suidan GL, Demers M, Herr N, Carbo C, Brill A, Cifuni SM, Mauler M, Cicko S, Bader M, Idzko M, Bode C, Wagner DD. Platelet serotonin promotes the recruitment of neutrophils to sites of acute inflammation in mice. Blood. 2013;121(6): 1008-15.

[104] Marcus AJ, Silk ST, Safier LB, Ullman HL. Superoxide production and reducing activity in human platelets. J Clin Invest. 1977;59(1):149-58.

[105] Kraemer BF, Campbell RA, Schwertz H, Cody MJ, Franks Z, Tolley ND, Kahr WH, Lindemann S, Seizer P, Yost CC, Zimmerman GA, Weyrich AS. Novel anti-bacterial activities of β-defensin 1 in human platelets: suppression of pathogen growth and signaling of neutrophil extracellular trap formation. PLoS Pathog. 2011;7(11):e1002355.

[106] Nishinaka Y, Arai T, Adachi S, Takaori-Kondo A, Yamashita K. Singlet oxygen is essential for neutrophil extracellular trap formation. Biochem Biophys Res Commun. 2011;413(1):75-9.

[107] Massberg S, Grahl L, von Bruehl ML, Manukyan D, Pfeiler S, Goosmann C, Brinkmann V, Lorenz M, Bidzhekov K, Khandagale AB, Konrad I, Kennerknecht E, Reges K, Holdenrieder S, Braun S, Reinhardt C, Spannagl M, Preissner KT, Engelmann B.

Reciprocal coupling of coagulation and innate immunity via neutrophil serine proteases. Nat Med. 2010;16(8):887-96.

[108] Thomas GM, Carbo C, Curtis BR, Martinod K, Mazo IB, Schatzberg D, Cifuni SM, Fuchs TA, von Andrian UH, Hartwig JH, Aster RH, Wagner DD. Extracellular DNA traps are associated with the pathogenesis of TRALI in humans and mice. Blood. 2012;119(26):6335-43.

[109] Caudrillier A, Kessenbrock K, Gilliss BM, Nguyen JX, Marques MB, Monestier M, Toy P, Werb Z, Looney MR. Platelets induce neutrophil extracellular traps in transfusion-related acute lung injury. J Clin Invest. 2012;122(7):2661-71.

[110] Fuchs TA, Kremer Hovinga JA, Schatzberg D, Wagner DD, Lämmle B. Circulating DNA and myeloperoxidase indicate disease activity in patients with thrombotic microangiopathies. Blood. 2012;120(6):1157-64.

[111] Gardiner EE, Andrews RK. Neutrophil extracellular traps (NETs) and infection-related vascular dysfunction. Blood Rev. 2012;26(6):255-9.

[112] Andrews DA, Low PS. Role of red blood cells in thrombosis. Curr Opin Hematol. 1999;6(2):76-82.

[113] Wohner N, Sótonyi P, Machovich R, Szabó L, Tenekedjiev K, Silva MM, Longstaff C, Kolev K. Lytic resistance of fibrin containing red blood cells. Arterioscler Thromb Vasc Biol. 2011;31(10):2306-13.

[114] Laktionov PP, Tamkovich SN, Rykova EY, Bryzgunova OE, Starikov AV, Kuznetsova NP, Vlassov VV. Cell-surface-bound nucleic acids: Free and cell-surface-bound nucleic acids in blood of healthy donors and breast cancer patients. Ann N Y Acad Sci. 2004;1022:221-7.

[115] Goel MS, Diamond SL. Adhesion of normal erythrocytes at depressed venous shear rates to activated neutrophils, activated platelets, and fibrin polymerized from plasma. Blood. 2002;100(10):3797-803.

[116] von Brühl ML, Stark K, Steinhart A, Chandraratne S, Konrad I, Lorenz M, Khandoga A, Tirniceriu A, Coletti R, Köllnberger M, Byrne RA, Laitinen I, Walch A, Brill A, Pfeiler S, Manukyan D, Braun S, Lange P, Riegger J, Ware J, Eckart A, Haidari S, Rudelius M, Schulz C, Echtler K, Brinkmann V, Schwaiger M, Preissner KT, Wagner DD, Mackman N, Engelmann B, Massberg S. Monocytes, neutrophils, and platelets cooperate to initiate and propagate venous thrombosis in mice in vivo. J Exp Med. 2012;209(4):819-35.

[117] Higuchi DA, Wun TC, Likert KM, Broze GJ Jr. The effect of leukocyte elastase on tissue factor pathway inhibitor. Blood. 1992;79(7):1712-9.

[118] Kambas K, Mitroulis I, Apostolidou E, Girod A, Chrysanthopoulou A, Pneumatikos I, Skendros P, Kourtzelis I, Koffa M, Kotsianidis I, Ritis K. Autophagy mediates the

delivery of thrombogenic tissue factor to neutrophil extracellular traps in human sepsis. PLoS One. 2012;7(9):e45427.

[119] Maugeri N, Brambilla M, Camera M, Carbone A, Tremoli E, Donati MB, de Gaetano G, Cerletti C. Human polymorphonuclear leukocytes produce and express functional tissue factor upon stimulation. J Thromb Haemost. 2006;4(6):1323-30.

[120] Müller I, Klocke A, Alex M, Kotzsch M, Luther T, Morgenstern E, Zieseniss S, Zahler S, Preissner K, Engelmann B. Intravascular tissue factor initiates coagulation via circulating microvesicles and platelets. FASEB J. 2003;17(3):476-8.

[121] Zillmann A, Luther T, Müller I, Kotzsch M, Spannagl M, Kauke T, Oelschlägel U, Zahler S, Engelmann B. Platelet-associated tissue factor contributes to the collagen-triggered activation of blood coagulation. Biochem Biophys Res Commun. 2001;281(2):603-9.

[122] Engelmann B, Massberg S. Thrombosis as an intravascular effector of innate immunity. Nat Rev Immunol. 2013;13(1):34-45.

[123] Kannemeier C, Shibamiya A, Nakazawa F, Trusheim H, Ruppert C, Markart P, Song Y, Tzima E, Kennerknecht E, Niepmann M, von Bruehl ML, Sedding D, Massberg S, Günther A, Engelmann B, Preissner KT. Extracellular RNA constitutes a natural procoagulant cofactor in blood coagulation. Proc Natl Acad Sci U S A. 2007;104(15): 6388-93.

[124] Müller F, Mutch NJ, Schenk WA, Smith SA, Esterl L, Spronk HM, Schmidbauer S, Gahl WA, Morrissey JH, Renné T. Platelet polyphosphates are proinflammatory and procoagulant mediators in vivo. Cell. 2009;139(6):1143-56.

[125] Martinod K, Demers M, Fuchs TA, Wong SL, Brill A, Gallant M, Hu J, Wang Y, Wagner DD. Neutrophil histone modification by peptidylarginine deiminase 4 is critical for deep vein thrombosis in mice. Proc Natl Acad Sci U S A. 2013;110(21):8674-9.

[126] Chang X, Yamada R, Sawada T, Suzuki A, Kochi Y, Yamamoto K. The inhibition of antithrombin by peptidylarginine deiminase 4 may contribute to pathogenesis of rheumatoid arthritis. Rheumatology (Oxford). 2005;44(3):293-8.

[127] Pemberton AD, Brown JK, Inglis NF. Proteomic identification of interactions between histones and plasma proteins: implications for cytoprotection. Proteomics. 2010;10(7):1484-93.

[128] Yeromonahos C, Polack B, Caton F. Nanostructure of the fibrin clot. Biophys J. 2010 Oct 6;99(7):2018-27.

[129] Weisel JW. The electron microscope band pattern of human fibrin: various stains, lateral order, and carbohydrate localization. J Ultrastruct Mol Struct Res. 1986;96(1-3): 176-88.

[130] Yang Z, Mochalkin I, Doolittle RF. A model of fibrin formation based on crystal structures of fibrinogen and fibrin fragments complexed with synthetic peptides. Proc Natl Acad Sci U S A. 2000;97(26):14156-61.

[131] Guthold M, Liu W, Stephens B, Lord ST, Hantgan RR, Erie DA, Taylor RM Jr, Superfine R. Visualization and mechanical manipulations of individual fibrin fibers suggest that fiber cross section has fractal dimension 1.3. Biophys J. 2004;87(6):4226-36.

[132] Giannitsis DJ, St Pekker. Role of leukocyte nuclei in blood coagulation. Naturwissenschaften. 1974;61(12):690.

[133] Kheiri SA, Fasy TM, Billett HH. Effects of H1 histones and a monoclonal autoantibody to H1 histones on clot formation in vitro: possible implications in the antiphospholipid syndrome. Thromb Res. 1996;82(1):43-50.

[134] Ammollo CT, Semeraro F, Xu J, Esmon NL, Esmon CT. Extracellular histones increase plasma thrombin generation by impairing thrombomodulin-dependent protein C activation. J Thromb Haemost. 2011;9(9):1795-803.

[135] Takano S, Kimura S, Ohdama S, Aoki N. Plasma thrombomodulin in health and diseases. Blood. 1990;76(10):2024-9.

[136] Glaser CB, Morser J, Clarke JH, Blasko E, McLean K, Kuhn I, Chang RJ, Lin JH, Vilander L, Andrews WH, et al. Oxidation of a specific methionine in thrombomodulin by activated neutrophil products blocks cofactor activity. A potential rapid mechanism for modulation of coagulation. J Clin Invest. 1992;90(6):2565-73.

[137] Komissarov AA, Florova G, Idell S. Effects of extracellular DNA on plasminogen activation and fibrinolysis. J Biol Chem. 2011;286(49):41949-62.

[138] Plow EF. The major fibrinolytic proteases of human leukocytes. Biochim Biophys Acta. 1980;630(1):47-56.

[139] Zeng B, Bruce D, Kril J, Ploplis V, Freedman B, Brieger D. Influence of plasminogen deficiency on the contribution of polymorphonuclear leucocytes to fibrin/ogenolysis: studies in plasminogen knock-out mice. Thromb Haemost. 2002;88(5):805-10.

[140] Kolev K, Machovich R. Molecular and cellular modulation of fibrinolysis. Thromb Haemost. 2003;89(4):610-21.

[141] Das R, Burke T, Plow EF. Histone H2B as a functionally important plasminogen receptor on macrophages. Blood. 2007;110(10):3763-72.

[142] Kolev K, Tenekedjiev K, Komorowicz E, Machovich R. Functional evaluation of the structural features of proteases and their substrate in fibrin surface degradation. J Biol Chem. 1997;272(21):13666-75.

[143] Machovich R, Owen WG. An elastase-dependent pathway of plasminogen activation. Biochemistry. 1989;28(10):4517-22.

[144] Masson-Bessière C, Sebbag M, Girbal-Neuhauser E, Nogueira L, Vincent C, Senshu T, Serre G. The major synovial targets of the rheumatoid arthritis-specific antifilaggrin autoantibodies are deiminated forms of the alpha-and beta-chains of fibrin. J Immunol. 2001;166(6):4177-84.

[145] Sanchez-Pernaute O, Filkova M, Gabucio A, Klein M, Maciejewska-Rodrigues H, Ospelt C, Brentano F, Michel BA, Gay RE, Herrero-Beaumont G, Gay S, Neidhart M, Juengel A. Citrullination enhances the pro-inflammatory response to fibrin inrheumatoid arthritis synovial fibroblasts. Ann Rheum Dis. 2013;72(8):1400-6.

[146] Lacks SA. Deoxyribonuclease I in mammalian tissues. Specificity of inhibition by actin. J Biol Chem. 1981;256(6):2644-8.

[147] Napirei M, Ricken A, Eulitz D, Knoop H, Mannherz HG. Expression pattern of the deoxyribonuclease 1 gene: lessons from the Dnase1 knockout mouse. Biochem J. 2004;380(Pt 3):929-37.

[148] Takeshita H, Yasuda T, Nakajima T, Hosomi O, Nakashima Y, Kishi K. Mouse deoxyribonuclease I (DNase I): biochemical and immunological characterization, cDNA structure and tissue distribution. Biochem Mol Biol Int. 1997;42(1):65-75.

[149] Shiokawa D, Tanuma S. Characterization of human DNase I family endonucleases and activation of DNase gamma during apoptosis. Biochemistry. 2001;40(1):143-52.

[150] Napirei M, Ludwig S, Mezrhab J, Klöckl T, Mannherz HG. Murine serum nucleases--contrasting effects of plasmin and heparin on the activities of DNase1 and DNase1-like 3 (DNase1l3). FEBS J. 2009;276(4):1059-73.

[151] Farrera C, Fadeel B. Macrophage clearance of neutrophil extracellular traps is a silent process. J Immunol. 2013;191(5):2647-56.

[152] Napirei M, Wulf S, Mannherz HG. Chromatin breakdown during necrosis by serum Dnase1 and the plasminogen system. Arthritis Rheum. 2004;50(6):1873-83.

[153] Harvima RJ, Yabe K, Fräki JE, Fukuyama K, Epstein WL. Hydrolysis of histones by proteinases. Biochem J. 1988;250(3):859-64.

[154] Esmon CT. Molecular circuits in thrombosis and inflammation. Thromb Haemost. 2013;109(3):416-20.

[155] Papayannopoulos V, Zychlinsky A. NETs: a new strategy for using old weapons. Trends Immunol. 2009;30(11):513-21.

Chapter 3

S100A10: A Key Regulator of Fibrinolysis

Alexi P. Surette and David M. Waisman

Additional information is available at the end of the chapter

http://dx.doi.org/10.5772/57378

1. Introduction

Regulation of fibrinolytic activity can be achieved by several mechanisms, ranging from regulating the production and localization of the plasminogen activators and their inhibitors, the degradation and inactivation of plasmin via autoproteolysis, and the synthesis and localization of the cell surface receptors for plasminogen. Binding of the inactive zymogen plasminogen to its cell surface receptors has been shown to significantly increase the rate of its conversion to the active serine-protease plasmin by co-localizing plasminogen with its activators, the tissue-type plasminogen activator (tPA) and the urokinase-type plasminogen activator (uPA) [1–3].One such cell surface plasminogen receptor is S100A10 (p11) [4]. S100A10, a member of the S100 protein family, was initially discovered as an annexin A2 (p36) binding partner [5–7]. S100A10 has also been found to interact with other cellular proteins including the Rho GTPase-activating protein DLC1 [8], cytosolic phospholipase A2 [9], the serotonin 1B receptor [10] and various ion channels, including the potassium channel TASK-1 [11], the sodium channel Na(V)1.8 [12] and the calcium channels TRPV5 and TRPV6 [13]. However, the major binding partners of S100A10 on the cell surface are tPA and plasminogen [14]. The focus of this review will be to discuss the role that extracellular S100A10 plays in regulating the conversion of plasminogen to plasmin and the physiological consequences of that process (Figure 1).

S100A10 is found on the cell surface as part of the annexin A2 heterotetramer complex (AIIt) [15]. AIIt is composed of two annexin A2 (p36) subunits along with two S100A10 subunits which form a $p36_2$ /$p11_2$ complex. Initially, annexin A2 was proposed to exist as a monomer on the cell surface where it functioned as a plasminogen receptor [16,17]. The possibility that S100A10 was present on the cell surface was ruled out by these investigators who reported that S100A10 was not present on the cell surface [18]. Subsequently, it was firmly established that S100A10 was present on the cell surface and this S100A10 was shown to exist as a complex with annexin A2 [15]. In view of this report, the proposed role of annexin A2 as a plasminogen

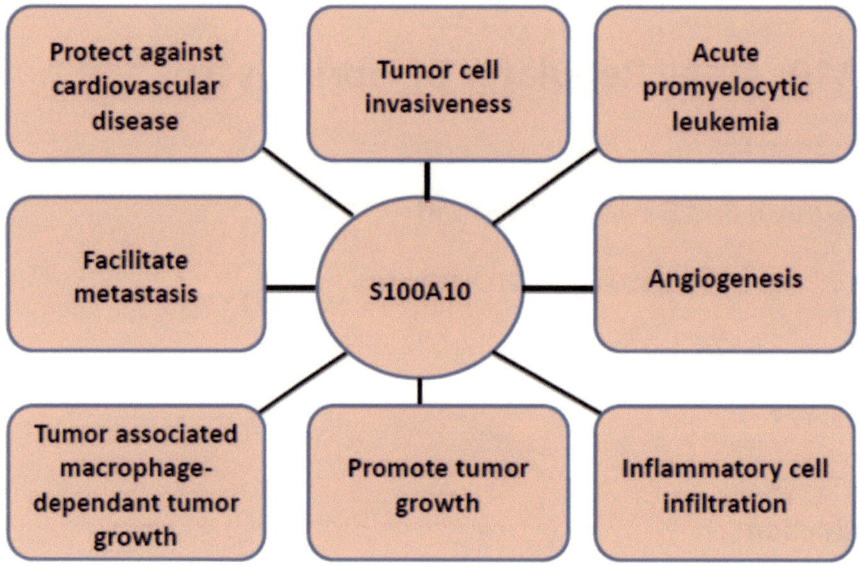

Figure 1. Roles of cell surface S100A10 in pathological processes. S100A10 on the cell surface participates in several pathological processes. S100A10 mediated fibrinolysis can have protective effects against cardiovascular disease and can participate in necessary inflammatory processes. Conversely, S100A10 mediated fibrinolysis may also participate in pathological inflammation and promote tumorigenesis through several mechanisms, including TAM infiltration, angiogenesis, tumor cell invasiveness and metastasis.

receptor was revised and it was reported that within the $p36_2p11_2$ complex, annexin A2 acted as the plasminogen receptor [19]. However, more rigorous studies have indicated that while annexin A2 does in fact anchor the $p36_2/p11_2$ complex to the cell surface in a calcium dependent fashion, S100A10 acts as the plasminogen receptor [14,15,20,21] (Figure 2).

Several cell surface proteins have been identified as plasminogen receptors, including histone 2B [22,23], integrin $\alpha_M\beta_2$ [24], α-enolase [25], cytokeratin-B [26,27] and Plg-R_{TK} [28]. All of these cell surface plasminogen receptors contain carboxyl-terminal lysines, which interact with the kringle domains of plasminogen [29–33]. Within the $p36_2/p11_2$ complex only S100A10 contains a carboxyl-terminal lysine. Binding studies using surface plasmon resonance demonstrated that S100A10 binds to plasminogen (K_d=1.81 μM) while annexin A2 does not bind plasminogen. Interestingly, the $p36_2/p11_2$ complex binds plasminogen with higher affinity (K_d=0.11 μM) than S100A10 alone, indicating that annexin A2 may induce a conformational change in S100A10 that facilitates the interaction of S100A10 with tPA or plasminogen. Treatment of both S100A10 and the $p36_2/p11_2$ complex with carboxypeptidase B, which removes carboxyl-terminal lysines, abolished plasminogen binding, indicating that plasminogen binding to the $p36_2/p11_2$ complex was dependent on the carboxyl-terminal lysine present on S100A10 [4,34]. S100A10 increased the rate of tPA dependent plasmin activation 46-fold while the $p36_2/p11_2$ complex increased the rate of activation 77-fold. Annexin A2, on the other hand, only increased the rate of activation 2-fold, indicating that S100A10 participates in plasminogen binding and subsequent generation of plasmin [21]. In the original studies in which purified annexin A2

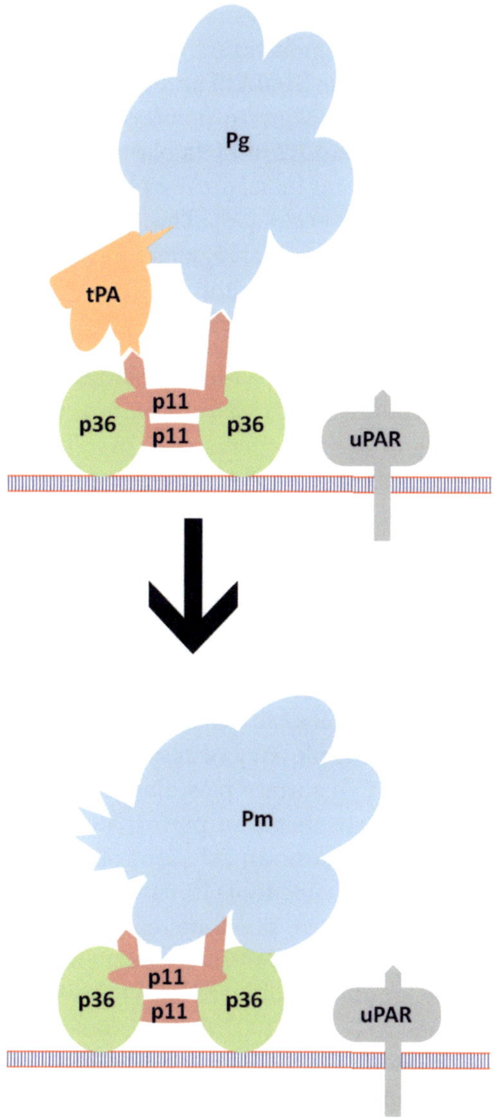

Figure 2. Model depicting AIIt dependant plasmin generation AIIt is composed of two annexin A2 (p36) monomers and two S100A10 (p11) monomers. Annexin A2 anchors AIIt to the cell membrane through phospholipid binding sites. Plasminogen (Pg) and tPA bind to S100A10 in a carboxyl-terminal lysine dependant fashion. AIIt also co-localizes with uPAR on the cell membrane. Binding of plasminogen to S100A10 therefore brings it into close proximity with the plasminogen activators tPA and uPA, accelerating proteolytic activation of plasminogen into the active serine protease plasmin (Pm). Plasmin binds to AIIt through annexin A2 and S100A10 in a non-carboxyl-terminal lysine dependant fashion.

was demonstrated to bind plasminogen, carboxypeptidase B treatment of this annexin A2 was observed to block plasminogen binding. Since annexin A2 does not possess a carboxyl-terminal lysine, a cleavage event at Lys307-Arg308 of annexin A2 was postulated to occur, thereby exposing the prerequisite carboxyl-terminal lysine for plasminogen binding [35]. However, this cleavage event has never been demonstrated to occur *in vitro* or *in vivo.* In contrast, carboxyl-terminal lysines are present on S100A10 and therefore do not require post-translational modification. Furthermore, Plow's group demonstrated that an antibody generated against the K327-D338 region of annexin A2 inhibits plasmin generation, suggesting that the carboxyl-terminus of annexin A2 remains intact during plasmin generation and therefore that the putative cleavage event does not occur [36]. The crystal structure of annexin A2 has revealed that the amino- and carboxyl-terminal regions of annexin A2 are present in a cleft in the concave surface of annexin A2 in close proximity to S100A10. Surprisingly the possibility that the annexin A2 antibody might affect the conformation of S100A10 was not considered.

In addition to binding plasminogen, the carboxyl-terminal lysines of S100A10 form the binding site for tPA [21]. Since the $p36_2$ /$p11_2$ complex also co-localizes with the uPA receptor, uPAR, at the cell surface [15], binding of plasminogen to S100A10 brings plasminogen into close proximity to both plasminogen activators on the cell surface, thereby dramatically increasing the rate of conversion of plasminogen to plasmin.

2. Role of S100A10 in fibrinolysis

Conversion of plasminogen to plasmin contributes to the maintenance of vascular patency, as the serine-protease plasmin Is the principle enzyme responsible for degrading fibrin, the main protein component of blood clots. Cell surface plasminogen receptors, which play a critical role in the activation of plasminogen, therefore participate in the clearance of potentially dangerous blood clots. The advent of annexin A2 (annexin A2–/–) and S100A10 knock-out (S100A10–/–) mice have provided valuable tools to investigate the *in vivo* role of the $p36_2$ / $p11_2$ complex in fibrinolysis. As discussed, previous reports had suggested that annexin A2 was responsible for the generation of plasmin and subsequent fibrinolysis [16,35,37]. However, since annexin A2 is responsible for stabilization of S100A10 levels [38], loss of annexin A2 can be regarded as loss of both annexin A2 and S100A10. For example, studies conducted with the annexin A2 knockout mouse and with shRNA knockdown of annexin A2 in cultured cells have established that the S100A10 levels are uniquely sensitive to the annexin A2 levels and that depletion of cellular annexin A2 results in the concomitant depletion of S100A10 [8,38,39]. It is therefore impossible to determine whether annexin A2 or S100A10 is responsible for plasmin generation in the annexin A2 knockout mouse model.

Since annexin A2 is present on the cell surface of S100A10–/– endothelial cells [39], we can conclude that alterations in plasminogen binding and plasmin activation in this model are due to loss of S100A10. The S100A10–/– mouse is therefore helpful in clarifying the mechanism by which the $p36_2$ /$p11_2$ complex participates in fibrinolysis and neoangiogenesis [39]. This model revealed a significant increase in fibrin deposits in the lung, liver, kidney and spleen of the S100A10–/– mouse [39]. S100A10 was also shown to play an important role in the clearance of microvascular thrombi as the S100A10-/- mouse had an impaired ability to clear blood clots induced by the thrombin-like enzyme batroxobin. Clots formed after the experimental induction of vascular damage using the tail-clip assay were also more stable in the S100A10–/–mouse. Since the wild-type and S100A10–/– mice shared similar coagulation parameters, the observed reduction in bleeding time after tail clipping of the S100A10–/– mice was due to decreased fibrinolysis of the tail clip-induced blood clot. The time between cessation of bleeding and the initiation of subsequent episodes of bleeding, the rebleeding time, was of shorter duration and less frequent with the S100A10$^{-/-}$ mice, thus the clots formed by the S100A10–/– mice were more stable than the wild-type mice, again due to a decreased rate of fibrinolysis. S100A10 therefore plays a critical role in the fibrinolytic surveillance system which functions to maintain vascular patency. Failure of this system contributes to the pathogenesis of cardiovascular disease, including deep vein thrombosis, stroke, atherosclerosis and coronary heart disease.

Endothelial cells, which line the interior lumen of blood vessels, play a critical role in maintaining vascular patency by participating in the regulation of plasmin generation. Loss of S100A10 in endothelial cells results in a 40-50% decrease in plasminogen binding and activation, suggesting that endothelial cell S100A10 is crucial for vascular fibrinolysis and therefore plays a key role in the fibrinolytic surveillance system [39].

Other work using the S100A10–/– mouse demonstrated the role S100A10 plays in plasminogen-dependent macrophage invasion. Such invasion is critical in physiological and pathological inflammation as macrophages utilize proteases to remodel the extracellular matrix (ECM) in order to move through tissue barriers to reach sites of infection. Murine macrophages lacking S100A10 have an impaired ability to invade into the peritoneal cavity in response to inflammatory stimulation [40]. The presence of S100A10, but not annexin A2 alone, is associated with plasminogen dependent invasion by macrophages, providing further evidence that the S100A10 subunit of the $p36_2$ /$p11_2$ complex is responsible for plasmin generation.

3. Role of the $p36_2$ /$p11_2$ complex in hyperhomocysteinemia

Hyperhomocysteinemia, a condition where elevated levels of homocysteine are found in the blood, has been identified as an independent risk factor for cardiovascular disease [41–44]. Several groups have reported that elevated homocysteine levels results in endothelial cell dysfunction [45–49] and a hyperthrombotic state [41,50–52], which may provide a mechanism by which hyperhomocysteinemia contributes to cardiovascular disease. One mechanism by which homocysteine may promote a hyperthrombotic state is through an interaction with annexin A2 [42,52,53]. Homocysteine, a reactive thiol-containing amino acid produced during the conversion of methionine to cysteine [54], was postulated to form a disulfide bond with extracellular annexin A2 at Cys-8 [55]. This interaction was reported to interfere with tPA binding to annexin A2 [55], thus preventing tPA mediated plasmin generation and fibrinolysis, resulting in the accumulation of blood clots. The report of tPA forming a covalent bond with annexin A2 contradicts other reports that demonstrate tPA binding to the cell surface in a carboxyl-terminal lysine dependent fashion [56]. Results from our laboratory suggested that highly purified annexin A2 fails to bind to tPA [4]. A subsequent *in vivo* murine study by the

Hajjar group expanded on how homocysteine may target annexin A2 to inhibit fibrinolysis. They purified annexin A2 from control mice and mice on a hyperhomocysteinemic diet. A comparison of this purified annexin A2 revealed that the annexin A2 isolated from the mice on a hyperhomocysteinemic diet failed to stimulate tPA-dependent plasmin activation, ie. it was totally inactive. They concluded that elevated serum homocysteine formed a disulfide bond with extracellular annexin A2 resulting in inhibition of annexin A2-dependent plasmin generation [57]. The authors failed to note that 95% of annexin A2 is present intracellularly [17] and that only 5% of the total annexin A2 would be available to interact with homocysteine present in the blood. Thus even if all of the extracellular annexin A2 was modified by homocysteine, it is unclear how a population consisting of 5% extracellular homocysteine-modified annexin A2 and 95% unmodified intracellular annexin A2 could be completely inactive. Since the vast majority of the annexin A2 purified from murine lungs is intracellular, homocysteine would therefore have to label all or most of the intracellular annexin A2 in order to explain the *in vitro* results. Such labelling could also, theoretically, impact not only other annexin A2 functions but should also affect other redox-sensitive proteins and transcription factors which could contribute to endothelial cell dysfunction. It is also unclear how extracellular levels of homocysteine, which in the mouse model are unlikely to exceed 100 uM, could affect intracellular proteins since the intracellular levels of the homocysteine-reactive molecule, glutathione, is present intracellularly at levels of 10 mM. However, it seems implausible for homocysteine to label such a significant portion of intracellular annexin A2 as most homocysteine is bound to plasma proteins [58] and the effective free homocysteine concentration would be insufficient to label intracellular proteins to this extent. It therefore remains unclear how the reported interaction of annexin A2 with homocysteine may contribute to impaired fibrinolysis. Interestingly, a recent report appears to contradict the Hajjar model for homocysteinemia. The Lentz group investigated transgenic mice deficient for the cystathionine β-synthase (CBS), the enzyme responsible for metabolizing homocysteine to cystathionine. In humans, CBS deficiency causes severe hyperhomocysteinemia and this animal model is therefore representative of human disease. Loss of CBS did in fact result in endothelial dysfunction in these animals. However, CBS deficiency did not result in a prothrombotic phenotype. In fact the CBS-null animals displayed normal rates of fibrinolysis [59]. Since these authors were unable to reproduce the findings of the Hajjar study [57,60], they speculated that the prothrombotic phenotype observed in diet-induced hyperhomocysteinemia might not be due to elevated homocysteine but possibly due to other dietary metabolites.

The difficulty in reproducing the Hajjar study was recently discussed by Jakubowski [61]. He pointed out that if homocysteinylation of annexin A2 generates a prothrombotic phenotype, it should be observed in any model of hyperhomocysteinemia, regardless of whether the model is dietary or genetic. He proposed that annexin A2 homocysteinylation for an unknown reason did not occur in the genetic model of hyperhomocysteinemia. These data therefore suggest that annexin A2 does not play a physiologically relevant role in hyperhomocysteinemia in humans.

In humans, CBS deficiency results in severe hyperhomocysteinemia, where plasma homocysteine levels are in excess of 100μM. Treatment of these patients with B vitamins reduces plasma homocysteine to 30-80μM, which is still higher than the normal 10μM, and reduces the risk of thrombotic events significantly [62]. Mild to moderate hyperhomocysteinemia, where plasma homocysteine levels vary from 16-100μM [63], is more common and can be influenced by diet and lifestyle. Treatment of mild to moderate hyperhomocysteinemia with B vitamins results in a decrease in serum homocysteine to normal levels. This decrease, however, does not correspond with decreased cardiovascular disease [64–68]. These human studies support the notion that hyperhomocysteinemia does not create a prothrombotic state and brings into question whether homocysteine targets annexin A2 in order to create a prothrombotic state. Therefore, the current evidence. The current evidence repudiates the theory that the pathological effects of hyperhomocysteinemia are due to targeting of cell surface annexin A2 and the subsequent loss of tPA binding potential resulting in impaired fibrinolysis.

4. Role of S100A10 in cancer

Alterations in fibrinolytic activity contribute to the pathogenesis of a wide variety of diseases. Excessive fibrinolytic activity has been associated with the pathogenesis of acute promyelocytic leukemia (APL) [69]. APL is caused by a chromosomal translocation that results in the presence of the PML-RAR-α fusion protein. Treatment with all-*trans* retinoic acid (ATRA) has greatly improved outcomes for patients with APL, in part by decreasing the hyper-fibrinolytic state associated with the disease. A role for annexin A2 in the pathogenesis of APL was proposed based on the discovery that annexin A2 levels increased as a result of this fusion protein and treatment with ATRA reduced annexin A2 levels, potentially resulting in reduced fibrinolytic activity [70,71]. Subsequent studies indicated that annexin A2 was actually present in a complex with S100A10 on the cell surface of most cells, that annexin A2 stabilized S100A10 protein levels [72] and that the S100A10 subunits of the $p36_2p11_2$ complex were responsible for plasminogen binding and activation [15,21], our group decided to explore if annexin A2 existed as a complex with S100A10 on the surface of APL cells and if so whether this S100A10 contributed to the hyper-fibrinolytic state presented in APL. We established the presence of S100A10 as a $p36_2p11_2$ complex on the surface of APL cells. Next, we showed that treatment of NB4 cells, an APL cell line, with ATRA resulted in decreased total and cell surface annexin A2 and S100A10 protein levels while mRNA levels were not affected. α-enolase and histone H2B, two other myeloid cell plasminogen receptors, were unaffected by ATRA treatment, providing further evidence that the $p36_2p11_2$ complex was the primary plasminogen receptor that contributed to hyperfibrinolysis in APL. Interestingly, the drop in S100A10 protein levels preceded that of annexin A2. This delay was observed in total protein levels as well as in cell surface protein levels, providing an opportunity to observe whether fibrinolyic activity decreased with loss of cell surface S100A10 alone or whether loss of the complete $p36_2p11_2$ complex was required to decrease fibrinolytic activity following ATRA treatment. Decreases in plasminogen binding, plasmin generation and plasminogen dependent cell invasion were not dependent on the loss of cell surface annexin A2, as these decreases only corresponded with loss of cell surface S100A10. Further evidence that S100A10 was responsible for increased fibrinolysis in APL cells was provided by silencing S100A10 expression using shRNA. Loss of

S100A10 following shRNA expression did not alter cell surface annexin A2 levels but significantly impacted plasminogen binding, plasmin generation and invasion. In order to further explore the relationship between PML-RAR-α and $p36_2p11_2$ complex levels, PML-RAR-α expression was induced in the U937/PR-9 cell line, a myeloid cell line with a $ZnSO_4$ inducible PML-RAR-α promoter. Induction of PML-RAR-α did in fact increase total and cell surface annexin A2 and S100A10 protein levels, yet this effect was not transcriptionally regulated as mRNA levels for each of these proteins were not impacted by PML-RAR-α expression. This increase in the $p36_2p11_2$ complex levels resulted in increased fibrinolytic activity. This provided a clear link between PML-RAR-α expression and increased levels of the $p36_2p11_2$ complex. Subsequent depletion of S100A10 by shRNA in these cells mimicked the previous results observed in the NB4 cells, as plasminogen binding, plasmin stimulation and invasion were decreased with the loss of S100A10 while cell surface annexin A2 levels were unaltered [69]. This study clarified how the $p36_2p11_2$ complex participates in APL hyperfibrinolyis and demonstrates how elevation in S100A10 contributed to the pathogenesis of APL.

Plasmin proteolytic activity has long been associated with tumorigenesis [73,74]. Plasmin mediated proteolysis remodels the tumor microenvironment to permit tumor growth and degrades the basement membrane to permit cancer cell invasion through the stroma and metastasis to other organs. Plasmin directly degrades basement membrane matrix components such as fibronectin [75] and laminin [76] while also activating other proteases, including matrix metalloproteinases (MMP) -1 and -9 [77–80], to trigger a proteolytic cascade necessary for invasion through the basement membrane. Expression of the uPA-uPAR system is considered a prognostic biomarker for several types of malignancies, including breast carcinoma [81], gastric cancer [82], prostate cancer [83] and lung cancer [84]. As components of the plasmin generating system, such as uPAR, are also associated with tumor progression, the key question has been whether the $p36_2p11_2$ complex mediates plasmin generation by cancer cells and if so, does plasmin generated by the $p36_2p11_2$ complex contribute to tumor growth, invasion and metastasis. Multiple reports demonstrated increased annexin A2 expression in a variety of malignancies, which was frequently associated with poor prognosis [85–88]. These reports, however, did not investigate whether S100A10 levels were also associated with these malignancies. As work demonstrating that the carboxyl-terminal lysine of S100A10 was responsible for plasminogen binding and plasmin generation emerged, studies were conducted to observe whether S100A10-dependent plasmin generation contributed to increased invasiveness and tumorigenesis of cancer cells. Our laboratory reported that loss of S100A10 decreased the ability of HT-1080 fibrosarcoma cells [89] and CCL-222 colorectal cancer [90] to invade through an extracellular matrix and that S100A10-depleted cells displayed decreased plasminogen binding, plasmin generation and plasminogen-dependent cellular invasion. In the study with HT-1080 cells, loss of S100A10 significantly decreased the ability of these cancer cells to form metastatic lung foci while over-expression of S100A10 in these same cells increased the metastatic potential, as demonstrated by increased development of metastatic lung foci. More recently, the Zimonjic group reported that DLC1, a Rho GTPase-activating protein and known tumor suppressor, interacted with S100A10 in non small cell lung carcinoma cell lines. DLC1 competed with S100A10 for a common binding site on annexin A2. The DLC1-S100A10 interaction resulted in depletion of S100A10 protein levels as DLC1 prevented the inhibition of ubiquitin-dependent degradation of S100A10 by annexin A2. Depletion of S100A10 protein levels as a result of this interaction with DLC1 attenuated plasmin generation, migration, invasion through a matrigel extracellular matrix barrier and soft agar colony formation. Part of DLC1's tumor suppressor activity is therefore due to its role in decreasing S100A10 protein levels. Since DLC1-S100A10 interaction did not alter annexin A2 protein levels, this study provided further evidence that S100A10 dependent plasmin generation contributes to oncogenesis [8]. Tumor suppressor proteins such as DLC1 function by preventing normal cells from converting into cancer cells ie. they block the process of oncogenesis. Conceptually, this study was important because it linked the aberrant regulation of S100A10 protein levels with the process of oncogenesis.

In human studies, S100A10 has been identified as a tumor biomarker in several different malignancies. For example, S100A10 is associated with aggressive anaplastic carcinoma [91,92], as a marker for renal cell carcinoma [93], advanced diffuse large B-cell lymphoma [94], colorectal cancer [95], non-small cell lung carcinoma [96] and late stage aggressive gallbladder cancer [97]. Additionally, the S100A10 gene location has been identified as genomic region susceptible to epigenetic changes associated with cancer development, indicating the mechanisms associated with regulating S100A10 expression may be associated with malignancy [98]. Such associations between S100A10 levels and cancer development may correlate with cell culture and mouse studies suggesting S100A10 dependent plasmin generation facilitates tumor progression and metastasis.

Numerous studies have found associations between annexin A2 expression and tumorigenesis. These studies have proposed varying mechanisms by which annexin A2 may contribute to cancer development. Many groups maintain that annexin A2 directly interacts with plasminogen and this interaction leads to plasmin generation and subsequent plasmin mediated invasion and tumor growth. However, the majority of these studies fail to investigate whether S100A10 levels fluctuate with varying levels of annexin A2 [99–104], as would be expected by the reports demonstrating that annexin A2 protects S100A10 from ubiquitin dependent degradation [8]. Other studies have found that annexin A2 contributes to tumor progression by mechanisms other than increased plasmin generation. Annexin A2 regulates cell cycle progression by preventing G2 arrest in p53-dependent and -independent mechanisms in non-small cell lung cancer cells [105]. This provided a potential mechanism by which annexin A2 contributes to cell proliferation, which had been reported in several previous reports [102,106–109]. Annexin A2 may also contribute to tumorigenesis by protecting cancer cells from oxidative damage. Depletion of annexin A2 lead to increased levels of reactive oxygen species (ROS) and subsequent increased activation of ROS-induced proapoptotic kinases and cellular damage and resulting death. This study also demonstrated that annexin A2 increased cancer cell growth by preventing cellular protein oxidation, and elevations of reduced annexin A2 in human tumor samples correlated with reduced protein oxidation [110]. In addition to protein oxidation, ROS are also capable of mediating DNA damage [111]. Genotoxic agents, which are used in some chemotherapies, can cause DNA damage and subsequent cell death. Some genotoxic agents directly target and damage DNA, while other rely on the production of intracellular ROS that results from their metabolism [112]. Annexin

A2 levels increase in response to increased ROS [110]. Following increased ROS levels as a result of treatment with genotoxic agents, annexin A2 accumulates in the nucleus. Increased nuclear annexin A2 levels protected the cells from DNA damage following treatment with various genotoxic agents [113]. Elevated levels of annexin A2, through its redox functions, may therefore protect cancer cells from chemotherapeutic treatment. These studies demonstrate non-plasmin dependent mechanisms by which annexin A2 may directly contribute to tumor progression and poor prognosis (Figure 3).

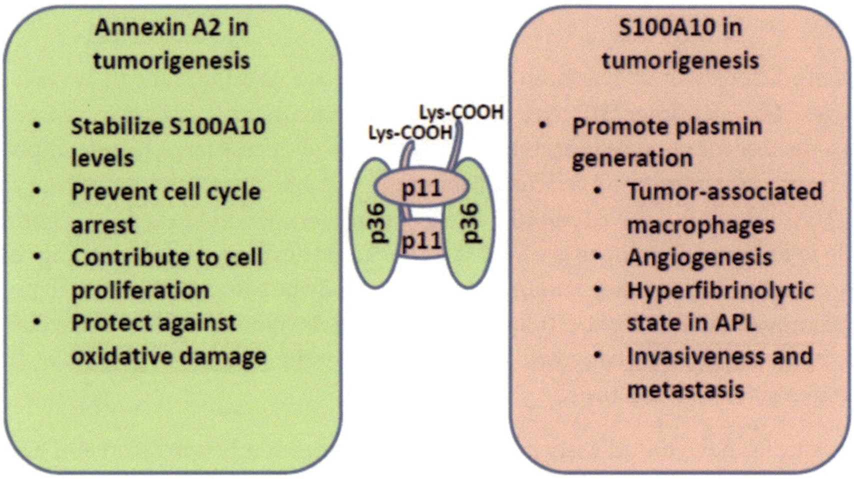

Figure 3. Roles of annexin A2 and S100A10 in tumorigenesis. Annexin A2 and S100A10 may promote tumorigenesis through several mechanisms. Annexin A2 contributes to tumorigenesis by stabilizing S100A10 levels, prevents cell cycle arrest, promotes cell proliferation and protects cancer cells from oxidative damage. S100A10 participates in tumorigenesis primarily by promoting plasmin generation, which contributes to TAM infiltration, angiogensis, invasiveness and metastasis and the hyperfibrinolytic state present in APL.

Tumor development and growth is a dynamic process that is dependent on stromal cells in addition to the cancer cells themselves. Tumor-associated macrophage (TAM) have been demonstrated to participate in tumor development [114], and increased TAM density within a solid tumor is associated with poor prognosis [115]. TAM infiltration into a growing tumor is dependent on the presence of S100A10 on the cell surface, presumably requiring the plasmin generated by the presence of S100A10 to remodel the ECM of the growing tumor and infiltrate into it. Tumor growth is impaired in S100A10−/− mice, and this impairment is due to an inability of TAM to invade into a growing tumor. Introduction of macrophages containing S100A10 into S100A10−/− mice rescued tumor growth, as did injection of S100A10 containing macrophages directly into growing tumors in S100A10−/− mice [116].

Angiogenesis, the process where a growing tumor is vascularized by endothelial cells in order to obtain a blood supply, has also been demonstrated to utilize the protease plasmin for proper angiogenesis associated ECM remodelling [117]. S100A10 dependent plasminogen activation promotes angiogenesis, as shown by decreased angiogenesis in tumors grown in the

http://dx.doi.org/10.5772/57378

S100A10−/− mouse and by a decreased ability of endothelial cells lacking S100A10 to invade through matrigel, an ECM substrate similar to that found in solid tumors [39]. These results clarify a previous study where annexin A2 dependent plasmin generation was postulated to contribute to angiogenesis [37]. Therefore, this study merely recapitulated the importance of annexin A2 in the regulation of S100A10 levels and how this function of annexin A2 often leads to the misassignment of S100A10-dependent functions to annexin A2.

Recently, both components of the $p36_2p11_2$ complex were demonstrated to mediate cell-cell interactions. S100A10 on the surface of endothelial cells was shown to bind to annexin A2 on the surface of breast cancer cells, indicating an additional mechanism by which these proteins may contribute to angiogenesis [118]. S100A10 dependent plasminogen binding and subsequent plasmin generation therefore contributes to tumor growth my a variety of different mechanisms, ranging from cancer cell remodelling of the tumor microenvironment to TAM and endothelial cell invasion into a growing tumor.

5. Conclusion

The involvement of S100A10 in the fibrinolytic surveillance system has been well documented. The recent demonstration of the regulation of S100A10 protein levels by oncogenes and tumor suppressor proteins suggest that S100A10 also plays a central role in cellular transformation. Since S100A10 is predominately an intracellular protein, proper spatio-temporal regulation of this protein is critical to the progression of pathological processes. Therefore, through its ability to bind plasminogen and tPA, S100A10 participates in hemostasis and oncogenesis and this makes S100A10 an attractive therapeutic target for diseases ranging from cancer to cardiovascular disease.

Acknowledgements

Supported by the Heart and Stroke Foundation of Nova Scotia

Author details

Alexi P. Surette[1] and David M. Waisman[1,2*]

*Address all correspondence to: david.waisman@dal.ca

1 Department of Pathology, Dalhousie University, Halifax, NS, Canada

2 Department of Biochemistry & Molecular Biology, Halifax, NS, Canada

References

[1] Herren T, Swaisgood C, Plow EF. Regulation of plasminogen receptors. Front Biosci J Virtual Libr. 2003 Jan 1;8:d1–8.

[2] Collen D. The Plasminogen (Fibrinolytic) System. Thromb Haemost. 1999 Aug;82(2): 259–70.

[3] Plow EF, Felez J, Miles LA. Cellular regulation of fibrinolysis. Thromb Haemost. 1991 Jul 12;66(1):32–6.

[4] MacLeod TJ, Kwon M, Filipenko NR, Waisman DM. Phospholipid-associated annexin A2-S100A10 heterotetramer and its subunits: characterization of the interaction with tissue plasminogen activator, plasminogen, and plasmin. J Biol Chem. 2003 Jul 11;278(28):25577–84.

[5] Gerke V, Weber K. Calcium-dependent conformational changes in the 36-kDa subunit of intestinal protein I related to the cellular 36-kDa target of Rous sarcoma virus tyrosine kinase. J Biol Chem. 1985 Feb 10;260(3):1688–95.

[6] Gerke V, Weber K. Identity of p36K phosphorylated upon Rous sarcoma virus transformation with a protein purified from brush borders; calcium-dependent binding to non-erythroid spectrin and F-actin. EMBO J. 1984 Jan;3(1):227–33.

[7] Gerke V, Weber K. The regulatory chain in the p36-kd substrate complex of viral tyrosine-specific protein kinases is related in sequence to the S-100 protein of glial cells. EMBO J. 1985 Nov;4(11):2917–20.

[8] Yang X, Popescu NC, Zimonjic DB. DLC1 interaction with S100A10 mediates inhibition of in vitro cell invasion and tumorigenicity of lung cancer cells through a RhoGAP-independent mechanism. Cancer Res. 2011 Apr 15;71(8):2916–25.

[9] Bailleux A, Wendum D, Audubert F, Jouniaux A-M, Koumanov K, Trugnan G, et al. Cytosolic phospholipase A2-p11 interaction controls arachidonic acid release as a function of epithelial cell confluence. Biochem J. 2004 Mar 1;378(Pt 2):307–15.

[10] Svenningsson P, Chergui K, Rachleff I, Flajolet M, Zhang X, El Yacoubi M, et al. Alterations in 5-HT1B receptor function by p11 in depression-like states. Science. 2006 Jan 6;311(5757):77–80.

[11] Girard C, Tinel N, Terrenoire C, Romey G, Lazdunski M, Borsotto M. p11, an annexin II subunit, an auxiliary protein associated with the background K+ channel, TASK-1. EMBO J. 2002 Sep 2;21(17):4439–48.

[12] Okuse K, Malik-Hall M, Baker MD, Poon W-YL, Kong H, Chao MV, et al. Annexin II light chain regulates sensory neuron-specific sodium channel expression. Nature. 2002 Jun 6;417(6889):653–6.

[13] Van de Graaf SFJ, Hoenderop JGJ, Gkika D, Lamers D, Prenen J, Rescher U, et al. Functional expression of the epithelial Ca(2+) channels (TRPV5 and TRPV6) requires association of the S100A10-annexin 2 complex. EMBO J. 2003 Apr 1;22(7):1478–87.

[14] MacLeod TJ, Kwon M, Filipenko NR, Waisman DM. Phospholipid-associated annexin A2-S100A10 heterotetramer and its subunits: characterization of the interaction with tissue plasminogen activator, plasminogen, and plasmin. J Biol Chem. 2003 Jul 11;278(28):25577–84.

[15] Kassam G, Choi KS, Ghuman J, Kang HM, Fitzpatrick SL, Zackson T, et al. The role of annexin II tetramer in the activation of plasminogen. J Biol Chem. 1998 Feb 20;273(8):4790–9.

[16] Cesarman GM, Guevara CA, Hajjar KA. An endothelial cell receptor for plasminogen/tissue plasminogen activator (t-PA). II. Annexin II-mediated enhancement of t-PA-dependent plasminogen activation. J Biol Chem. 1994 Aug 19;269(33):21198–203.

[17] Hajjar KA, Guevara CA, Lev E, Dowling K, Chacko J. Interaction of the fibrinolytic receptor, annexin II, with the endothelial cell surface. Essential role of endonexin repeat 2. J Biol Chem. 1996 Aug 30;271(35):21652–9.

[18] Hajjar KA, Guevara CA, Lev E, Dowling K, Chacko J. Interaction of the fibrinolytic receptor, annexin II, with the endothelial cell surface. Essential role of endonexin repeat 2. J Biol Chem. 1996 Aug 30;271(35):21652–9.

[19] Cesarman-Maus G, Hajjar KA. Molecular mechanisms of fibrinolysis. Br J Haematol. 2005 May;129(3):307–21.

[20] Kwon M, MacLeod TJ, Zhang Y, Waisman DM. S100A10, annexin A2, and annexin a2 heterotetramer as candidate plasminogen receptors. Front Biosci J Virtual Libr. 2005 Jan 1;10:300–25.

[21] Kassam G, Le BH, Choi KS, Kang HM, Fitzpatrick SL, Louie P, et al. The p11 subunit of the annexin II tetramer plays a key role in the stimulation of t-PA-dependent plasminogen activation. Biochemistry (Mosc). 1998 Dec 1;37(48):16958–66.

[22] Das R, Burke T, Plow EF. Histone H2B as a functionally important plasminogen receptor on macrophages. Blood. 2007 Nov 15;110(10):3763–72.

[23] Herren T, Burke TA, Das R, Plow EF. Identification of histone H2B as a regulated plasminogen receptor. Biochemistry (Mosc). 2006 Aug 8;45(31):9463–74.

[24] Pluskota E, Soloviev DA, Bdeir K, Cines DB, Plow EF. Integrin alphaMbeta2 orchestrates and accelerates plasminogen activation and fibrinolysis by neutrophils. J Biol Chem. 2004 Apr 23;279(17):18063–72.

[25] Miles LA, Dahlberg CM, Plescia J, Felez J, Kato K, Plow EF. Role of cell-surface lysines in plasminogen binding to cells: identification of alpha-enolase as a candidate plasminogen receptor. Biochemistry (Mosc). 1991 Feb 12;30(6):1682–91.

[26] Hembrough TA, Li L, Gonias SL. Cell-surface cytokeratin 8 is the major plasminogen receptor on breast cancer cells and is required for the accelerated activation of cell-associated plasminogen by tissue-type plasminogen activator. J Biol Chem. 1996 Oct 11;271(41):25684–91.

[27] Gonias SL, Hembrough TA, Sankovic M. Cytokeratin 8 functions as a major plasminogen receptor in select epithelial and carcinoma cells. Front Biosci J Virtual Libr. 2001 Nov 1;6:D1403–1411.

[28] Andronicos NM, Chen EI, Baik N, Bai H, Parmer CM, Kiosses WB, et al. Proteomics-based discovery of a novel, structurally unique, and developmentally regulated plasminogen receptor, Plg-RKT, a major regulator of cell surface plasminogen activation. Blood. 2010 Feb 18;115(7):1319–30.

[29] Hajjar KA. Cellular receptors in the regulation of plasmin generation. Thromb Haemost. 1995 Jul;74(1):294–301.

[30] Miles LA, Castellino FJ, Gong Y. Critical role for conversion of glu-plasminogen to Lys-plasminogen for optimal stimulation of plasminogen activation on cell surfaces. Trends Cardiovasc Med. 2003 Jan;13(1):21–30.

[31] Hajjar KA, Nachman RL. Endothelial cell-mediated conversion of Glu-plasminogen to Lys-plasminogen. Further evidence for assembly of the fibrinolytic system on the endothelial cell surface. J Clin Invest. 1988 Nov;82(5):1769–78.

[32] Miles LA, Plow EF. Receptor mediated binding of the fibrinolytic components, plasminogen and urokinase, to peripheral blood cells. Thromb Haemost. 1987 Oct 28;58(3):936–42.

[33] Castellino FJ, McCance SG. The kringle domains of human plasminogen. Ciba Found Symp. 1997;212:46–60; discussion 60–65.

[34] Fogg DK, Bridges DE, Cheung KK-T, Kassam G, Filipenko NR, Choi K-S, et al. The p11 subunit of annexin II heterotetramer is regulated by basic carboxypeptidase. Biochemistry (Mosc). 2002 Apr 16;41(15):4953–61.

[35] Hajjar KA, Jacovina AT, Chacko J. An endothelial cell receptor for plasminogen/tissue plasminogen activator. I. Identity with annexin II. J Biol Chem. 1994 Aug 19;269(33):21191–7.

[36] Das R, Burke T, Plow EF. Histone H2B as a functionally important plasminogen receptor on macrophages. Blood. 2007 Nov 15;110(10):3763–72.

[37] Ling Q, Jacovina AT, Deora A, Febbraio M, Simantov R, Silverstein RL, et al. Annexin II regulates fibrin homeostasis and neoangiogenesis in vivo. J Clin Invest. 2004 Jan; 113(1):38–48.

[38] He K-L, Deora AB, Xiong H, Ling Q, Weksler BB, Niesvizky R, et al. Endothelial cell annexin A2 regulates polyubiquitination and degradation of its binding partner S100A10/p11. J Biol Chem. 2008 Jul 11;283(28):19192–200.

[39] Surette AP, Madureira PA, Phipps KD, Miller VA, Svenningsson P, Waisman DM. Regulation of fibrinolysis by S100A10 in vivo. Blood. 2011;118(11):3172 –3181.

[40] O'Connell PA, Surette AP, Liwski RS, Svenningsson P, Waisman DM. S100A10 regulates plasminogen-dependent macrophage invasion. Blood. 2010 Aug 19;116(7):1136–46.

[41] Tofler GH, D'Agostino RB, Jacques PF, Bostom AG, Wilson PWF, Lipinska I, et al. Association between increased homocysteine levels and impaired fibrinolytic potential: potential mechanism for cardiovascular risk. Thromb Haemost. 2002 Nov;88(5): 799–804.

[42] Hajjar KA. Homocysteine: a sulph'rous fire. J Clin Invest. 2001 Mar;107(6):663–4.

[43] Karolczak K, Olas B. Mechanism of action of homocysteine and its thiolactone in hemostasis system. Physiol Res Acad Sci Bohemoslov. 2009;58(5):623–33.

[44] Lentz SR. Mechanisms of homocysteine-induced atherothrombosis. J Thromb Haemost JTH. 2005 Aug;3(8):1646–54.

[45] Cai H, Harrison DG. Endothelial dysfunction in cardiovascular diseases: the role of oxidant stress. Circ Res. 2000 Nov 10;87(10):840–4.

[46] Zhang C, Cai Y, Adachi MT, Oshiro S, Aso T, Kaufman RJ, et al. Homocysteine induces programmed cell death in human vascular endothelial cells through activation of the unfolded protein response. J Biol Chem. 2001 Sep 21;276(38):35867–74.

[47] Jacobsen DW, Catanescu O, Dibello PM, Barbato JC. Molecular targeting by homocysteine: a mechanism for vascular pathogenesis. Clin Chem Lab Med CCLM FESCC. 2005;43(10):1076–83.

[48] Tousoulis D, Bouras G, Antoniades C, Marinou K, Miliou A, Papageorgiou N, et al. The activation of endothelin-1 pathway during methionine-induced homocysteinemia mediates endothelial dysfunction in hypertensive individuals. J Hypertens. 2010 May;28(5):925–30.

[49] Moshal KS, Sen U, Tyagi N, Henderson B, Steed M, Ovechkin AV, et al. Regulation of homocysteine-induced MMP-9 by ERK1/2 pathway. Am J Physiol Cell Physiol. 2006 Mar;290(3):C883–891.

[50] Dionisio N, Jardín I, Salido GM, Rosado JA. Homocysteine, intracellular signaling and thrombotic disorders. Curr Med Chem. 2010;17(27):3109–19.

[51] Khajuria A, Houston DS. Induction of monocyte tissue factor expression by homocysteine: a possible mechanism for thrombosis. Blood. 2000 Aug 1;96(3):966–72.

[52] Ling Q, Hajjar KA. Inhibition of endothelial cell thromboresistance by homocysteine. J Nutr. 2000 Feb;130(2S Suppl):373S–376S.

[53] Hajjar KA. Homocysteine-induced modulation of tissue plasminogen activator binding to its endothelial cell membrane receptor. J Clin Invest. 1993 Jun;91(6):2873–9.

[54] Selhub J. Homocysteine metabolism. Annu Rev Nutr. 1999;19:217–46.

[55] Hajjar KA, Mauri L, Jacovina AT, Zhong F, Mirza UA, Padovan JC, et al. Tissue plasminogen activator binding to the annexin II tail domain. Direct modulation by homocysteine. J Biol Chem. 1998 Apr 17;273(16):9987–93.

[56] Félez J, Miles LA, Fábregas P, Jardí M, Plow EF, Lijnen RH. Characterization of cellular binding sites and interactive regions within reactants required for enhancement of plasminogen activation by tPA on the surface of leukocytic cells. Thromb Haemost. 1996 Oct;76(4):577–84.

[57] Jacovina AT, Deora AB, Ling Q, Broekman MJ, Almeida D, Greenberg CB, et al. Homocysteine inhibits neoangiogenesis in mice through blockade of annexin A2-dependent fibrinolysis. J Clin Invest. 2009 Nov;119(11):3384–94.

[58] Kang SS, Wong PW, Becker N. Protein-bound homocyst(e)ine in normal subjects and in patients with homocystinuria. Pediatr Res. 1979 Oct;13(10):1141–3.

[59] Dayal S, Chauhan AK, Jensen M, Leo L, Lynch CM, Faraci FM, et al. Paradoxical absence of a prothrombotic phenotype in a mouse model of severe hyperhomocysteinemia. Blood. 2012 Mar 29;119(13):3176–83.

[60] Dayal S, Wilson KM, Leo L, Arning E, Bottiglieri T, Lentz SR. Enhanced susceptibility to arterial thrombosis in a murine model of hyperhomocysteinemia. Blood. 2006 Oct 1;108(7):2237–43.

[61] Jakubowski H. Homocysteine in Protein Structure/Function and Human Disease: Chemical Biology of Homocysteine-containing Proteins. Springer; 2013.

[62] Yap S, Boers GHJ, Wilcken B, Wilcken DEL, Brenton DP, Lee PJ, et al. Vascular Outcome in Patients With Homocystinuria due to Cystathionine β-Synthase Deficiency Treated Chronically A Multicenter Observational Study. Arterioscler Thromb Vasc Biol. 2001 Dec 1;21(12):2080–5.

[63] Eikelboom JW, Lonn E, Genest J, Hankey G, Yusuf S. Homocyst(e)ine and Cardiovascular Disease: A Critical Review of the Epidemiologic Evidence. Ann Intern Med. 1999 Sep 7;131(5):363–75.

[64] Clarke R, Halsey J, Lewington S, Lonn E, Armitage J, Manson JE, et al. Effects of lowering homocysteine levels with B vitamins on cardiovascular disease, cancer, and cause-specific mortality: Meta-analysis of 8 randomized trials involving 37 485 individuals. Arch Intern Med. 2010 Oct 11;170(18):1622–31.

[65] Bønaa KH, Njølstad I, Ueland PM, Schirmer H, Tverdal A, Steigen T, et al. Homocysteine lowering and cardiovascular events after acute myocardial infarction. N Engl J Med. 2006 Apr 13;354(15):1578–88.

[66] Lonn E, Yusuf S, Arnold MJ, Sheridan P, Pogue J, Micks M, et al. Homocysteine lowering with folic acid and B vitamins in vascular disease. N Engl J Med. 2006 Apr 13;354(15):1567–77.

[67] Den Heijer M, Willems HPJ, Blom HJ, Gerrits WBJ, Cattaneo M, Eichinger S, et al. Homocysteine lowering by B vitamins and the secondary prevention of deep vein thrombosis and pulmonary embolism: A randomized, placebo-controlled, double-blind trial. Blood. 2007 Jan 1;109(1):139–44.

[68] Study of the Effectiveness of Additional Reductions in Cholesterol and Homocysteine (SEARCH) Collaborative Group, Armitage JM, Bowman L, Clarke RJ, Wallendszus K, Bulbulia R, et al. Effects of homocysteine-lowering with folic acid plus vitamin B12 vs placebo on mortality and major morbidity in myocardial infarction survivors: a randomized trial. JAMA J Am Med Assoc. 2010 Jun 23;303(24):2486–94.

[69] O'Connell PA, Madureira PA, Berman JN, Liwski RS, Waisman DM. Regulation of S100A10 by the PML-RAR-α oncoprotein. Blood. 2011 Apr 14;117(15):4095–105.

[70] Menell JS, Cesarman GM, Jacovina AT, McLaughlin MA, Lev EA, Hajjar KA. Annexin II and bleeding in acute promyelocytic leukemia. N Engl J Med. 1999 Apr 1;340(13):994–1004.

[71] Liu Y, Wang Z, Jiang M, Dai L, Zhang W, Wu D, et al. The expression of annexin II and its role in the fibrinolytic activity in acute promyelocytic leukemia. Leuk Res. 2011 Jul;35(7):879–84.

[72] Puisieux A, Ji J, Ozturk M. Annexin II up-regulates cellular levels of p11 protein by a post-translational mechanisms. Biochem J. 1996 Jan 1;313 (Pt 1):51–5.

[73] Mignatti P, Rifkin DB. Biology and biochemistry of proteinases in tumor invasion. Physiol Rev. 1993 Jan;73(1):161–95.

[74] Markus G, Kohga S, Camiolo SM, Madeja JM, Ambrus JL, Karakousis C. Plasminogen activators in human malignant melanoma. J Natl Cancer Inst. 1984 Jun;72(6): 1213–22.

[75] Tapiovaara H, Alitalo R, Vaheri A. Plasminogen activation on tumor cell surface and its involvement in human leukemia. Adv Cancer Res. 1996;69:101–33.

[76] Andreasen PA, Kjøller L, Christensen L, Duffy MJ. The urokinase-type plasminogen activator system in cancer metastasis: A review. Int J Cancer. 1997;72(1):1–22.

[77] Davis GE, Pintar Allen KA, Salazar R, Maxwell SA. Matrix metalloproteinase-1 and -9 activation by plasmin regulates a novel endothelial cell-mediated mechanism of

collagen gel contraction and capillary tube regression in three-dimensional collagen matrices. J Cell Sci. 2001 Mar;114(Pt 5):917–30.

[78] Gong Y, Hart E, Shchurin A, Hoover-Plow J. Inflammatory macrophage migration requires MMP-9 activation by plasminogen in mice. J Clin Invest. 2008 Sep;118(9): 3012–24.

[79] Mazzieri R, Masiero L, Zanetta L, Monea S, Onisto M, Garbisa S, et al. Control of type IV collagenase activity by components of the urokinase-plasmin system: a regulatory mechanism with cell-bound reactants. EMBO J. 1997 May 1;16(9):2319–32.

[80] Pepper MS. Role of the Matrix Metalloproteinase and Plasminogen Activator-Plasmin Systems in Angiogenesis. Arter Thromb Vasc Biol. 2001 Jul 1;21(7):1104–17.

[81] Duffy MJ, O'siorain L, O'grady P, Devaney D, Fennelly JJ, Lijnen HJ. Urokinase-plasminogen activator, a marker for aggressive breast carcinomas. Preliminary report. Cancer. 1988;62(3):531–3.

[82] Ding Y, Zhang H, Zhong M, Zhou Z, Zhuang Z, Yin H, et al. Clinical significance of the uPA system in gastric cancer with peritoneal metastasis. Eur J Med Res. 2013 Aug 28;18(1):28.

[83] Kumano M, Miyake H, Muramaki M, Furukawa J, Takenaka A, Fujisawa M. Expression of urokinase-type plasminogen activator system in prostate cancer: Correlation with clinicopathological outcomes in patients undergoing radical prostatectomy. Urol Oncol Semin Orig Investig. 2009 Mar;27(2):180–6.

[84] Smith HW, Marshall CJ. Regulation of cell signalling by uPAR. Nat Rev Mol Cell Biol. 2010 Jan 1;11(1):23–36.

[85] Chiang Y, Davis RG, Vishwanatha JK. Altered expression of annexin II in human B-cell lymphoma cell lines. Biochim Biophys Acta. 1996 Oct 11;1313(3):295–301.

[86] Emoto K, Yamada Y, Sawada H, Fujimoto H, Ueno M, Takayama T, et al. Annexin II overexpression correlates with stromal tenascin-C overexpression: a prognostic marker in colorectal carcinoma. Cancer. 2001 Sep 15;92(6):1419–26.

[87] Emoto K, Sawada H, Yamada Y, Fujimoto H, Takahama Y, Ueno M, et al. Annexin II overexpression is correlated with poor prognosis in human gastric carcinoma. Anticancer Res. 2001 Apr;21(2B):1339–45.

[88] Vishwanatha JK, Chiang Y, Kumble KD, Hollingsworth MA, Pour PM. Enhanced expression of annexin II in human pancreatic carcinoma cells and primary pancreatic cancers. Carcinogenesis. 1993 Dec;14(12):2575–9.

[89] Choi K-S, Fogg DK, Yoon C-S, Waisman DM. p11 regulates extracellular plasmin production and invasiveness of HT1080 fibrosarcoma cells. FASEB J Off Publ Fed Am Soc Exp Biol. 2003 Feb;17(2):235–46.

[90] Zhang L, Fogg DK, Waisman DM. RNA interference-mediated silencing of the S100A10 gene attenuates plasmin generation and invasiveness of Colo 222 colorectal cancer cells. J Biol Chem. 2004 Jan 16;279(3):2053–62.

[91] Rust R, Visser L, van der Leij J, Harms G, Blokzijl T, Deloulme JC, et al. High expression of calcium-binding proteins, S100A10, S100A11 and CALM2 in anaplastic large cell lymphoma. Br J Haematol. 2005 Dec;131(5):596–608.

[92] Ito Y, Arai K, Nozawa R, Yoshida H, Higashiyama T, Takamura Y, et al. S100A10 expression in thyroid neoplasms originating from the follicular epithelium: contribution to the aggressive characteristic of anaplastic carcinoma. Anticancer Res. 2007 Aug;27(4C):2679–83.

[93] Domoto T, Miyama Y, Suzuki H, Teratani T, Arai K, Sugiyama T, et al. Evaluation of S100A10, annexin II and B-FABP expression as markers for renal cell carcinoma. Cancer Sci. 2007 Jan;98(1):77–82.

[94] Nishiu M, Yanagawa R, Nakatsuka S, Yao M, Tsunoda T, Nakamura Y, et al. Microarray analysis of gene-expression profiles in diffuse large B-cell lymphoma: identification of genes related to disease progression. Jpn J Cancer Res Gann. 2002 Aug; 93(8):894–901.

[95] Shang J, Zhang Z, Song W, Zhou B, Zhang Y, Li G, et al. S100A10 as a novel biomarker in colorectal cancer. Tumour Biol J Int Soc Oncodevelopmental Biol Med. 2013 Jul 5;

[96] Remmelink M, Mijatovic T, Gustin A, Mathieu A, Rombaut K, Kiss R, et al. Identification by means of cDNA microarray analyses of gene expression modifications in squamous non-small cell lung cancers as compared to normal bronchial epithelial tissue. Int J Oncol. 2005 Jan 1;26(1):247–58.

[97] Tan Y, Ma S-Y, Wang F-Q, Meng H-P, Mei C, Liu A, et al. Proteomic-based analysis for identification of potential serum biomarkers in gallbladder cancer. Oncol Rep. 2011 Oct;26(4):853–9.

[98] Leśniak W. Epigenetic regulation of S100 protein expression. Clin Epigenetics. 2011 Aug 1;2(2):77–83.

[99] Sharma MR, Koltowski L, Ownbey RT, Tuszynski GP, Sharma MC. Angiogenesis-associated protein annexin II in breast cancer: selective expression in invasive breast cancer and contribution to tumor invasion and progression. Exp Mol Pathol. 2006 Oct;81(2):146–56.

[100] Sharma M, Blackman MR, Sharma MC. Antibody-directed neutralization of annexin II (ANX II) inhibits neoangiogenesis and human breast tumor growth in a xenograft model. Exp Mol Pathol. 2012 Feb;92(1):175–84.

[101] Zhang H-J, Yao D-F, Yao M, Huang H, Wang L, Yan M-J, et al. Annexin A2 silencing inhibits invasion, migration, and tumorigenic potential of hepatoma cells. World J Gastroenterol WJG. 2013 Jun 28;19(24):3792–801.

[102] Wu B, Zhang F, Yu M, Zhao P, Ji W, Zhang H, et al. Up-regulation of Anxa2 gene promotes proliferation and invasion of breast cancer MCF-7 cells. Cell Prolif. 2012 Jun;45(3):189–98.

[103] Zhao P, Zhang W, Tang J, Ma X-K, Dai J-Y, Li Y, et al. Annexin II promotes invasion and migration of human hepatocellular carcinoma cells in vitro via its interaction with HAb18G/CD147. Cancer Sci. 2010 Feb;101(2):387–95.

[104] Wang Y, Lv H, Li Z, Li C, Wu X. Effect of shRNA mediated down-regulation of Annexin A2 on biological behavior of human lung adencarcinoma cells A549. Pathol Oncol Res POR. 2012 Apr;18(2):183–90.

[105] Wang C-Y, Chen C-L, Tseng Y-L, Fang Y-T, Lin Y-S, Su W-C, et al. Annexin A2 silencing induces G2 arrest of non-small cell lung cancer cells through p53-dependent and -independent mechanisms. J Biol Chem. 2012 Sep 21;287(39):32512–24.

[106] Chiang Y, Schneiderman MH, Vishwanatha JK. Annexin II expression is regulated during mammalian cell cycle. Cancer Res. 1993 Dec 15;53(24):6017–21.

[107] Bao H, Jiang M, Zhu M, Sheng F, Ruan J, Ruan C. Overexpression of Annexin II affects the proliferation, apoptosis, invasion and production of proangiogenic factors in multiple myeloma. Int J Hematol. 2009 Sep 1;90(2):177–85.

[108] Zhang J, Guo B, Zhang Y, Cao J, Chen T. Silencing of the annexin II gene down-regulates the levels of S100A10, c-Myc, and plasmin and inhibits breast cancer cell proliferation and invasion. Saudi Med J. 2010 Apr;31(4):374–81.

[109] Chiang Y, Rizzino A, Sibenaller ZA, Wold MS, Vishwanatha JK. Specific down-regulation of annexin II expression in human cells interferes with cell proliferation. Mol Cell Biochem. 1999 Sep 1;199(1-2):139–47.

[110] Madureira PA, Hill R, Miller VA, Giacomantonio C, Lee PWK, Waisman DM. Annexin A2 is a novel cellular redox regulatory protein involved in tumorigenesis. Oncotarget. 2011 Dec;2(12):1075–93.

[111] Cooke MS, Evans MD, Dizdaroglu M, Lunec J. Oxidative DNA damage: mechanisms, mutation, and disease. FASEB J. 2003 Jul 1;17(10):1195–214.

[112] Mah L-J, El-Osta A, Karagiannis TC. γH2AX: a sensitive molecular marker of DNA damage and repair. Leukemia. 2010 Apr;24(4):679–86.

[113] Madureira PA, Hill R, Lee PWK, Waisman DM. Genotoxic agents promote the nuclear accumulation of annexin A2: role of annexin A2 in mitigating DNA damage. PloS One. 2012;7(11):e50591.

[114] Siveen KS, Kuttan G. Role of macrophages in tumour progression. Immunol Lett. 2009 Apr 27;123(2):97–102.

[115] Lissbrant IF, Stattin P, Wikstrom P, Damber JE, Egevad L, Bergh A. Tumor associated macrophages in human prostate cancer: relation to clinicopathological variables and survival. Int J Oncol. 2000 Sep;17(3):445–51.

[116] Phipps KD, Surette AP, O'Connell PA, Waisman DM. Plasminogen Receptor S100A10 Is Essential for the Migration of Tumor-Promoting Macrophages into Tumor Sites. Cancer Res. 2011 Nov 1;71(21):6676 –6683.

[117] Oh C-W, Hoover-Plow J, Plow EF. The role of plasminogen in angiogenesis in vivo. J Thromb Haemost JTH. 2003 Aug;1(8):1683–7.

[118] Myrvang HK, Guo X, Li C, Dekker LV. Protein interactions between surface Annexin A2 and S100A10 mediate adhesion of breast cancer cells to microvascular endothelial cells. FEBS Lett. 2013 Aug 27;

Chapter 4

Comparative Fibrinolysis

Emma Beatriz Casanave and Juan Tentoni

Additional information is available at the end of the chapter

http://dx.doi.org/10.5772/57359

1. Introduction

Haemostasis prevents leaks or obstructions within the blood vessels following three interrelated sequences: formation of the haemostatic plug, platelet consolidation and dissolution of fibrin clot by the fibrinolytic system (Juhan-Vague and Hans 2003; Van Cott and Laposata 2001; Vasse 2008). Coagulation factors circulate in the blood as proenzymes until they are activated by vascular damage (Lane et al. 2005; Owens and Mackman 2010). These enzymes amplified and disseminated the sequence and then are stopped by natural inhibitors (Mulder et al. 2010; Middeldorp 2011) and the fibrinolytic system (Greenberg and Orthner 1999; Levi et al. 2012). Cellular phospholipids make the process much more efficient (Hoffman 2003; Gentry 2004; Rivera et al. 2009).Activated Factor XIIIa stabilizes the polymer (Sidelmann et al. 2000; Greenberg and Lai 2003; Muszbek et al. 2011). Plasminogen (Plg) is the key in thrombus lysis; and is synthesized in mammals principally by the liver (Stafford 1964; Degen 2001; Zhang et al. 2002; Zorio et al. 2008). Natural Plg activators are: tissue plasminogen activator (tPA) and urokinase (uPA) (Fleming and Melzig 2012); streptokinase (SK) acts as in an exogenous path (Sazonova et al. 2009). Free Plm is very active and degrades other proteins, such as complement, fibrinogen (Fbg), factors II, V and VIII or activates metallo-proteases involved in tissue remodeling by degradation of cellular matrix (Collen 2001; Parfyonova et al. 2002; Dewyer et al. 2007).The main inhibitors of Plm are the alpha2 plasmin inhibitor (α2PI) (Menoud et al. 1996; Fraser et al. 2011) and Plasminogen activator inhibitor type 1 (PAI-1) (Declerk et al. 1998; Vaughan 2005). Thrombin activatable fibrinolysis inhibitor (TAFI) is a link between the two systems, it is activated by thrombin generated during coagulation, and suppresses fibrinolysis (Marx 2004; Hilmayer et al. 2006; Milijic et al. 2010).

2. Selection of animal model in fibrinolysis, a challenge

There is a growing homology in the components of the fibrinolytic system along zoological evolution. Fibrinolysis is present in all vertebrates but invertebrates generally only have clumping of blood corpuscles (Withers 1992). Vertebrates factors involved in coagulation and fibrinolysis have evolved from common ancestral proteins and fibrinolytic ones seem to be related to digestive proteolytic enzymes used by rudimentary microorganisms to be released and disseminated, avoiding the host´s nonspecific defense and immunity response (Patthy 1990; Gladysheva et al, 2003; Opal and Esmon 2003; Levi et al. 2012).

Insects have rich sources of pharmacological active substances that may have medical value: The venom of *Lonomia oblique* caterpillar may induce a hemorrhagic syndrome in humans, and blood incoagulability in laboratory animals (Prezoto et al. 2002). Bee venom of *Bombus ignites* contains a Kunitz type serine protease inhibitor (Bi-KTI) that acts as an antifibrinolytic agent inhibiting plasmin (Choo et al 2012). In nature, there are many animals adapted to a diet of fresh blood, and they had to evolve mechanisms to control their host coagulation processes, to maintain the blood in a fluid state during intake and subsequent digestion (Tanaka-Azevedo et al 2010). A variety of coagulation inhibitors have been isolated from blood sucking animals such as ticks (Jacobs et al 1990; Waxman et al 1990), leeches (Sawyer 1986, 1991), hookworms (Cappello et al 1995) and bats (Gardell et al 1991).

Very little is known about the fibrinolytic system and its component concentrations in animals and the relevance of these models for human health is questioned due to many reasons: interspecies differences (Siller-Matula et al. 2008; Ralph and Brainard 2012), lack of reliable results (Vap et al. 2012), use of diagnostic equipment designed only for human care, inadequate relationship of test reagent to clotting factor concentration (Ravanat et al. 1995; Jagadeeswaran and Sheehan 1999; Kubalek et al. 2002, Münster et al. 2002; Gentry 2004; Weir-M et al. 2004). Also, anatomical features of the animal chosen can make it really difficult to obtain good quality blood samples (Saito et al. 1976; Meinkoth and Allison 2007). For example, vessel size and blood flow are important determinants of vascular function when mouse model is used for human research of aorta (Fay et al 2007).

3. Objective of this chapter

In this chapter we summarize the actual knowledge about fibrinolytic assays among different animal species and we compare these findings with healthy adult human beings.

4. Fibrinolytic parameters

A review of laboratory tests was conducted in a phylogenetic order: fish, amphibians, reptiles, birds and mammals. It was designed to assess the fibrinolytic system in its various stages: global (whole blood lysis time WBLT, whole blood diluted lysis time WDLT, euglobulin lysis time ELT), specific (Plg, PAI-1, tPA, α2PI and the thrombin-activatable fibrinolysis inhibitor TAFI) and degradation products generated from the degradation of fibrinogen / fibrin FDP, D Dimer DD, and Plm-α2PI, tPA-PAI-1, uPA-PAI-1 complexes (Blanco 2003; Urano and Suzuki 2011).

The results of these assays are summarized in Tables 1, 2, 3, 4, 5, 6, 7, 8, 9 and 10 (Tentoni et al, 2010).

In fishes the information is insufficient (Tables 1 and 2). WBLT is undetectable in lamprey and black fish, while lysis is fast in dog fish. The genes encoded for Plg and tPA were identified in the blowfish *Fugu rubripes* (Jiang and Doolittle 2003). Rats with diets based on fish oil decrease the fibrinolytic activity due to an increase of PAI-1 (Sano et al. 2003), whereas dietary supplementation with fish protein increases fibrinolysis by increasing tPA in blood (Murata et al. 2004).

In amphibians (Tables 1 to 3), the marine toad *Bufo marinus* and the tree frog *Hyla caerula* show spontaneous WBLT (Hackett and Lapage 1961, Hackett and Hann 1964), while it does not occur in the common frog *Rana temporaria*, leopard frog *Rana pipiens* or the clawed toad *Xenopuslaevis*(Table 2),but can be induced if possible inhibitors are removed, which suggests a large concentration of antifibrinolytic agents. The existence of a protein similar to Plg in *Rana tigrina* and *Xenopus laevis* is explained by the fibrinolysis produced after the addition of uPA (Srivastava et al. 1981).

There is no evidence of a fibrinolytic system in reptiles, lizards (Trachydosaurus rugosus rugosus, Tiliqua scincoides, Amphibolorus barbatus, Varanus acanthrus, Iguana iguana), turtles (Chelodina longicollis), crocodiles (Crocodylus porosus) or pitons (Liasis spp, Morelia spp) (Tables 1 and 10). A strong circulating antithrombin protects these vertebrates from intravascular thrombosis (Hackett and Hann 1964; Kubalek et al. 2002), however low concentrations of α2PI were detected in the circulation of the snake Bitis arietans using a chromogenic method (Table 10).

Snake venoms are mixtures of many peptides which affect the blood coagulation and fibrinolysis pathways such as Plg activators (Kini 2005; Miller et al 2009) and fibrinogen degradators (Meyer 2000). Recently a non hemorrhagic metalloproteinase (BleucMP) was purified from *Bothrops leucurus* snake venom by two chromatographic steps procedure on DEAE-Sephadex A-25, which has an efficient proteolytic action over fibrinogen (Sérgio et al 2011).

Birds are deficient in Factors XI and XII so the clotting times exceeding 70 minutes (Wartelle 1957; Soulier et al. 1959, Bigland 1964). Fibrinolysis can be activated with the saliva of the vampire *Diaemus youngui* (Cartwright and Hawkye 1969), but not with SK (Cliffton and Cannamela 1951). Plg concentration in quails is indetectable due the chromogenic assay is activated with SK instead of uPA. Vultures have the highest reported value DD concentration among the animals with reduced levels of Fbg and clotting factors, remaining a disseminated intravascular coagulation in man, with the advantage of being easily reversible (Weir-M et al. 2004).

The WDLT in the *Halichoerus grypus* is lower than in humans (Table 3), suggesting the existence of an active fibrinolytic system.The Plg activity in *Balaenoptera borealis*is cannot be activated by SK but reacts against rabbit antibody antiPlg (Robinson et al. 1969).

FDP was undetectable in the *Mirounga angustirostris* elephant seal (Table 1 and 6).

Plg activators similar to tPA were discovered in the South American vampire bat´s *Desmodus rotundus* saliva (Verstraete 1995) and they all need fibrin as a cofactor (Schleuning et al. 1992).These activators do not degrade Fbg, or cause neuronal damage such as tPA does (Grandjean et al. 2004) and also have a prolonged plasma half-life (Zavalova et al. 2002).

In dogs (Tables 1, 3, 4, 5, 6, 7 and 10), except for the Plg when it is measured by activation with SK, the values of all the fibrinolytic assays are quite similar to the values in humans, as reported by Wohl et al. (1983).

In cats (Tables 1, 3, 5, 9 and 10) there is a marked difference in functional PAI-1 activity when compared to man, and its Plg cannot be activated with tPA but with uPA (Welles 1996).

In studied rodents, the fibrinolytic system is quite similar to that in humans, but Plg is poorly activated with SK; Plg, tPA, uPA and PAI-1 have been described in *Mus musculus* mouse (Tables 1, 7 and 8), the first two having high sequence homology with their human counterpart (Poplis and Castellino 2002). Interesting enough, PAI-1 deficient mice present a mild hyperfibrinolytic state in adulthood, whereas Plg deficiency predisposes to severe thrombosis (Eitzman et al. 2000; Mackman 2005). The main inhibitors of fibrinolysis in mice are α2PI and TAFI (Marx et al. 2000). In rodent capybara *Hydrochaeris hydrochaeris* (Tables 1 and 5), Plg cannot be activated even with 500 U/mL of SK (Leitao et al, 2000).

Rat (Tables 1, 3, 4, 5, 7, 8, 9 and 10), guinea pigs (Tables 4, 5 and 10) and rabbits (Tables 1, 3, 4, 5, 7, 9 y 10) are the most employed animal models in fibrinolytic research.

Plg cannot be activated with SK in cattle (Tables 1, 5, 6 and 10), pigs (Tables 1, 5, 7 and 10) and sheep (Tables 5, 7 and 10), (Cliffton and Cannamella 1953; Korninger and Colleen 1981; Wohl et al 1983; Zhang et al 2012). Horses (Tables 1, 5, 6, 7, 9 and 10) have higher levels of functional PAI-1 and α2PI when compared to humans (Barton et al. 1998). The fibrinolytic activity in llama is similar to that of horses and other domestic species (Morin et al 1995).

In armadillos *Chaetophractus villosus* our research group found prolonged WBLT and WDLT with PAI-1 functional activity four times greater than in man; this high concentration of inhibitor can be successfully removed with the ELT technique, despite the anticoagulant used (citrate/oxalate). The α2PI concentration is similar to that measured in humans. DD was undetectable in the immunological test (Tentoni et al., 2008). Nevertheless we found FXIII activity in this mammal, with a range from 32 to 78 percent (%) in relation to the calibration curve obtained with a pool of healthy humans platelets poor plasma using Berichrom chromogenix assay (Dade Behring). The fibrin plug was resistant to urea 5M for more than 36 hours; its coagulation factors depend on the vitamin K cycle because the oral administration of 0.28 mg/kg/day of acenocumarol increased baseline values of Prothrombin time PT ($p<0.01$) and activated Partial Thromboplastin time aPTT ($p<0.05$). When PTT-LA reagent is used in aPTT assays in armadillos, the typical shortened values of this specie (20 seconds) increases (26-30 seconds) (Tentoni et al., unpublished), as observed in pigs by Velik-Salchner et al. (2006).

Species	Fbg (mg/dL)	Author
human	188 - 381	Williams *et al*, 2005
armadillo[a]	211 - 333	Casanave *et al*, 2006
armadillo[a´]	258 - 380	Tentoni *et al*, 2008
whale[b]	147	Saito *et al*, 1976
iguana[c]	420 - 440	Kubalek *et al*, 2002
cat[d]	50 - 165	O´Rourke *et al*, 1982
cat	150 - 400	Herring and McMichael, 2012
eagle[e]	80 - 160	García-Montijano *et al*, 2002
frog[f]	590 - 990	Coppo *et al*, 2005
dolphin[g]	269 - 417	Tibbs *et al*, 2005
mouse[h]	200 - 260	Tsakiris *et al*, 1999
dog	141 - 227	Mischke *et al*, 2000
dog	179. - 329	Machida *et al*, 2010
dog	150 - 400	Herring and McMichael, 2012
rat	168 - 192	Honda *et al*, 2008
japanese quail[i]	140 - 260	Belleville *et al*, 1982
pig[j]	181 - 534	Velik-Salchner *et al*, 2006
pig	130 - 170	Schöchl *et al*, 2011
rabbit[k]	257 - 286	Marval *et al*, 1992
cow[l]	125 - 697	Heuwieser *et al*, 1989
sheep	178 - 215	Wilhelmi *et al*, 2012
horse[m]	78 - 156	Barton *et al*, 1998
monkey[n]	119 - 239	Suzuki *et al*, 1977
elephant seal[o]	50 - 162	Gulland *et al*, 1996
capybara[p]	124	Leitâo *et al*, 1999
ostrich[q]	172 - 356	Frost *et al*, 1999
caiman[r]	430 - 1500	Arocha-Piñango *et al*, 1982.
marine fish[s]	220 - 280	Pavlidis *et al*, 1999
asian elephant[t]	412 - 510	Gentry *et al*, 1996
vulture[u]	< 20	Weir-M *et al*, 2004
llama[v]	140 - 300	Morin *et al*, 1995

A Chaetophractus villosus (n:20); a´ (n:24); b Balaenoptera borealis (n:1); c Iguana iguana (n:26); d (n:21); e Aquila adalberti (n:12); f Rana catesbeiana (n:302); g Tursiops truncatus (n:17); h Mus musculus; i Coturnix coturnix japonica ; j(n: 80); k New Zealand rabbits (n:102); l (n:90); m foals (n:53); n Macaca fuscata (n:52); o Mirounga angustirostris (n:19); p Hydrochaeris hydrochaeris (n:2); q Struthio camelus (n:30); r Caiman crocodilus; s Dentex dentex; t Elephas maximus; u Coragyps atratus (n:2); v (n: 46 adult females); < less than.

Table 1. Fibrinogen (Fbg) concentration values in different vertebrates

Species	WBLT (hours)	Author
human	"/> 24	Conard, 1976
lamprey[a]	nd	Hawkey, 1971
black fish[b]	nd	Hawkey, 1971
common frog[c]	nd	
leopard frog[d]	nd	Blofield, 1965
clawed toad[e]	nd	
domestic birds	nd	Niewiarowski & Latallo, 1959
dogfish[f]	2 – 4	Hawkey, 1971 Doolittle & Surgernor, 1962
japanese quail[g]	"/> 72	Belleville *et al*, 1982
armadillo	"/> 72	Tentoni *et al*, 2008

a Petromyzon marinus; b Tautoga onitis; c Rana temporaria; d Rana pipiens; e Xenopus lavéis; f Mustelus canis; g Coturnix coturnix japonica (n:10 adult males); nd: not detectable; > more than.

Table 2. Whole blood lysis time (WBLT) values in different vertebrates

Species	WDLT (hours)	Author
human	> 20	Fearnley *et al*, 1957
tiger frog[a]	> 48	Srivastava *et al*, 1981
seal[b]	5.9 – 8.5	Lohman *et al*, 1998
dog[c]	> 20	
rat[d]	> 20	Hedlin *et al*, 1972
rabbit[e]	> 20	
rabbit[f]	> 30	Hassett *et al*, 1986
cat[g]	nd	Welles *et al*, 1994
armadillo	> 72	Tentoni *et al*, 2008

nd: not detectable; a *Rana tigrina* (n:6) measured at 4 and 37ºC; at 22ºC WDLT range was 31.5-45.3 hours; b *Halichoerus grypus* (n:2, both females), before immersion; c (n:3); d (n:6); e (n:4); f New Zealand male rabbits (n:4); g (n:15); > more than.

Table 3. Whole blood diluted lysis time (WDLT) values in different vertebrates

Species	ELT (minutes)	Author
human	"/> 120	Kowalski *et al*, 1959
armadillo[a]	15.4 – 45.6	Bermúdez, 2003
armadillo [a´]	24.5 - 93	Tentoni *et al*, 2008
tiger frog[b]	nd	Srivastava *et al*, 1981
japanese quail[c]	nd	Belleville *et al*, 1982
dog	21 - 109	Hedlin *et al*, 1972
guinea pig[d]	< 90	Kaspareit *et al*, 1988
rabbit	270 - 450	Hassett *et al*, 1986
monkey[e]	240	Suzuki et al, 1977
vulture[f]	nd	Weir-M *et al*, 2004
rat	105 - 145	Groza *et al*, 1988

a *Chaetophractus villosus* using citrated plasma (n:20, 10 females and 10 males); a´ using oxalated plasma; b *Rana tigrina* (n:6); c *Coturnix coturnix japonica* (n:10 young males); d *Cavia porcellus* (n:45); e *Macaca fuscata*; f *Coragyps atratus* (n:2); nd: not detectable; > more than; < less than.

Table 4. Euglobulin lysis time (ELT) values in different vertebrates

<table>
<tr><th>Species</th><th>Plg (%)</th><th>Author</th></tr>
<tr><td>human</td><td>80 - 120</td><td>Perkins, 1999</td></tr>
<tr><td>japanese quail[a]</td><td>0</td><td>Belleville et al, 1982</td></tr>
<tr><td>dog</td><td>102 - 115 #</td><td>Lanevschi et al, 1996b</td></tr>
<tr><td>dog</td><td>3,2 - 4,4</td><td>Karges et al, 1994</td></tr>
<tr><td>cat</td><td>50 - 200</td><td>O´Rourke et al, 1982</td></tr>
<tr><td>cat</td><td>94 - 122</td><td rowspan="4">Karges et al, 1994</td></tr>
<tr><td>rat</td><td>6 - 14</td></tr>
<tr><td>guinea pig[b]</td><td>0.4 – 6.1</td></tr>
<tr><td>rabbit</td><td>2</td></tr>
<tr><td>rabbit</td><td>147 - 217 #</td><td>Marval et al, 1992</td></tr>
<tr><td>rabbit</td><td>84 - 108 #</td><td>Hassett et al, 1986</td></tr>
<tr><td>sheep</td><td>0.7 – 1.5</td><td rowspan="2">Karges et al, 1994</td></tr>
<tr><td>cow</td><td>0</td></tr>
</table>

Species	Plg (%)	Author
monkey[c]	24 - 39	
monkey[d]	164 #	Suzuki *et al*, 1977
capybara[e]	0	Leitâo *et al*, 2000
pig	2.1 – 5.2	Karges *et al*, 1994
pig	0	Hahn *et al*, 1996
horse[f]	66.5 – 98.1	Barton *et al*, 1998
whale[g]	112 #	Saito *et al*, 1976
armadillo	28 - 40	Tentoni *et al*, 2008

Results are expressed as percent for Plg activity in relation to the calibration curve obtained with a pool of healthy humans platelets poor plasma, using a chromogenix assay after activation with SK.

a *Coturnix coturnix japonica* (n:10 young males); b *Cavia porcellus*; c *Macaca fascicularis*; d *Macaca fuscata*; e *Hydrochaeris hydrochaeris*, it was impossible to activate its Plg with 500 U/mL of SK; f neonatal foals, Plg calibration curve was performed using equine pooled plasma; g *Balaenoptera borealis* (n:1); # Plg measured using uPAas activator.

Table 5. Plasminogen (Plg) activity values in different vertebrates

Species	FDP (µg/mL)	Author
human	< 10	Amiral *et al*, 1990
dog	< 5	Boisvert *et al*, 2001
dog	< 5	Stokol, 2003
dog	< 5	Griffin *et al*, 2003
dog	0 – 1.18	Machida *et al*, 2010
dog	< 10	Herring & McMichael, 2012
cat	< 10	Herring & McMichael, 2012
horse	5.5 – 10.9	Barton *et al*, 1998
horse	< 10	Stokol *et al*, 2005
elephant seal[a]	0	Gulland *et al*, 1996
dolphin[b]	< 10	Tibbs *et al*, 2005
cow	< 5	Irmak & Turgut, 2005
armadillo	0 - 10	Tentoni *et al*, 2008

A *Mirounga angustirostris*; b *Tursiops truncatus* (n: 12); < less than.

Table 6. Fibrin fibrinogen degradation products (FDP) concentration values in different mamals

Species	DD (µg/mL)	Author
human	< 0.50	Estève *et al*, 1996
dog	0.08 – 0.39	Stokol *et al*, 2000b
dog	0.02 – 0.28	Caldin *et al*, 2000
dog	< 0.25	Nelson, 2005
dog	< 0.25	Herring & McMichael, 2012
cat	< 0.25	Herring & McMichael, 2012
rat	0.18	Asakura *et al*, 2002
rat	< 0.02	Ravanant *et al*, 1995
hen	< 0.02	
rabbit	< 0.02	
sheep	< 0.02	
monkey[a]	< 0.05	
mouse	< 0.02	
mouse	0	Tsakiris *et al*, 1999
pig	0	Roussi *et al*, 1996
pig	< 0.01	Schöchl *et al*, 2011
horse[b]	0.46 – 0.92	Monreal *et al*, 2000
horse	0 – 0.91	Machida *et al*, 2010
horse	< 0.50	Stokol *et al*, 2005
ostrich	0.25	Frost *et al*, 1999
vulture	"/> 1	Weir-M *et al*, 2004
armadillo	nd	Tentoni *et al*, 2008
dolphin	< 0.50	Tibbs *et al*, 2005

A *Papio papio*; b (n: 30); nd: not detectable; < less than; > more than.

Table 7. D Dimer (DD) concentration values in different vertebrates.

Species	PAI-1 immunologic (ng/mL)	Author
human	4 – 43	Declerck *et al*, 1988
mouse[a]	1.3 – 2.5	Tsakiris *et al*, 1999
mouse	1 – 2	Matsuo *et al*, 2007
pig	0	Roussi *et al*, 1996

Species	PAI-1 immunologic (ng/mL)	Author
pig[b]	5.6 – 9.0	Schöchl *et al*, 2011
armadillo	1.0 – 2.2	Tentoni *et al*, 2008
rat	3.9	Nieuwenhuys *et al*, 1998

A *Mus musculus* (n: 160); b measured with Porcine PAI-1 Activity Assay

Table 8. Immunological Plasminogen activator inhibitor type 1 (PAI-1) concentration in different mammals

Species	PAI-1 functional (U/mL)	Author
human	< 10	Van Cott & Laposata, 2001
cat	0	Welles, 1996
rabbit	0.06 – 0.16	Hassett *et al*, 1986
horse	19.6 – 42.2	Barton *et al*, 1998
armadillo	24.8 – 37.7	Tentoni *et al*, 2008
rat	1.0	Nobukata *et al*, 2000
rat	4.9 – 7.4	Emeis *et al*, 1992

Results are expressed as units of PAI-1 present in plasma in relation to the calibration curve obtained with a commercial standard when using immunological test; < less than

Table 9. Functional Plasminogen activator inhibitor type 1 (PAI-1) concentration in different mammals

Species	α_2PI (%)	Author
Human	70 - 130	Teger-Nilsson *et al*, 1977
japanese quail[a]	65 - 85	Belleville *et al*, 1982
ostrich[b]	115.6	Frost *et al*, 1999
hen	109.4	
snake[c]	10	
Sheep	68.8	
whale[d]	50	Saito *et al*, 1976
dog	96 - 103	Lanevschi *et al*, 1996b
dog	92 - 94	Karges *et al*, 1994
cat	70 - 86	
rat	118 - 138	

Species	α_2PI (%)	Author
guinea pig[e]	91 - 101	
sheep	90 - 109	
pig	63 - 104	
monkey[f]	82 - 99	
rabbit	91 - 108	
rabbit	66 - 92	Hassett *et al*, 1986
pig	87 - 127	Hahn *et al*, 1996
rat	120	Nobukata *et al*, 2000
horse	154 - 240	Barton *et al*, 1998
cow	80 - 94	Daugschies *et al*, 1998
armadillo	72 - 101	Tentoni *et al*, 2008

Results are expressed as percent for α_2PI activity in relation to the calibration curve obtained with a pool of healthy humans platelets poor plasma, using a chromogenix assay after activation with an excess of Plm.

a Coturnix coturnix japonica; b Struthio camelus; c Bitis arietans; d Balaenoptera borealis (n:1); e Cavia porcellus; f Macaca fascicularis.

Table 10. alpha2 plasmin inhibitor activity (α_2PI) in different vertebrates

5. Conclusions

The information summarized in this chapter helps the choice of appropriate animal experimental models for studying fibrinolysis and the correct extrapolation of animal results toward humans. Previous work from our laboratory, has identified the choice of the armadillo as an animal model because it adapts well to captivity conditions, endures repeated blood sampling, shows excellent tolerance to cardiac puncture and recovers quickly from anaesthesia (Bermúdez et al. 2004; Casanave et al. 2005; 2006). *Chaetophractus villosus* has a hypercoagulable and hypofibrinolytic profile (Tentoni et al., 2008) as pigs, which are frequently used as an animal model in human research. Finally, the study of animals' haemostatic mechanisms is important in the field of zoology, for the advancement of scientific knowledge and in biomedicine, helping to select a suitable experimental animal model.

Acknowledgements

This work was supported by Secretaría General de Ciencia y Tecnología, Universidad Nacional del Sur (SGCyT-UNS), Project 24/B152 and by Agencia Nacional de Promoción Científica y Tecnológica (ANPCyT), PICTR 74/02, Argentina.

Author details

Emma Beatriz Casanave[1,2] and Juan Tentoni[3*]

*Address all correspondence to: juan.tentoni@uns.edu.ar

1 Cátedra de Fisiología Animal, Departamento de Biología, Bioquímica y Farmacia, Universidad Nacional del Sur. San Juan, Bahía Blanca, Argentina

2 Consejo Nacional de Investigaciones Científicas y Técnicas (CONICET), Buenos Aires, Argentina

3 Cátedra del Practicanato Profesional Bioquímico, Departamento de Biología, Bioquímica y Farmacia, Universidad Nacional del Sur, San Juan, Bahía Blanca, Argentina

References

[1] Amiral J, Grosley M, Mimilla F, Plassart V, Chambrette B. Monoclonal antibodies to different neo-epitopes on fibrinogen and fibrin degradation products. Blood Coagul. Fibrinolysis 1990;1(4-5):447-52.

[2] Arocha-Piñango CL, Gorzula SJ, Ojeda A.The blood clotting mechanism of spectacled Caiman *Caiman crocodilus.* Molecular Physiology 1982;2:161-70.

[3] Asakura H, Suga Y, Aoshima K, Ontachi Y, Mizutani T, Kato M, Saito M, Morishita E, Yamazaki M, Takami A, Miyamoto K, Nakao S. Marked difference in pathophysiology between tissue factor and lipopolysaccharide-induced disseminated intravascular coagulation models in rats. Crit. Care Med. 2002;30(1):161-4.

[4] Barton MH, Morris DD, Norton N, Prasse KW.Hemostatic and fibrinolytic indices in neonatal foals with presumed septicemia. J. Vet. Intern. Med.1998;12:26-35.

[5] Belleville J, Cornillon B, Paul J, Baguet J, Clendinnen G, Eloy R. Haemostasis, blood coagulation and fibrinolysis in the japanese quail. Comparative Biochemistry and Physiology. 1998;71:219-30.

[6] Bermúdez PM. Estudio experimental de la hemostasia en el armadillo *Chaetophractus villosus* (Mammalia, Dasypodidae). Thesis. Universidad Nacional del Sur. Bahía Blanca, Argentina; 2003.

[7] Bermúdez PM, Polini NN, Casanave EB. A study of platelets in the armadillo *Chaetophractus villosus* (Xenarthra, Dasypodidae). Platelets 2004;15(5):279-85.

[8] Bigland CH. Blood clotting times of five avian species. Poultry Science 1964;43:1035-9.

[9] Blanco A. Evaluación del mecanismo fibrinolítico. In: Fundamentos para el manejo práctico en el laboratorio de hemostasia. 1st edition, Grupo Cooperativo Argentino de Hemostasia y Trombosis, Federación Bioquímica de la Provincia de Buenos Aires, Argentina; 2003. p 425-34.

[10] Blofield A. A spontaneously active fibrinolytic system in *Xenopus laevis* which is further activated by human urokinase. Nature 1965;206(985):736-7.

[11] Boisvert AM, Swenson CL, Haines CJ. Serum and plasma latex agglutination tests for detection of fibrin(ogen) degradation products in clinically ill dogs. Veterinary Clinical Pathology 2001;30(3):133-6.

[12] Caldin M, Furlanello T, Lubas G.Validation of an immunoturbidimetric D dimer assay in canine citrated plasma. Veterinary Clinical Pathology 2000;29(2):51-4.

[13] Cappello M, Vlasuk GP, Bergum PW, Huang S, Hotez PJ. Ancylostoma caninum anticoagulant peptide: a hookworm-derived inhibitor of human coagulation factor Xa. Proceedings of the NationalAcademy of Sciences of the United States of America1995;92(13):6152–6.

[14] Cartwright T The Plasminogen Activator of vampire bat saliva blood 1974; 43 (3): 317-326

[15] Cartwright T, Hawkey C. Activation of the blood fibrinolytic mechanism in birds by saliva of the vampire bat (*Diaemus youngi*). J Physiol 1969;201(1):45-6.

[16] Casanave EB, Bermúdez PM, Polini NN. Principal coagulation factors and natural anticoagulants in the armadillo *Chaetophractus villosus* (Mammalia, Xenarthra, Dasypodidae). Comparative Clinical Pathology 2006;14(4):210-6.

[17] Casanave EB, Bermúdez PM, Polini NN. Haemostatic mechanisms of the armadillo *Chaetophractus villosus* (Xenarthra, Dasypodidae). Comparative Clinical Pathology 2005;13(4):171-5.

[18] Choo YM, Lee KS, Yoon HJ, Qiu Y, Wan H, Sohn MR, Sohn HD, Jin BR. Antifibrinolytic role of a bee venom serine protease inhibitor that acts as a Plasmin Inhibitor. PLoS One 2012;7(2):e32269. doi:10.1371/journal.pone.0032269.

[19] Cliffton EE, Cannamela DA. Variations in proteolytic activity of serum of animals including man. Proc. Soc. Exp. Biol. Med.1951;77(2):305-8.

[20] ClifftonEE, Cannamela, DA(1953). Proteolytic and fibrinolyticactivity of serum: activation by streptokinase and staphylokinase indicating dissimilarity of enzymes. *Blood 1953*;8:554–62.

[21] Collen D. Role of the plasminogen system in fibrin-homeostasis and tissue remodeling. Ham-Wasserman Lecture Hematology: American Society of Hematology, Education Program 2001;1-9.

[22] Conard J. Plasma plasminogen activator-clot lysis assay techniques. In Davidson JF, Samama MM, Desnoyers PC (eds): Progress in Chemical Fibrinolysis and Thrombolysis 1976;2:15-6. Raven Press, New York. USA.

[23] Coppo JA, Mussart NB, Fioranelli SA, Zeinsteger PA.Blood and urine physiological values in captive bullfrog, *Rana catesbeiana* (Anura: Ranidae). Analecta Veterinaria 2005;25(1):15-7.

[24] Daugschies A, Rupp U, Rommel M. Blood clotting disorders during experimental sarcocystiosis in calves. International Journal for Parasitology 1998;28:1187-94.

[25] Declerck PJ, Alessi MC, Verstreken M, Kruithof EK, Juhan-Vague I, Collen D. Measurement of plasminogen activator inhibitor 1 in biologic fluids with a murine monoclonal antibody-based enzyme-linked immunosorbent assay. Blood 1998;71(1):220-5.

[26] Degen JL. Genetic interactions between the coagulation and fibrinolytic systems. Thromb. Haemost. 2001;86(1):130-7.

[27] Dewyer NA, Sood V, Lynch EM, Luke CE, Upchurch GR Jr, Wakefield TW, Kunkel S, Henke PK. Plasmin inhibition increases MMP-9 activity and decreases vein wall stiffness during venous thrombosis resolution. J. Surg. Res.2007;142(2):357-63.

[28] Dukes HH, Swenson MJ. Coagulación de la sangre. In: Fisiología de los animales domésticos. 4th edition. Ediciones Aguilar. México; 2000. p: 78-97.

[29] Eitzman DT, Westrick RJ, Nabel EG, Ginsburg D. Plasminogen activator inhibitor-1 and vitronectin promote vascular thrombosis in mice. Blood 2000;95:577-80.

[30] Emeis JJ, Van den Hoogen C. Pharmacological modulation of the endotoxin-induced increase in plasminogen activator inhibitor activity in rats. Blood Coagul Fibrinolysis 1992;3(5):575-81.

[31] Estève F, Grimaux M, Migaud-Fressart M, Stötzer KE, Amiral J. Individual and quantitative rapid testing of D. Dimer using an automated system. XIIIth International Congress on Fibrinolysis and Thrombolysis. Barcelona, Spain; 1990.

[32] Fay WP, Garg N, Sunkar M. Vascular functions of the plasminogen activation system. Arterioscler. Thromb. Vasc. Biol.2007;27:1231-7.

[33] Fearnley GR, Balmforth G, Fearnley E. Evidence of a diurnal fibrinolytic rhythm; with a simple method of measuring natural fibrinolysis. Clin. Sci.1957;16:645-50.

[34] Fleming M, Melzig MF. Serine-proteases as plasminogen activators in terms of fibrinolysis. J. Pharm. Pharmacol.2012;64(8):1025-39.

[35] Fraser SR, Booth NA, Mutch NJ. The antifibrinolytic function of factor XIII is exclusively expressed through α2-antiplasmin cross-linking. Blood 2011;117(23):6371-74.

[36] Frost CL, Naudè RJ, Oelofsen W, Jacobson B. Comparative blood coagulation studies in the ostrich. Immunopharmacology 1999;45:75-81.

[37] García-Montijano M, García A, Lemus JA, Montesinos A, Canales R, Luaces I, Pereira P. Blood chemistry, protein electrophoresis, and hematologic values of captive spanish imperial eagles (*Aquila adalberti*). Journal of Zoo Medicine 2002;33(2):112-7.

[38] Gardell SJ, Ramjit DR, Stabilito II. Effective thrombolysis without marked plasminemia after bolus intravenous administration of vampire bat salivary plasminogen activator in rabbits. Circulation1991;84(1):244–53.

[39] Gentry PA. Comparative aspects of blood coagulation. The Veterinary Journal 2004;168: 238-51.

[40] Gentry PA, Ross ML, Yamada Y.Blood coagulation profile of the Asian elephant (*Elephas maximus*). Zoo. Biology 1996;15(4):413-423.

[41] Gladysheva IP, Turner RB, Sazonova IY, Liu L, Reed GL. Coevolutionary patterns in plasminogen activation. Proc. Natl.Acad. Sci. U.S.A.2003;100:9168–72.

[42] Grandjean C, McMullen PC, Newschwander G. Vampire bats yield potent clot buster for ischemic stroke. J Cardiovasc Nurs 2004;19:417-20.

[43] Greenberg CS, Lai T-S.Fibrin formation and stabilization. Thrombosis and Hemorrhage. In: Thrombosis and Hemorrhage. Third edition, edited by Loscalzo-Schafer, Lippincott, Williams and Wilkins. USA; 2003. p: 81-104.

[44] Greenberg CS, Orthner CL. Blood coagulation and fibrinolysis. In: Wintrobe´s Clinical Hematology. 10 th edition. Williams and Wilkins eds. Maryland. USA; 1999. p: 684-764.

[45] Griffin A, Callan MB, Shofer FS, Giger U. Evaluation of a canine D-dimer point-of-care test kit for use in samples obtained from dogs with disseminated intravascular coagulation, thromboembolic disease, and hemorrhage. AJVR 2003;64(12):1562-9.

[46] Groza P, Artino-Radulescu M, Nicolescu E.Blood coagulation and fibrinolysis after confinement hypokinesia. Physiologie 1988;25(4):161-8.

[47] Gulland FMD, Werner L, O´Neill S, Lowenstine LJ, Trupkiewitz J, Smith D, Royal B, Strubel I. Baseline coagulation assay values for northern elephant seals (*Mirounga angustirostris*), and disseminated intravascular coagulation in this species. Journal of Wildlife Diseases1996;32(3):536-40.

[48] Hackett E, Hann C. Erythrocytes and the liquefying of clotted amphibian blood in vitro. Nature 1964;204: 590-1.

[49] Hackett E, Lepage R. The clotting of the blood of an amphibian, Bufo marinus Linn. Aust J. Exp. Biol. Med. Sci. 1961;39:57-65.

[50] Hahn N, Popov-Cenic S, Dorer A. Basiswerte von Blutgerinnungsparametern des Hausschweins (*Sus scrofa domesticus*).[Basic values of blood coagulation parameters in pigs (*Sus scrofa domesticus*)]. Berl Münch Tierärztl Wochenschr.1996;109(1):23-7.

[51] Hassett MA, Krishnamurti C, Barr CF, Alving BM. The rabbit as a model for studies of fibrinolysis. Thrombosis Research 1986;43:313-23.

[52] Hawkey C. Fibrinolysis in animals. Proc. Roy. Soc. Med.1971;64:925-6.

[53] Hedlin AM, Monkhouse FC, Milojevic SM. A comparative study of fibrinolytic activity in human, rat, rabbit, and dog blood. Canadian Journal of Physiology and Pharmacology 1972;50(1):11-6.

[54] Herring J, McMichael M. Diagnostic approach to small animal bleeding disorders. Topics in Companion Animal Medicine 2012;27(2):73-80.

[55] Heuwieser W, Biesel M, Grunert E.Physiological coagulation profile of dairy cattle. J. Vet. Med.1989;36:24-31.

[56] Hillmayer K., Macovei A., Pauwels D., Compernolle G., Declerck P.J., Gils A. Characterization of rat thrombin-activatable fibrinolysis inhibitor (TAFI) -a comparative study assessing the biological equivalence of rat, murine and human TAFI. J. Thromb. Haemost. 2006;4:2470-77.

[57] Hoffman M. A cell-based model of coagulation and the role of factor VIIa. Blood Rev. 2003; 17(Suppl. 1): S1-5.

[58] Honda T, Honda K, Kokubun C, Nishimura T, Hasegawa M, Nishida A, Inui T, Kitamura K (2008). Time-course changes of haematology and clinical chemistry values in pregnant rats. J. Toxicol. Sci. 33(3):375-80.

[59] Irmak K, Turgut K. Disseminated intravascular coagulation in cattle with abomasal displacement. Vet. Res. Communications 2005;29:61-8.

[60] Jacobs JW, Cupp EW, Sardana M, Friedman PA. Isolation and characterization of a coagulation factor Xa inhibitor from black fly salivary glands. Thrombosis and Haemostasis1990; 64 (2):235–8.

[61] Jagadeeswaran P, Sheehan JP (1999). Analysis of blood coagulation in the zebrafish. Blood Cells, 25: 239-49.

[62] Jiang Y, Dollittle RF. The evolution of vertebrate blood coagulation as viewed from a comparison of puffer fish and sea squirt genomes. Proc. Natl. Acad. Sci. 2003; 100(13): 7527-32.

[63] Juhan-Vague I, Hans M. From fibrinogen to fibrin and its dissolution. Bull. Acad. Natl. Med.2003;187(1): 69-84.

[64] Karges HE, Funk KA, Ronneberger H. Activity of coagulation and fibrinolysis parameters in animals. Arzneim-Forsch/Drug Res 1994;44:793-7.

[65] Kaspareit J, Messow C, Edel J. Blood coagulation studies in guinea pigs (*Cavia porcellus*). Lab. Anim.1988;22(3):206-11.

[66] Kini RM. Serine proteases affecting blood coagulation and fibrinolysis from snake venoms. Pathophysiol. Haemost. Thromb.2005;34:200–04.

[67] Korninger C, Collen D. Studies on the specific fibrinolytic effect of humanextrinsic (tissue-type) plasminogen activator in human blood and in variousanimal species *in vitro*. Thromb. Haemost.1981:46(2):561–5.

[68] Kowalski E, Kopec M, Niewiarowski S. An evaluation of the euglobulin method for the determination of fibrinolysis. J. Clin. Path.1959;12:215-8.

[69] Kubalek S, Mischke R, Fehr M. Investigations on blood coagulation in the green Iguana (*Iguana iguana*). J. Vet. Med. A 2002;49(4):210-6.

[70] Lane DA, Philippou H, Huntington JA. Directing thrombin. Invited review, section Hemostasis, Thrombosis and Vascular Biology. From ImperialCollegeLondonUniversity of Cambridge, UK;2005. p: 1-20.

[71] Lanevschi A, Kramer JW, Greene SA, Meyers KM. Fibrinolytic activity in dogs after surgically induced trauma. Am J Vet Res 1996b;57(8): 1137-40.

[72] Leitâo DPS, Polizello ACM, Rothschild Z. Coagulation and fibrinolysis in capybara (*Hydrochaeris hydrochaeris*), a close relative of the guinea-pig (*Cavia Porcellus*). Comparative Biochemistry and Physiology Part A 2000;125:113-20.

[73] Levi M, van der Poll T, Schultz M. New insights into pathways that determine the link between infection and thrombosis. Neth. J. Med.2012;70(3):114-20.

[74] Levi M, van der Poll T, Schultz M. Systemic versus localized coagulation activation contributing to organ failure in critically ill patients. Semin. Immunopathol. 2012;34:167-79.

[75] Lohman S, Folkow LP, Osterud B, Sager G. Changes in fibrinolytic activity in diving grey seals. Comparative Biochemistry and Physiology Part A 1998;120:693-8.

[76] Machida T,Kokubu H, Matsuda K, Miyoshi K, Uchida E. Clinical use of D-Dimer measurement for the diagnosis of disseminated intravascular coagulation in dogs. J. Vet. Med. Sci.2010;72(10):1301–6.

[77] Mackman N. Tissue-Specific Hemostasis in mice.Arterioscler Thromb. Vasc. Biol. 2005;25:2273-81.

[78] Markland FS. Snake venoms and the hemostatic system. Toxicon 1998;36(12): 1749-800.

[79] Marval E, Garcia L, Candela DE, Arocha-Piñango CL. Valores normales de hemoglobina, hematocrito, factores de coagulación y fibrinolisis en conejos Nueva Zelanda blancos. Sangre (Barc.)1992;37(5):355-61.

[80] Marx PF. Thrombin-activatable-fibrinolysis inhibitor. Curr. Med. Chem.2004;11(17): 2335-48.

[81] Marx PF, Wagenaar GTM, Reijerkerk A, Tiekstra MJ, van Rossum AGSH, Gebbink MFBG, Meijers JCM. Characterization of mouse thrombin-activatable fibrinolysis inhibitor. Thromb. Haemost.2000;83: 297-303.

[82] Matsuo O, Lijnen HR, Ueshima S, Kojima S, Smyth SS. A guide to murine fibrinolytic factor structure, function, assays, and genetic alterations. Journal of Thrombosis and Haemostasis 2007;5:680-9.

[83] Meinkoth JH, Allison RW. Sample collection and handling: getting accurate results. Vet. Clin. North Am. Small Anim. Pract.2007;37(2):203-19.

[84] Menoud PA, Sappino N, Boudal-Khoshbeen M, Vassalli JD, Sappino AP.The kidney is a major site of alpha (2)-antiplasmin production. Journal of Clinical Investigation 1996;97:2478-84.

[85] Meyer DJ. Evaluación de la hemostasia: anormalidades de la coagulación y las plaquetas. In: El laboratorio en Medicina Veterinaria. Interpretación y diagnóstico. 2nd. ed. Intermédica. Buenos Aires. Argentina; 2000. p119-48.

[86] Middeldorp S. Evidence-based approach to thrombophilia testing. J. Thromb. Thrombolysis 2011;31:275-81.

[87] Milijic P, Heylen E, Willemse J, Djordjevic V, Radojkovic D, Colovic M, Elezovic I, Hendriks D. Thrombin activatable fibrinolysis inhibitor (TAFI): a molecular link between coagulation and fibrinolysis. Srp. Arh. Celok. Lek.2010;138 Suppl. 1: 74-8.

[88] Miller EKI, Trabi M, Masci PP, Lavin MF, de Jersey J, et al. Crystalstructure of textilinin-1, a Kunitz-type serine protease inhibitor from the venom of the Australian common brown snake (Pseudonaja textiles). FEBS J. 2009; 276:3163–75.

[89] Mischke R. Hemostasis. In: Diagnóstico Clínico de Laboratorio en Veterinaria. Translated from 4th German edition. Editores Médicos SA. España; 2000. p: 92-111.

[90] Monreal L, Anglés A, Espada Y, Monasterio J, Monreal M. Hypercoagulation and hypofibrinolysis in horses with colic and DIC. Equine Vet. J. Suppl. 2000;(32):9-25.

[91] Morin DE, Yamada M, Gentry PA. Procoagulant, anticoagulant and fibrinolytic activities in llama plasma. Comp. Clin. Pathology 1995;5:125-9.

[92] Mulder R, Ki ten Kate M, Kluin- Nelemans HC, Mulder AB. Low cut-off values increase diagnostic performance of protein S assays. Thromb. Haemost. 2010;104:618-25.

[93] Münster AM, OlsenAK, Bladbjerg EM. Usefulness of human coagulation and fibrinolysis assays in domestic pigs. Comp. Med. 2002;52:39-43.

[94] Murata M, Sano Y, Bannai S, Ishihara K, Matsushima R, Uchida M.Fish protein stimulated the fibrinolysis in rats. Ann. Nutr. Metab.2004;48:348-56.

[95] Muszbek L, Bereczky Z, Bagoly Z, Komáromi I, Katona E. Factor XIII: a coagulation factor with multiple plasmatic and cellular functions. Physiological Review 2011;91(3):931-72.

[96] Nelson OL. Use of the D-dimer assay for diagnosing thromboembolic disease in the dog. J. Am. Anim. Hosp. Assoc. 2005;41:145-9.

[97] Nieuwenhuys CM, Béguin S, Offermans RF, Emeis JJ, Hornstra G, Haemskerk JW. Hypocoagulant and lipid-lowering effects of dietary n-3 polyunsaturated fatty acids with unchanged platelet activation in rats. Arteroscler. Thromb. Vasc. Biol.1998;18(9): 1480-9.

[98] Niewiaroski S, Latallo Z. Comparative studies of the fibrinolytic system of sera of various vertebrates. Thromb. Diath. Haemorrh. 1959;3:404-417.

[99] Nobukata H, Ishikawa T, Obata M, Shibutani Y. Age-related changes in coagulation, fibrinolysis, and platelet aggregation in male WBN/Kob rats. Thrombosis Research 2000;98:507-16.

[100] O'Rourke L, Feldman BF, Ito RK. Coagulation, fibrinolysis, and kinin generation in adult cats. Am. J. Vet. Res. 1982;43:1478-80.

[101] Opal SM, Esmon CT. Bench-to-bedside review: Functional relationships between coagulation and the innate immune response and their respective roles in the pathogenesis of sepsis.Critical Care 2003;7:23-38.

[102] Owens III AP, Mackman N. Tissue factor and thrombosis: The clot starts here. Thrombosis and Haemostasis 2010;104:432-9.

[103] Parfyonova YV, Plekhanova OS, Tkachuk VA (2002).Plasminogen activators in vascular remodeling and angiogenesis. Biochemistry (Moscow) 2002;67:119-34.

[104] Patthy L. Evolution of blood coagulation and fibrinolysis. Blood Coagulation and Fibrinolysis 1990:1:153-66.

[105] Pavlidis M, Berry M, Kokkari C, Kentouri M. Prothrombin time, activated partial thromboplastin time and fibrinogen values in Mediterranean marine teleosts. Fish Physiology and Biochemistry 1999;21(4):335-43.

[106] Perkins SL. Normal blood and bone marrow values in humans. In: Wintrobe's Clinical Hematology, Appendix A. 10th edition. Williams and Wilkins eds. Maryland. USA; 1999. p:2738-48.

[107] Poplis VA, Castellino FJ. Gene targeting of components of the fibrinolytic system. Thrombosis and Haemostasis 2002;87(1):22-31.

[108] Prezoto BC, Maffei FHA, Mattar L, Chudzinski-Tavassi AM, Curi PR. Antithrombotic effect of *Lonomia oblique* caterpillar bristle extract on experimental venous thrombosis. *Brazilian Journal of Medical and Biological Research* 2002;35(6):703–12.

[109] Ralph AG, Brainard BM. Update on disseminated intravascular coagulation: when to consider it, when to expect it, when to treat it. Top Companion Anim. Med. 2012;27(2):65-72.

[110] Ravanat C, Freund M, Dol F, Cadroy Y, Roussi J, Incardona F, Maffrand JP, Boneu B, Drouet L, Legrand C, Herbert J-M, Cazenave JP. Cross-reactivity of human molecular markers for detection of prethrombotic states in various animal species. Blood Coagulation and Fibrinolysis 1995;6:446-55.

[111] Rivera J, Lozano ML, Navarro-Núñez L, Vicente V. Platelet receptors and signaling in the dynamics of thrombus formation. Review article. Haematologica 2009;94:700-11.

[112] Robinson AJ, Kropatkin M, Aggeler PM.Hageman factor (factor XII) deficiency in marine mammals. Science 1969;166(911):1420-2.

[113] Roussi J, André P, Samama M, Pignaud G, Bonneau M, Laporte A, Drouet L.Platelet functions and haemostasis parameters in pigs: absence of side effects of a procedure of general anaesthesia. Thromb. Res.1996;81(3):297-305.

[114] Saito H, Poon MC, Goldsmith GH, Ratnoff OD, Arnason Ù. Studies on the blood clotting and fibrinolytic system in the plasma from a sei (baleen) whale. Proceedings of the Society for Experimental Biology and Medicine 1976;152:503-7.

[115] Sano Y, Sato K, Uchida M, Murata M.Blood coagulation and fibrinolysis of rats fed fish oil: reduced coagulation factors especially involved in intrinsic pathway and increased activity of plasminogen activator inhibitor. Biosci. Biotechnol. Biochem. 2003;67:2100-5.

[116] Sawyer RT. Leech Biology and Behaviour, vol. 1 *Anatomy, Physiology, and Behaviour,* Clarendon Press, Oxford, 418 pp. 1986.

[117] Sawyer RT. Thrombolytics and anticoagulants from leeches. Nature Biotechnology1991;9(6):513–8.

[118] Sazonova IY, Mc Namee RA, Houng AK, King SM, Hedstrom L, Reed GL. Reprogrammed streptokinases develop fibrin-targeting and dissolve blood clots with more potency than tissue plasminogen activator. J. Thromb. Haemost. 2009;7(8):1321-28.

[119] Schleuning WD, Alagon A, Boidol W, Bringmann P, Petri T, Kratzschmar J, Haendler B, Langer G, Baldus B, Wuit W, *et al.*Plasminogen activators from the saliva of *Desmodus rotundus* (common vampire bat): unique fibrin specificity. Ann. N Y Acad. Sci. 1992;667:395-403.

[120] Schöchl H,Solomon C, Schulz A, Voelckel W, Hanke A. Thromboelastometry (TEM®) findings in disseminated intravascular coagulation in a pig model of endotoxinemia. Mol. Med.2011;17(34):266-72.

[121] Sérgio M, Gomes R, de Queiroz MR, Mamede CCN, Mendes MM, Hamaguchi A,Homsi-Brandeburgo MI, Sousa MV, Aquino EN, Castro MS, de Oliveira F, Rodri-

gues VM. Purification and functional characterization of a new metalloproteinase (BleucMP) from *Bothrops leucurus* snake venom. Comparative Biochemistry and Physiology, Part C 2011;153:290–300.

[122] Sidelmann JJ, Gram J, Jespersen J, Kluft C. Fibrin clot formation and lysis: basic mechanisms. Semin. Thromb. Hemost. 2000;26:605-18.

[123] Siller-Matula JM, Plasenzotti R, Spiel A, Quehenberger P, Jilma B. Thromb. Haemost. 2008;100: 397-404.

[124] Soulier JP, Wartelle O, Ménaché D. Hageman trait and PTA deficiency; the role of contact of blood with glass. British Journal of Haematology 1959;5:121-38.

[125] Srivastava VM, Dube B, Dube RK, Agarwal GP, Ahmad N. Blood fibrinolytic system in *Rana tigrina.* Thromb. Haemost. 1981;45(3):252-4.

[126] Stafford JL. The fibrinolytic mechanism in haemostasis: A review. J Clin Path 1964;17:520-30.

[127] Stokol T (2003). Plasma D-dimer for the diagnosis of thromboembolic disorders in dogs. Vet. Clin. Small Anim. 2003;33:1419-35.

[128] Stokol T, Brooks MB, Erb HN, Mauldin GE. D-dimer concentrations in healthy dogs and dogs with disseminated intravascular coagulation. American Journal Vet. Res. 2000b;61:393-8.

[129] Stokol T, Erb HN, De Wilde L, Tornquist SJ, Brooks M. Evaluation of latex agglutination kits for detection of fibrin(ogen) degradation products and D-dimer in healthy horses and horses with severe colic. Veterinary Clinical Pathology 2005;34 (4):375-82.

[130] Suzuki K, Egawa H, Hashimoto S. Comparative studies of coagulative and fibrinolytic faculties between the Japanese monkey and the human. Thrombosis and Haemostasis 1977;37(2):233-42.

[131] Tanaka-Azevedo M, Morais-Zani K, Torquato RJS, Tanaka AS. Thrombin Inhibitors from different animals. Hindawi Publishing Corporation Journal of Biomedicine and Biotechnology, 2010;2010, Article ID 641025, doi:10.1155/2010/641025.

[132] Teger-Nilsson AC, Friberger P, Gyzander E. Determination of a new rapid plasmin inhibitor in human blood by means of a plasmin specific tripeptide substrate. Scand. J. Clin. Lab. Invest.1977;37:403-9.

[133] Tentoni J, Polini NN, Casanave EB. Fibrinolytic system of the armadillo *Chaetophractus villosus* (Xenarthra, Dasypodidae). Comparative Clinical Pathology 2008;17:193-6.

[134] Tentoni J.; Polini NN.; Casanave EB. Comparative vertebrate Fibrinolysis. Comparative Clinical Pathology 2010;19(3):225-34.

[135] Tibbs RF, Elghetany MT, Tran LT, Van Bonn W, Romano T, Cowan DF. Characterization of the coagulation system in healthy dolphins: the coagulation factors, natural

anticoagulants, and fibrinolytic products Comparative Clinical Pathology 2005;14: 95-8.

[136] Tsakiris DA, Scudder L, Hodivala-Dilke K, Inés RO. Hemostasis in the mouse (*Mus musculus*): a review. Thromb. Haemost.1999;81:177-88.

[137] Urano T, Suzuki Y. [Parameters related to fibrinolysis and their meanings]. Rinsho Byori.2011;59(7):703-8.

[138] van Cott EM, Laposata M. Coagulation, fibrinolisis and hipercoagulation. In: Henry JB ed. Clinical diagnosis and management by laboratory methods. 20thedition, W.B. Saunders Co; 2001. p642-59.

[139] Vap LM, Harr KE, Arnold JE, Freeman KP, Getzy K, Lester S, Friedichs KR. ASVCP quality assurance guidelines: control of preanalytical and analytical factors for hematology for mammalian and non mammalian species, hemostasis, and cross matching in veterinary laboratories. Vet. Clin. Pathol. 2012;41(1):8-17.

[140] Vasse M. Protein Z, a protein seeking a pathology. Thromb. Haemost. 2008;100:548-556.

[141] Vaughan DE. PAI-1 and atherothrombosis. J. Thromb. Haemost. 2005;3(8):1879-83.

[142] Velik-Salchner C, Schnürer C, Fries D, Müssigang PR, Moser PL, Streif W, Kolbitsch C, Lorenz IH.Normal values for thrombelastography (ROTEM®) and selected coagulation parameters in porcine blood. Thrombosis Research 2006;117:597-602.

[143] Verstraete M. The fibrinolytic system: from Petri dishes to genetic engineering. Thrombosis and Haemostasis 1995;74:25-35.

[144] Wartelle O. Mecanisme de la coagulation chez la poule. L´étude des elements du complex prothrombique et de la thromboplastino-formation. Révue d´Hématologie 1957;12:351-87.

[145] Waxman L, Smith DE, Arcuri KE, Vlasuk GP. Tick anticoagulant peptide (TAP) is a novel inhibitor of blood coagulation factor Xa. Science1990;248(4955):593–6.

[146] Weir-M J, Acurero Z, Salas-A R, Arteaga-Vizcaino M.Blood coagulation factors in the black headed vulture (*Coragyps atratus*), a potential animal model for the study of haemostasis. Thrombosis Research 2004;113(3-4):269-73.

[147] Welles EG. Antithrombotic and fibrinolytic factors. A review. Veterinary Clinics of North America: Small Animal Practice 1996;26:1111-27.

[148] Welles EG, Boudreaux MK, Crager CS, Tyler JW.Platelet function and antithrombin, plasminogen, and fibrinolytic activities in cats with heart disease. Am. J. Vet. Res. 1994;55:619-27.

[149] Wilhelmi MH, Tiede A, Teebken OM, Bisdas T, Haverich A, Mischke R. Ovine blood: establishment of a list of reference values relevant for blood coagulation in sheep. ASAIO Journal (American Society for Artificial Internal Organs) 2012;58(1):79-82.

[150] Williams WJ, Lichtman MA, Beutler E, Kipps TJ. Manual de Hematología. 6th edition. Marbán SL eds. Madrid. España; 2005. 558 pp.

[151] Withers PC (1992). Blood. In: Comparative Animal Physiology, Saunders College Publishing 1992. p727-76

[152] Wohl RC, Sinio L, Summaria L, Robbins KC.Comparative activation kinetics of mammalian plasminogens. Biochimica et Biophysica Acta 1983;745:20-31.

[153] Zhang Y, Gladysheva IP, Houng AK, Reed GL. *Streptococcus uberis* plasminogen activator (SUPA) activates human plasminogen through novel species-specific and fibrin-targeted mechanisms. The Journal of Biological Chemistry 2012;287 (23):19171-6.

[154] Zavalova LL, Basanova AV, Baskova IP. Fibrinogen-Fibrin System Regulators from Bloodsuckers. Biochemistry (Moscow) 2002; 67(1):135-42.

[155] Zhang L, Seiffert D, Fowler BJ, Jenkins GR, Thinnes TC, Loskutoff DJ, Parmer RJ, Miles LA. Plasminogen has a broad extrahepatic distribution. Thromb. Haemost. 2002:87(3): 493-501.

[156] Zorio E; Gilabert-Estellés J, España F, Ramón LA, Cosin R, Estellés A. Fibrinolisis: the key to new pathogenetic mechanism. Curr. Med. Chem. 2008;15:923-9.

Chapter 5

Thrombolytic/Fibrinolytic Mechanism of Natural Products

Eduardo Fuentes, Luis Guzmán, Marcelo Alarcón,
Rodrigo Moore and Iván Palomo

Additional information is available at the end of the chapter

http://dx.doi.org/10.5772/57608

1. Introduction

Morphological and angiographic studies have demonstrated that the formation of thrombi at sites of atherosclerotic lesions is the major cause of the development of clinical complications of atherosclerosis, which are leading contributors to morbidity and mortality throughout the industrialized world [1]. Thrombogenicity of the atherosclerotic plaque is determined mainly by the stability of a fibrous cap and contents of tissue factor in its core, which activates the coagulation cascade when exposed to flowing blood. These elements interact with each other and with the blood vessel wall and under physiological conditions the blood flow to tissues is unimpaired by clotting [2]. Under pathophysiological conditions, activation of blood coagulation occurs primary through interaction of platelets, vessel wall and plasma proteins (so-called primary haemostasis). In this sense, there is evidence in the cardiology literature that the combination of thrombolysis with antiplatelet agents speeds and augments thrombolysis and seems to improve survival [3]. Moreover, epidemiologic studies have provided evidence that foods (fruit and vegetables) with the experimentally proven thrombolytic/fibrinolytic effect could reduce the risk of thrombosis [4].

This chapter discusses the involvement of coagulation and fibrinolytic system components in thrombosis, and possible mechanisms of thrombolytic/fibrinolytic effects of natural products.

2. Coagulation and fibrinolytic system components in thrombosis

Thrombosis is associated with activation of several enzymatic cascades, including the coagulation, fibrinolysis, complement, and kinin systems. Thus, plasma markers of coagulation and fibrinolysis have proven to be sensitive in the initial diagnosis of acute deep venous thrombosis [5]. Nowadays, the use of oral anticoagulants in secondary prevention is widely reported, but inconveniences arising from the need for its stringent control and the thin line between good therapy and incorrect therapy necessitate the search for new anticoagulants with higher specificity and with no need for such strict controls and follow up.

Coagulation components. Coagulation is the process by which blood forms clots. It is an important part of haemostasis; this begins almost immediately after an injury to the blood vessel that has damaged the endothelium lining the vessel. The cessation of blood loss from a damaged vessel begins with the junction of platelet to the subendothelial matrix and subsequent activation of the coagulation system which stabilizes the platelet-rich clot and fibrin. This process fails to stop the bleeding and begins the process of repairing a damaged vessel. Disorders in coagulation can lead to an increased risk of bleeding (hemorrhage) or obstructive clotting (thrombosis). For this reason there must be different mechanisms of regulation of this phenomenon, for example serine protease inhibitors. A major class of serine protease inhibitors regulating procoagulant enzymes is the serpin superfamily [6].

The principal inhibitor of procoagulant enzymes such as thrombin and factor Xa is the serpin antithrombin. There are, however, other serpins that act to control coagulation enzymes, such as heparin cofactor II (HCII), protease nexin I (PN1) and protein C inhibitor (PCI) [6]. Some serpins act to control the action of anticoagulant enzymes, such as activated protein C. Many of the serpins that control enzymes in the coagulation system are under the control of glycosaminoglycans such as heparin, heparan sulfate and dermatan sulfate which have been found to significantly accelerate the interaction between serpins and coagulation proteases, usually increasing the reaction rates from values that are not relevant under physiological conditions to rates that are relevant [5]. Another mechanism involving a serpin is the protein Z/Z-dependent protease inhibitor (PZ/ZPI) system that inhibits activated factors X, XI and IX by different mechanisms. ZPI is catalytically activated by PZ and in that way regulates the function of Xa factor on the surface of the membrane. PZ joins to a binding site which is located in the region of G helix [7]. For example, the ZPI inhibits prothrombinase activity (factor Xa complex) in the presence of phospholipids and calcium ions, the presence of PZ enhances this process 1000 times, but it also directly inhibits coagulation factor Xia [8]. In this same context, it has been recently demonstrated that residues of the C and D helices of ZPI are key to the interactions with heparin and modulate inhibitory function of serpins [9].

It has been recently demonstrated that coagulation systems may be regulated by MicroRNAs (miRNAs) that are an abundant class of small non-coding RNAs which are regulators in a growing number of physiological and pathological processes. However, their role in haemostasis, a complex physiological process involving a multitude of effectors, is just beginning to be characterized. For example miR-19, miR-20, and miR-106b regulate the tissue factor expression or it has been determined that there is an inverse correlation observed between miR-18a and miR-19b levels with antithrombin mRNA and miR-10b that regulate the expression of heparin. miR-15a, miR-21, miR-23b, miR-29c regulate de TFPI expression. The potential target of these miRNAs suggests that certain miRNAs may be involved in the regulation of selected haemostatic proteins and thereby regulate the clotting system [10, 11].

Fibrinolytic components. Fibrinolysis is a process by which fibrin is eliminated through activation of a blood protease cascade, and plasmin is responsible for such degradation. This process starts with the proteolitic cleavage of the plasminogen zymogen to convert it in plasmin through its tissue plasminogen activator (tPA) and urokinase plasminogen activator(uPA) [5]. Plasmin acts catalytically over fibrin exposing lysine residues of the new carboxyterminals which join to plasminogen and its activator in order to amplify fibrinolysis. Thrombin activatable fibrinolysis inhibitor (TAFI) is a key element in this process as it is able to control the plasmin activity by removing lysine residues in carboxyterminal region thereby preventing positive feedback of the system. In order for TAFI to exert its action over its substrate; it must be activated by the thrombin-thrombomodulin complex [12]. Very recently, it has been reported that the renin-angiotensin-aldosterone system is implied in fibrinolysis regulation; this effect is carried out through the angiotensin receptor type 1. The results of this study demonstrate that angiotensin-1-9 favours the development of venous thrombosis in rats decreasing the levels of plasminogen activator and increasing the levels of Plasminogen activator inhibitor 1 (PAI-1) [13]. PAI-1 also called serpin E1 is the main inhibitor of the plasminogen activator and it has been widely reported in the scientific literature as being responsible for thrombotic events and recurrent foetal loss [14]. The activation of the fibrinolytic system is essential to eliminate intravascular deposits of fibrin resulting from the physiological or pathological activation of the coagulation system, but the proper functioning of this system depends on its regulation. The fibrinolytic system is important not only in physiological processes but also in pathological ones, such as inflammation, tumour invasion or cardiovascular diseases.

3. Platelets and thrombolysis

The recognition of arterial thrombosis as the major causative factor in acute coronary syndromes, in particular acute myocardial infarction, was a major advance in cardiology in the 1980s [15]. Stroke is considered an independent entity by the World Health Organization classification, the current gold standard treatment of which is the intravenous application of thrombolytic therapy within a 4.5 h time window from the onset of stroke symptoms [16].

The main elements of thrombus include fibrin, thrombin, and platelets [17]. Current techniques to dissolve clot focus on the fibrin and prothrombin activation, fail to address the important effects of platelets; thrombolysis may dissolve the fibrin component of the clot but may have no effect on the platelet portion [18]. Fibrinolytic therapy has a potent platelet aggregating effect as does the exposure of the ruptured atherosclerotic plaque [19].

The use of thrombolytic agents, such as the recombinant tissue-type plasminogen activator (rt-PA), is well established in the strategy for treatment of acute myocardial infarction [20]. The insoluble fibrin fibre is hydrolyzed into fibrin degradation products by plasmin, which is generated from plasminogen by plasminogen activators, such as t-PA, urokinase, Hageman factor, and streptokinase plasminogen complex [21, 22].

However, larger thrombi have notoriously proven to be resistant to intravenous tPA lysis with recanalization rates in the range of only 13% to 20% [23]. Even if endovascular treatment of ischemic stroke is proven to improve clinical outcomes, there will still be many patients with residual partial or complete occlusion after intravenous tPA alone suffering ischemia, whereas waiting for catheter rescue [24]. Thrombolysis resistance has also been demonstrated in platelet-rich thrombi, as seen in postmortem microscopic examination of serial sections of coronary thrombus of patients with acute myocardial infarction and sudden death revealing that thrombus formed at the plaque fissure is very rich in platelets, whereas proximal and distal extensions of the thrombus are composed of erythrocyte-rich material [25].

Platelet activation plays a central role in thrombus formation and can be inhibited by many agents [26], even a weak antiplatelet agent such as aspirin is beneficial when given alone or in conjunction with reperfusion, such therapy may improve early coronary flow rates as well as stabilize or maintain subsequent perfusion and provide an incremental improvement in clinical outcomes [27]. Therefore, development of combination therapies for acute ischemic stroke that can be delivered quickly in the emergency setting is crucial. Ongoing strategies that are in either phase II or III clinical trials include thrombin-inhibition, sonothrombolysis, and platelet-inhibition [28].

With platelet activation, there is high affinity and binding to fibrinogen and von Willebrand factor; in addition, there is up-regulation of further platelet activation. Activated platelets can also facilitate thrombin generation by providing a catalytic surface and by releasing an activated form of factor V [29], resulting in more fibrin production. In addition, exposure of clot-bound thrombin by lytics converts more fibrinogen to fibrin, causing rethrombosis [30].

The active glycoprotein (GP) IIb/IIIa receptors bind fibrinogen, and this forms links between platelets causing aggregation. Hence GP IIb/IIIa antagonists such as abciximab are potent inhibitors of platelet aggregation. There is evidence in the cardiology literature that the combination of thrombolysis with a GP IIb/IIIa antagonist speeds and augments thrombolysis and seems to improve survival [31].

The $\alpha_{IIb}\beta_3$ integrin (GP IIb/IIIa) is found exclusively on platelets and megakaryocytes, with 70,000 to 90,000 receptors expressed on each platelet in the resting state. These heterodimeric molecules have large extracellular regions for cation-facilitated ligand binding and small intracytoplasmic tails mediating intracellular signal transduction [32]. Integrin binding affinity is dynamic and dependent on the receptor's conformational status. In the resting state, affinity for fibrinogen binding is low, platelet agonists, via "inside-to-outside" signals; trigger a change in the receptor's structure, transforming it to a high-affinity state [33, 34].

For platelet inhibition the most commonly used antiplatelet agent is aspirin, which inhibits platelet cyclooxygenase-1, and also, two distinct classes of antiplatelet agents with distinct mechanisms of action, glycoprotein IIb-IIIa antagonists (e.g., abciximab, eptifibatide) and antagonists of the platelet ADP receptor $P2Y_{12}$ (e.g., clopidogrel, prasugrel), have been used in acute coronary syndromes [35].

The advantage of blocking the GP IIb/IIIa receptor is that platelet to platelet binding through fibrinogen or von Willebrand factor is prevented, but platelet binding to the subendothelial elements, that is, the surface of the damaged vessel, remains intact. An initial layer of platelets is formed, resulting in hemostasis but not aggregation that can lead to local thrombosis or downstream embolization to the distal microcirculation. These drugs prevent not only local thrombosis attributable to platelet aggregation but also damage to the distal vascular bed by platelet embolization [36].

The results of the Combined Approach to Lysis Utilizing Eptifibatide and rt-PA in Acute Ischemic Stroke–Enhanced Regimen (CLEAR-ER) [37] a multicenter, double-blind, randomized phase II safety trial of intravenous tPA versus eptifibatide, sought to estimate the safety and efficacy of combination GP IIb/IIIa+reduced dose of intravenous tPA when delivered to hyperacute ischemic stroke, demonstrating that emergent adjunctive therapies are feasible within the first few hours of stroke onset and need to be further pursued as a means of amplifying the thrombolysis effect of intravenous tPA [38].

Combination therapy with a local fibrinolytic and systemic GP IIb/IIIa receptor inhibitors in the peripheral setting may represent a promising new means to accelerate reperfusion, prevent reocclusion, allow fibrinolytic dose reductions, and improve clinical outcomes [39].

4. Thrombolytic/fibrinolytic mechanisms of natural products

Thrombolytic drugs (tPA, streptokinase (SK), and uPA) have the ability to effectively dissolve blood clots; they differ in their detailed mechanisms in ways that alter their selectivity for fibrin clots. The SK binds equally to circulating and non-circulating plasminogen, produces significant fibrinogenolysis along with clot fibrinolysis [42]. For this reason, tPA is generally preferred as a thrombolytic agent over SK, especially when used for dissolving coronary and cerebral vascular thrombi. Because SK is derived from streptococci, patients who have had recent streptococci infections can require significantly higher doses of SK to produce thrombolysis.

Moreover, these drugs are not used in patients who have undergone surgery or those with a history of nervous lesions, gastrointestinal bleeding or hypertension [42]. The treatment with tPA is limited in platelet-rich thrombi that are highly resistant to lysis by t-PA [25]. Considerable efforts have been directed towards the discovery and development of natural products from various plants which have antiplatelet [43, 44], anticoagulant [45], antithrombotic [46] and thrombolytic activity [4]. Epidemiologic studies have provided evidence that foods with experimentally proven antithrombotic and thrombolytic effects could reduce the risk of thrombosis (Table 1) [47, 48, 49].

Studies from around the world have demonstrated the potent antiplatelet properties of Ginkgo, which inhibits platelet aggregation and thrombin activity [50, 51]. The extract was obtained by a polyphenolic method, the fibrinolytic effects of Streptokinase was compared with those of the Ginkgo extract using a fluorometric method. The study was performed in vitro on a labeled clot; fibrinogen was labeled with the fluorescent agent fluorescein isothiocyanate and precipitated in the presence of Ca^{2+}. The Streptokinase (100 U/mL to 1000 U/mL) and Ginkgo extract was added to labeled fibrin in a plasma environment. A linear relationship was observed between the Streptokinase and Ginkgo extract [42]. The results indicate that the effects of Ginkgo extract on the fibrinolytic system are similar to those of streptokinase [42]; hence, this herbal extract can be used as a complement to or as a substitute for streptokinase. In this sense, there is evidence that some natural products have fibrinolytic effects.

Other researchers have found that organic extracts of six Bangladeshi plants (Ageratum conyzoides L., Clausena suffruticosa, Leea indica (Burm.f.) Merr., Leucas aspera Willd., Senna sophera L. Roxb., and Solanum torvum Swartz), have thrombolytic activity. An in vitro thrombolytic model was used to check the clot lysis effect of the all these extracts [52]. The venous blood was allowed to form clots which were weighed and treated with the extract to disrupt the clots,the weight of clot before and after treatment provided a percentage of clot lysis. Among the herbs studied *Clausena suffruticosa, Leea indica* and *Leucas aspera* showed a very significant ($p < 0.0001$) percentage (%) of clot lysis compared to the reference drug streptokinase ($75.00 \pm 3.04\%$) [4].

Prasad, S. *et al* [53] have tried six herbal preparations (*Tinospora cordifolia, Rubia cordifolia, Hemidesmus indicus, Glycyrrhiza glabra Linn, Fagonia arabica* and *Bacopa monnieri Linn),* that have been used since ancient times for neuroprotection and for curing vascular diseases. For example, *Hemidesmus indicus* was reported to have antithrombotic activity [54] or *Fagonia arabica* is known to have a blood purifying property [55]. When compared with the clot lysis percentage obtained through water (negative control), a significant thrombolytic activity was observed after treating the clots with *Fagonia arabica* and *Bacopa monnieri* 75.6% and 41.8% clot lysis was obtained respectively (p value < 0.0001 &=0.0023 respectively). Chourasia, S.R. *et al* [55], found the same clot lysis percentage by streptokinase as well as *F. arabica.*

Yamada, K. *et al* [56] analyzed ten onion varieties, the antithrombotic activity of which was assessed in vivo by using a laser-induced thrombosis test in mice. Toyohira, showed significant antithrombotic activity both in vitro and in vivo. Toyohira showed thrombolytic activity in addition to the antiplatelet effect. Superkitamomiji, 2935A, and K83211 showed only thrombolytic activity.

Natto-extracts is soybeans fermented with Bacillus subtilis, Suzuki *et al* [57], investigated the effects of dietary supplementation with natto-extracts on neointima formation and on thrombolysis at the site of endothelial injury. In control animals, thrombolysis started from the center of the thrombus and mural thrombus remained attached on vessel wall. A supplementation with natto-extracts seems to have modulated the process of thrombolysis, which started from near the vessel walls and then thrombi detached from them.

Rajput, M.S. *et al* [58], explored the fibrinolytic potential of the methanolic extract of the fruits of *Lagenaria siceraria* (bottle gourd), the fibrinolytic activity was expressed as percentage of plasma clot liquefaction and was determined by plasma clot lysis at 37°C in 24 h. Treatment of plasma clot combined with methanolic extract showed a reduction by 54.72% which was significant when compared to the control (saline – 3.68%; $p < 0.01$).

Torres-Urrutia, C. *et al* [59] studied samples of 19 fruits and 26 vegetables. The extracts prepared from each sample included an aqueous (juice or pressed solubles) and/or methanol-soluble fraction. The extracts were evaluated for antiplatelet, anticoagulant, and fibrinolytic activity in vitro at a final concentration of 1 mg/ml, the fibrinolytic effect was determined with the euglobin clot lysis time and fibrin plate methods. Out of all fruits and vegetables the fibrinolytic activity was observed only in raspberries.

Bordia, A. *et al* [60], determined the effects of a preparation of dried garlic powder (Sapec) in 12 healthy subjects on fibrinolysis and platelet aggregation. Total euglobulin fibrinolytic activity and t-PA activity were significantly higher 4 and 6 h after garlic and placebo ingestion.

Ginger (Zingiber officinale) is a popular food spice and it is reported to contain antihistaminic and antioxidant factors. Verna, S.K. *et al* [61] studied the effect of ginger on fibrinolytic activity on 30 healthy adult with high fat diet. The ginger increased fibrinolysis activity by 31.5% in these patients compared with the placebo.

Morozova, E.N. *et al* [62]found a high fibrinolytic activity in *Flammulina velutipes* (also known as the golden needle mushroom), this was compared with those of *Aspergillus terricola* and *Streptomyces griseusproteinases*. Then Park, S.E. *et al* [63] purified a fibrinolytic enzyme from the culture supernatant by ion exchange and gel filtration chromatographies. This was the first study of fibrinolytic enzyme from mushrooms and their application as therapeutic agents. Other researchers also have isolated different enzymes with fibrinolytic activity from mushrooms [64, 65]. Also Kim *et al* [66], found fibrinolitic activity on *Cordyceps militaris* a medicinal mushroom, their results for the fibrinolysis pattern showed that enzyme rapidly hydrolyzed the fibrin and fibrinogen chains.

Choi, H.S *et al* [67], also isolated a protease with fibrinolitic properties from a Chinese herb (Spirodela polyrhiza), the homogenate of this herb was filtered and centrifuged, the supernatant was concentrated by ultrafiltration. The protease hydrolyzed not only fibrin but also fibrinogen, cleaving Aalpha and Bbeta without affecting the gamma chain of fibrinogen. The fibrinolytic activity was measured in the fibrin plate assay [68].

Another plant extract/product which has been identified to have fibrinolytic activity is *Ananas comosus,* this has a proteolytic enzyme called bromelain, which has displayed anti-inflammatory and analgesic properties in human and laboratory studies. It has been shown to increase fibrinolytic activity [69, 70].

Plant-derived medicines have a long history of use for the prevention and treatment of human diseases. Advances in phytochemistry and identification of plant compounds to cure certain diseases have renewed the interest in herbal medicines; about 30% of pharmaceuticals are prepared from plants worldwide. Some of these plant products are modified further with recombinant technology [71] to make them more effective and site specific. They may even be incorporated as a thrombolytic agent for the improvement of the patients suffering from atherothrombotic diseases [72, 73, 74, 75]. There are several thrombolytic drugs that have be reported to have adverse side effects,, sometimes the patients died due to bleeding and embolism [77, 78, 79, 80]. In this context, on the basis of the beneficial effects of clot dissolving properties of plant extracts/products, these agents should be considered as a complement to or as a substitute for thrombolytic drugs.

Name of Compound	Source	Effect	Mechanism of Action	References
Polyphenols	*Ginkgo biloba*	Antithrombotic	Fibrinolytic	[42]
Terpene lactones	*Ginkgo biloba*	Antithrombotic	Fibrinolytic	[81]
Sterols	*Bacopa monnieri Linn*	Antithrombotic	Fibrinolytic	[82]
Steroidal sapogenins	*Lagenaria siceraria*	Antithrombotic	Fibrinolytic	[83]
Hydroxycinnamic acid	*Ananas comosus*	Antithrombotic	Fibrinolytic	[84]

Table 1. Natural bioactive compound with antithrombotic and fibrinolytic activities.

Acknowledgements

This work was funded by the CONICYT REGIONAL / GORE MAULE / CEAP / R09I2001, Interdisciplinary Excellence Research Program on Healthy Aging (PIEI-ES), and supported by grant no. 1130216 (I.P., M.G., R.M., M.A., J.C.) from Fondecyt, Chile.

Author details

Eduardo Fuentes[1,2], Luis Guzmán[1], Marcelo Alarcón[1,2], Rodrigo Moore[1,2] and Iván Palomo[1,2*]

*Address all correspondence to: ipalomo@utalca.cl

1 Department of Clinical Biochemistry and Immunohematology, Faculty of Health Sciences, Interdisciplinary Excellence Research Program on Healthy Aging (PIEI-ES), Universidad de Talca, Talca, Chile

2 Centro de Estudios en Alimentos Procesados (CEAP), CONICYT-Regional, Gore Maule, Talca, Chile

References

[1] Libby, P.; Ridker, P.M.; Hansson, G.K. Progress and challenges in translating the biology of atherosclerosis. *Nature* 2011, *473*, 317-325.

[2] Ananyeva, N.M.; Kouiavskaia, D.V.; Shima, M.; Saenko, E.L. Intrinsic pathway of blood coagulation contributes to thrombogenicity of atherosclerotic plaque. *Blood* 2002, *99*, 4475-4485.

[3] Zinkstok, S.M.; Vermeulen, M.; Stam, J.; de Haan, R.J.; Roos, Y.B. Antiplatelet therapy in combination with rt-PA thrombolysis in ischemic stroke (ARTIS): rationale and design of a randomized controlled trial. *Cerebrovasc Dis* 2010, *29*, 79-81.

[4] Rahman, M.A.; Sultana, R.; Bin Emran, T.; Islam, M.S.; Chakma, J.S.; Rashid, H.U.; Hasan, C.M. Effects of organic extracts of six Bangladeshi plants on in vitro thrombolysis and cytotoxicity. *BMC Complement Altern Med* 2013, *13*, 25.

[5] Palomo I, F.P., Pereira J Sistyema de la coagulación y sistema fibrinolítico en Hematología fisiopatología y diagnóstico. *Editorial Universidad de Talca* 2005, 493-514.

[6] Huntington, J.A. Thrombin inhibition by the serpins. *J Thromb Haemost* 2013, *11 Suppl 1*, 254-264.

[7] Huang, X.; Yan, Y.; Tu, Y.; Gatti, J.; Broze, G.J., Jr.; Zhou, A.; Olson, S.T. Structural basis for catalytic activation of protein Z-dependent protease inhibitor (ZPI) by protein Z. *Blood* 2012, *120*, 1726-1733.

[8] Karimi, Z.; Falsafi-Zade, S.; Galehdari, H. The role of Ca(2+) ions in the complex assembling of protein Z and Z-dependent protease inhibitor: A structure and dynamics investigation. *Bioinformation* 2012, *8*, 407-411.

[9] Yang, L.; Ding, Q.; Huang, X.; Olson, S.T.; Rezaie, A.R. Characterization of the heparin-binding site of the protein z-dependent protease inhibitor. *Biochemistry* 2012, *51*, 4078-4085.

[10] Camaioni, C.; Gustapane, M.; Cialdella, P.; Della Bona, R.; Biasucci, L.M. Microparticles and microRNAs: new players in the complex field of coagulation. *Intern Emerg Med* 2013, *8*, 291-296.

[11] Stavik, B.; Skretting, G.; Olstad, O.K.; Sletten, M.; Dehli Vigeland, M.; Sandset, P.M.; Iversen, N. TFPI alpha and beta regulate mRNAs and microRNAs involved in cancer biology and in the immune system in breast cancer cells. *PloS one* 2012, *7*, e47184.

[12] Antovic, J.P.; Blomback, M. Thrombin-activatable fibrinolysis inhibitor antigen and TAFI activity in patients with APC resistance caused by factor V Leiden mutation. *Thromb Res* 2002, *106*, 59-62.

[13] Mogielnicki, A.; Kramkowski, K.; Hermanowicz, J.; Leszczynska, A.; Przyborowski, K.; Buczko, W. Angiotensin-(1-9) enhances stasis-induced venous thrombosis in the rat because of the impairment of fibrinolysis. *Journal of the renin-angiotensin-aldosterone system : JRAAS* 2013.

[14] Su, M.T.; Lin, S.H.; Chen, Y.C.; Kuo, P.L. Genetic association studies of ACE and PAI-1 genes in women with recurrent pregnancy loss: a systematic review and meta-analysis. *Thromb Haemost* 2013, *109*, 8-15.

[15] Skinner, M.P. Thrombosis and thrombolysis: platelet membrane glycoproteins. *Heart Lung Circ* 2007, *16*, 176-179.

[16] Hacke, W.; Kaste, M.; Bluhmki, E.; Brozman, M.; Davalos, A.; Guidetti, D.; Larrue, V.; Lees, K.R.; Medeghri, Z.; Machnig, T.; Schneider, D.; von Kummer, R.; Wahlgren, N.; Toni, D. Thrombolysis with alteplase 3 to 4.5 hours after acute ischemic stroke. *N Engl J Med* 2008, *359*, 1317-1329.

[17] Moliterno, D.J.; Topol, E.J. Conjunctive use of platelet glycoprotein IIb/IIIa antagonists and thrombolytic therapy for acute myocardial infarction. *Thrombosis and haemostasis* 1997, *78*, 214-219.

[18] Cannon, C.P. Overcoming thrombolytic resistance: rationale and initial clinical experience combining thrombolytic therapy and glycoprotein IIb/IIIa receptor inhibition for acute myocardial infarction. *J Am Coll Cardiol* 1999, *34*, 1395-1402.

[19] Combining thrombolysis with the platelet glycoprotein IIb/IIIa inhibitor lamifiban: results of the Platelet Aggregation Receptor Antagonist Dose Investigation and Reperfusion Gain in Myocardial Infarction (PARADIGM) trial. *J Am Coll Cardiol* 1998, *32*, 2003-2010.

[20] Huang, T.C.; Jordan, R.E.; Hantgan, R.R.; Alevriadou, B.R. Differential effects of c7E3 Fab on thrombus formation and rt-PA-Mediated thrombolysis under flow conditions. *Thrombosis research* 2001, *102*, 411-425.

[21] Kim, J.S.; Kim, J.E.; Choi, B.S.; Park, S.E.; Sapkota, K.; Kim, S.; Lee, H.H.; Kim, C.S.; Park, Y.; Kim, M.K.; Kim, Y.S.; Kim, S.J. Purification and characterization of fibrinolytic metalloprotease from Perenniporia fraxinea mycelia. *Mycol Res* 2008, *112*, 990-998.

[22] Bhargavi, P.L.; Prakasham, R.S. A fibrinolytic, alkaline and thermostable metalloprotease from the newly isolated Serratia sp RSPB11. *Int J Biol Macromol* 2013.

[23] Alexandrov, A.V.; Demchuk, A.M.; Burgin, W.S.; Robinson, D.J.; Grotta, J.C. Ultrasound-enhanced thrombolysis for acute ischemic stroke: phase I. Findings of the CLOTBUST trial. *J Neuroimaging* 2004, *14*, 113-117.

[24] Barreto, A.D.; Pedroza, C.; Grotta, J.C. Adjunctive Medical Therapies for Acute Stroke Thrombolysis: Is There a CLEAR-ER Choice? *Stroke* 2013, *44*, 2377-2379.

[25] Jang, I.K.; Gold, H.K.; Ziskind, A.A.; Fallon, J.T.; Holt, R.E.; Leinbach, R.C.; May, J.W.; Collen, D. Differential sensitivity of erythrocyte-rich and platelet-rich arterial thrombi to lysis with recombinant tissue-type plasminogen activator. A possible explanation for resistance to coronary thrombolysis. *Circulation* 1989, *79*, 920-928.

[26] Kessel, D.O.; Patel, J.V. Current trends in thrombolysis: implications for diagnostic and interventional radiology. *Clin Radiol* 2005, *60*, 413-424.

[27] Alexander, J.H.; Harrington, R.A. Adjunctive Antiplatelet Therapy in Acute Myocardial Infarction: The Road to Improved Infarct-Related Artery Patency. *J Thromb Thrombolysis* 1997, *4*, 353-355.

[28] Barreto, A.D.; Alexandrov, A.V. Adjunctive and alternative approaches to current reperfusion therapy. *Stroke* 2012, *43*, 591-598.

[29] Reverter, J.C.; Beguin, S.; Kessels, H.; Kumar, R.; Hemker, H.C.; Coller, B.S. Inhibition of platelet-mediated, tissue factor-induced thrombin generation by the mouse/human chimeric 7E3 antibody. Potential implications for the effect of c7E3 Fab treatment on acute thrombosis and "clinical restenosis". *J Clin Invest* 1996, *98*, 863-874.

[30] Becker, R.C. Thrombosis and the role of the platelet. *Am J Cardiol* 1999, *83*, 3E-6E.

[31] Ohman, E.M.; Kleiman, N.S.; Gacioch, G.; Worley, S.J.; Navetta, F.I.; Talley, J.D.; Anderson, H.V.; Ellis, S.G.; Cohen, M.D.; Spriggs, D.; Miller, M.; Kereiakes, D.; Yakubov, S.; Kitt, M.M.; Sigmon, K.N.; Califf, R.M.; Krucoff, M.W.; Topol, E.J. Combined accelerated tissue-plasminogen activator and platelet glycoprotein IIb/IIIa integrin receptor blockade with Integrilin in acute myocardial infarction. Results of a randomized, placebo-controlled, dose-ranging trial. IMPACT-AMI Investigators. *Circulation* 1997, *95*, 846-854.

[32] Wagner, C.L.; Mascelli, M.A.; Neblock, D.S.; Weisman, H.F.; Coller, B.S.; Jordan, R.E. Analysis of GPIIb/IIIa receptor number by quantification of 7E3 binding to human platelets. *Blood* 1996, *88*, 907-914.

[33] Chew, D.P.; Moliterno, D.J. A critical appraisal of platelet glycoprotein IIb/IIIa inhibition. *J Am Coll Cardiol* 2000, *36*, 2028-2035.

[34] Cierniewski, C.S.; Byzova, T.; Papierak, M.; Haas, T.A.; Niewiarowska, J.; Zhang, L.; Cieslak, M.; Plow, E.F. Peptide ligands can bind to distinct sites in integrin alphaIIbbeta3 and elicit different functional responses. *J Biol Chem* 1999, *274*, 16923-16932.

[35] Michelson, A.D. Advances in antiplatelet therapy. *Hematology Am Soc Hematol Educ Program* 2011, *2011*, 62-69.

[36] Topol, E.J.; Yadav, J.S. Recognition of the importance of embolization in atherosclerotic vascular disease. *Circulation* 2000, *101*, 570-580.

[37] Pancioli, A.M.; Adeoye, O.; Schmit, P.A.; Khoury, J.; Levine, S.R.; Tomsick, T.A.; Sucharew, H.; Brooks, C.E.; Crocco, T.J.; Gutmann, L.; Hemmen, T.M.; Kasner, S.E.; Kleindorfer, D.; Knight, W.A.; Martini, S.; McKinney, J.S.; Meurer, W.J.; Meyer, B.C.; Schneider, A.; Scott, P.A.; Starkman, S.; Warach, S.; Broderick, J.P. Combined Approach to Lysis Utilizing Eptifibatide and Recombinant Tissue Plasminogen Activator in Acute Ischemic Stroke-Enhanced Regimen Stroke Trial. *Stroke* 2013, *44*, 2381-2387.

[38] Pancioli, A.M.; Broderick, J.; Brott, T.; Tomsick, T.; Khoury, J.; Bean, J.; del Zoppo, G.; Kleindorfer, D.; Woo, D.; Khatri, P.; Castaldo, J.; Frey, J.; Gebel, J., Jr.; Kasner, S.; Kidwell, C.; Kwiatkowski, T.; Libman, R.; Mackenzie, R.; Scott, P.; Starkman, S.; Thurman, R.J. The combined approach to lysis utilizing eptifibatide and rt-PA in acute ischemic stroke: the CLEAR stroke trial. *Stroke* 2008, *39*, 3268-3276.

[39] Shlansky-Goldberg, R. Combination therapy in peripheral vascular disease: the rationale of using both thrombolytic and antiplatelet drugs. *J Am Coll Surg* 2002, *194*, S103-113.

[40] Palomo, I.; Fardella, P.; Pereira, J. Sistema de la Coagulación y Sistema Fibrinolítico. In *Hematología: Fisiopatología y Diagnóstico*; Palomo, I.; Pereira, J.; Palma, J., Eds.; Talca, 2005.

[41] Collen, D. The plasminogen (fibrinolytic) system. *Thromb Haemost* 1999, *82*, 259-270.

[42] Naderi, G.A.; Asgary, S.; Jafarian, A.; Askari, N.; Behagh, A.; Aghdam, R.H. Fibrinolytic effects of Ginkgo biloba extract. *Exp Clin Cardiol* 2005, *10*, 85-87.

[43] Demrow, H.S.; Slane, P.R.; Folts, J.D. Administration of wine and grape juice inhibits in vivo platelet activity and thrombosis in stenosed canine coronary arteries. *Circulation* 1995, *91*, 1182-1188.

[44] Briggs, W.H.; Folts, J.D.; Osman, H.E.; Goldman, I.L. Administration of raw onion inhibits platelet-mediated thrombosis in dogs. *J Nutr* 2001, *131*, 2619-2622.

[45] Leta, G.C.; Mourao, P.A.; Tovar, A.M. Human venous and arterial glycosaminoglycans have similar affinity for plasma low-density lipoproteins. *Biochim Biophys Acta* 2002, *1586*, 243-253.

[46] Rajapakse, N.; Jung, W.K.; Mendis, E.; Moon, S.H.; Kim, S.K. A novel anticoagulant purified from fish protein hydrolysate inhibits factor XIIa and platelet aggregation. *Life Sci* 2005, *76*, 2607-2619.

[47] Bordbar, S.; Anwar, F.; Saari, N. High-value components and bioactives from sea cucumbers for functional foods--a review. *Mar Drugs* 2011, *9*, 1761-1805.

[48] Chakrabarti, S.; Freedman, J.E. Review: Nutriceuticals as antithrombotic agents. *Cardiovasc Ther* 2010, *28*, 227-235.

[49] Phang, M.; Lazarus, S.; Wood, L.G.; Garg, M. Diet and thrombosis risk: nutrients for prevention of thrombotic disease. *Semin Thromb Hemost* 2011, *37*, 199-208.

[50] Kellermann, A.J.; Kloft, C. Is there a risk of bleeding associated with standardized Ginkgo biloba extract therapy? A systematic review and meta-analysis. *Pharmacotherapy* 2011, *31*, 490-502.

[51] Mahady, G.B. Ginkgo biloba for the prevention and treatment of cardiovascular disease: a review of the literature. *J Cardiovasc Nurs* 2002, *16*, 21-32.

[52] Prasad, S.; Kashyap, R.S.; Deopujari, J.Y.; Purohit, H.J.; Taori, G.M.; Daginawala, H.F. Development of an in vitro model to study clot lysis activity of thrombolytic drugs. *Thromb J* 2006, *4*, 14.

[53] Prasad, S.; Kashyap, R.S.; Deopujari, J.Y.; Purohit, H.J.; Taori, G.M.; Daginawala, H.F. Effect of Fagonia Arabica (Dhamasa) on in vitro thrombolysis. *BMC Complement Altern Med* 2007, *7*, 36.

[54] Mary, N.K.; Achuthan, C.R.; Babu, B.H.; Padikkala, J. In vitro antioxidant and antithrombotic activity of Hemidesmus indicus (L) R.Br. *J Ethnopharmacol* 2003, *87*, 187-191.

[55] Chourasia, S.R.; Kashyap, R.S.; Purohit, H.J.; Deopujari, J.Y.; Taori, G.M.; Daginawala, H.F. In-vitro clot lytic potential of Fagonia arabica: a comparative study of two methods. *Blood Coagul Fibrinolysis* 2011, *22*, 288-294.

[56] Yamada, K.; Naemura, A.; Sawashita, N.; Noguchi, Y.; Yamamoto, J. An onion variety has natural antithrombotic effect as assessed by thrombosis/thrombolysis models in rodents. *Thromb Res* 2004, *114*, 213-220.

[57] Suzuki, Y.; Kondo, K.; Matsumoto, Y.; Zhao, B.Q.; Otsuguro, K.; Maeda, T.; Tsukamoto, Y.; Urano, T.; Umemura, K. Dietary supplementation of fermented soybean, natto, suppresses intimal thickening and modulates the lysis of mural thrombi after endothelial injury in rat femoral artery. *Life Sci* 2003, *73*, 1289-1298.

[58] Rajput, M.S.; Mathur, V.; Agrawal, P.; Chandrawanshi, H.K.; Pilaniya, U. Fibrinolytic activity of kaempferol isolated from the fruits of Lagenaria siceraria (Molina) Standley. *Nat Prod Res* 2011, *25*, 1870-1875.

[59] Torres-Urrutia, C.; Guzman, L.; Schmeda-Hirschmann, G.; Moore-Carrasco, R.; Alarcon, M.; Astudillo, L.; Gutierrez, M.; Carrasco, G.; Yuri, J.A.; Aranda, E.; Palomo, I. Antiplatelet, anticoagulant, and fibrinolytic activity in vitro of extracts from selected fruits and vegetables. *Blood Coagul Fibrinolysis* 2011, *22*, 197-205.

[60] Legnani, C.; Frascaro, M.; Guazzaloca, G.; Ludovici, S.; Cesarano, G.; Coccheri, S. Effects of a dried garlic preparation on fibrinolysis and platelet aggregation in healthy subjects. *Arzneimittelforschung* 1993, *43*, 119-122.

[61] Pignon, J.M.; Henni, T.; Amselem, S.; Vidaud, M.; Duquesnoy, P.; Vernant, J.P.; Kuentz, M.; Cordonnier, C.; Rochant, H.; Goossens, M. Frequent detection of minimal residual disease by use of the polymerase chain reaction in long-term survivors after bone marrow transplantation for chronic myeloid leukemia. *Leukemia* 1990, *4*, 83-86.

[62] Morozova, E.N.; Falina, N.N.; Denisova, N.P.; Barkova, L.V.; Psurtseva, N.V. [Analysis of the component constitution and substrate specificity of a fibrinolytic preparation from the fungus Flammulina velutipes]. *Biokhimiia* 1982, *47*, 1181-1185.

[63] Park, S.E.; Li, M.H.; Kim, J.S.; Sapkota, K.; Kim, J.E.; Choi, B.S.; Yoon, Y.H.; Lee, J.C.; Lee, H.H.; Kim, C.S.; Kim, S.J. Purification and characterization of a fibrinolytic protease from a culture supernatant of Flammulina velutipes mycelia. *Biosci Biotechnol Biochem* 2007, *71*, 2214-2222.

[64] Kim, J.H.; Kim, Y.S. Characterization of a metalloenzyme from a wild mushroom, Tricholoma saponaceum. *Biosci Biotechnol Biochem* 2001, *65*, 356-362.

[65] Shin, H.H.; Choi, H.S. Purification and characterization of cysteine protease from Pleurotus ostreatus. *Biosci Biotechnol Biochem* 1998, *62*, 1416-1418.

[66] Kim, J.S.; Sapkota, K.; Park, S.E.; Choi, B.S.; Kim, S.; Nguyen, T.H.; Kim, C.S.; Choi, H.S.; Kim, M.K.; Chun, H.S.; Park, Y.; Kim, S.J. A fibrinolytic enzyme from the medicinal mushroom Cordyceps militaris. *J Microbiol* 2006, *44*, 622-631.

[67] Choi, H.S.; Sa, Y.S. Fibrinolytic and antithrombotic protease from Spirodela polyrhiza. *Biosci Biotechnol Biochem* 2001, *65*, 781-786.

[68] Jeon O. H.; Moon W. J.; Kim D. S. An anticoagulant/fibrinolytic protease from Lumbricus rubellus. *J. Biochem. Mol. Biol.* 1995, *28*, 138-1452.

[69] Taussig, S.J.; Batkin, S. Bromelain, the enzyme complex of pineapple (Ananas comosus) and its clinical application. An update. *J Ethnopharmacol* 1988, *22*, 191-203.

[70] Ako, H.; Cheung, A.H.; Matsuura, P.K. Isolation of a fibrinolysis enzyme activator from commercial bromelain. *Arch Int Pharmacodyn Ther* 1981, *254*, 157-167.

[71] Kowalski, M.; Brown, G.; Bieniasz, M.; Oszajca, K.; Chabielska, E.; Pietras, T.; Szemraj, Z.; Makandjou-Ola, E.; Bartkowiak, J.; Szemraj, J. Cloning and expression of a new recombinant thrombolytic and anthithrombotic agent-a staphylokinase variant. *Acta Biochim Pol* 2009, *56*, 41-53.

[72] Gillman, M.W.; Cupples, L.A.; Gagnon, D.; Posner, B.M.; Ellison, R.C.; Castelli, W.P.; Wolf, P.A. Protective effect of fruits and vegetables on development of stroke in men. *JAMA* 1995, *273*, 1113-1117.

[73] Joshipura, K.J.; Ascherio, A.; Manson, J.E.; Stampfer, M.J.; Rimm, E.B.; Speizer, F.E.; Hennekens, C.H.; Spiegelman, D.; Willett, W.C. Fruit and vegetable intake in relation to risk of ischemic stroke. *JAMA* 1999, *282*, 1233-1239.

[74] Liu, S.; Manson, J.E.; Lee, I.M.; Cole, S.R.; Hennekens, C.H.; Willett, W.C.; Buring, J.E. Fruit and vegetable intake and risk of cardiovascular disease: the Women's Health Study. *Am J Clin Nutr* 2000, *72*, 922-928.

[75] Bazzano, L.A.; He, J.; Ogden, L.G.; Loria, C.M.; Vupputuri, S.; Myers, L.; Whelton, P.K. Fruit and vegetable intake and risk of cardiovascular disease in US adults: the first National Health and Nutrition Examination Survey Epidemiologic Follow-up Study. *Am J Clin Nutr* 2002, *76*, 93-99.

[76] Baruah, D.B.; Dash, R.N.; Chaudhari, M.R.; Kadam, S.S. Plasminogen activators: a comparison. *Vascul Pharmacol* 2006, *44*, 1-9.

[77] Verstraete, M. Third-generation thrombolytic drugs. *Am J Med* 2000, *109*, 52-58.

[78] Gallus, A.S. Thrombolytic therapy for venous thrombosis and pulmonary embolism. *Baillieres Clin Haematol* 1998, *11*, 663-673.

[79] Sandercock, P.; Berge, E.; Dennis, M.; Forbes, J.; Hand, P.; Kwan, J.; Lewis, S.; Lindley, R.; Neilson, A.; Wardlaw, J. Cost-effectiveness of thrombolysis with recombinant tissue plasminogen activator for acute ischemic stroke assessed by a model based on UK NHS costs. *Stroke* 2004, *35*, 1490-1497.

[80] Capstick, T.; Henry, M.T. Efficacy of thrombolytic agents in the treatment of pulmonary embolism. *Eur Respir J* 2005, *26*, 864-874.

[81] Pietri, S.; Maurelli, E.; Drieu, K.; Culcasi, M. Cardioprotective and anti-oxidant effects of the terpenoid constituents of Ginkgo biloba extract (EGb 761). *J Mol Cell Cardiol* 1997, *29*, 733-742.

[82] Kojima, S.; Soga, W.; Hagiwara, H.; Shimonaka, M.; Saito, Y.; Inada, Y. Visible fibrinolysis by endothelial cells: effect of vitamins and sterols. *Biosci Rep* 1986, *6*, 1029-1033.

[83] Matsuura, H. Saponins in garlic as modifiers of the risk of cardiovascular disease. J Nutr 2001, 131, 1000S-1005S.

[84] Henry, B.L.; Thakkar, J.N.; Martin, E.J.; Brophy, D.F.; Desai, U.R. Characterization of the plasma and blood anticoagulant potential of structurally and mechanistically novel oligomers of 4-hydroxycinnamic acids. Blood Coagul Fibrinolysis 2009, 20, 27-34.

Section 2

Clinical Aspects of Fibrinolysis

Chapter 6

Clinical Application of Fibrinolytic Assays

Dominic Pepperell, Marie-Christine Morel-Kopp and Chris Ward

Additional information is available at the end of the chapter

http://dx.doi.org/10.5772/57316

1. Introduction

Haemostasis is a complex balance between thrombus formation and fibrinolysis. Research into bleeding and thrombotic conditions has lead over many years to a detailed knowledge of the role of the components of coagulation, and subsequently many clinical applications have been developed for the testing of platelets, clotting factors and coagulation inhibitors. However, the same cannot be said for the components of fibrinolysis. Fibrinolytic research over the last 30 years has not resulted in the translation of basic science into routine clinical tests of fibrinolytic factors [1, 2], except for D-dimer assays, which are an indirect marker of both thrombosis and fibrinolysis. This has occurred partly due to the difficulties with individual fibrinolytic factor assays, but also due to the inherent limitation of using a single factor assessment to quantify the complex and dynamic process of fibrinolysis.

An ideal assay that could provide an overall or 'global' assessment of haemostasis would take into account the interactions between the proteins of the coagulation and fibrinolytic pathways, blood cellular components and the vessel wall. Such an assay does not currently exist, but refinements of old techniques with updated technology and the development of new global assays have brought improvements in this regard. The ability to assess fibrinolysis is a major benefit of some of these global assays, and has led renewed interest in this field.

Potential clinical applications

There are multiple potential clinical situations in which the ability to detect hypo- or hyperfibrinolysis could in theory be useful. Hypofibrinolysis is a risk factor for thrombosis. Venous thromboembolism (VTE) is a common condition, with an incidence of approximately 1 in 1000 adults [3]. A potential benefit of detecting a fibrinolytic defect would be to identify individuals at higher risk of a first event, which could lead to different management strategies particularly in clinical scenarios such as pregnancy and the peri-operative period where the risk is already known to be higher. This is relevant because currently only approximately one quarter of patients have a detectable inherited or acquired thrombophilia on testing, and 20% of patients have no cause at all found for their first VTE [3-5]. In addition, recurrent VTE events occur in approximately 20-30% of patients within 5 years [4, 6], and identification of hypofibrinolysis as a risk factor might be useful in informing the duration of anticoagulation. Hypofibrinolysis may also be important in arterial thrombosis such as myocardial infarction, and the ability to detect patients who are at increased risk of infarction or stent occlusion due impaired clot lysis would be an important clinical application [7].

Hyperfibrinolysis can result in an increased bleeding risk during surgery and invasive procedures. As it is associated with increased morbidity and mortality, identifying hyperfibrinolysis is a key aim for fibrinolytic assays [8]. Particularly in major procedures such as liver transplant, cardiac valve repair or revascularisation surgery, challenges to the haemostatic system are complex and continuously evolving, and the ability to rapidly detect hyperfibrinolysis in these patients has lead to an improvement in their care [8-10]. Recently, attention has turned to the need for measuring fibrinolysis in trauma patients since the publication of a large multinational study revealed improvements in survival with the early administration of an anti-fibrinolytic drug [11]. Increased fibrinolysis can also be detected in some patients with inherited bleeding conditions such as haemophilia A, indicating that anti-fibrinolytics may also benefit these patients. Finally, disseminated intravascular coagulation (DIC) is a syndrome with abnormal activation of the both coagulation and fibrinolytic systems. Identifying hyperfibrinolysis in suspected cases could assist in the diagnosis of DIC, which otherwise requires complex scoring systems [12].

In this chapter we review assays of the individual factors of the fibrinolytic system and global tests which provide an overall assessment of the fibrinolysis. In each section we will outline the assay itself and its strengths and weakness, before reviewing the literature regarding its use and current or future clinical applications.

2. Fibrinolytic factors

2.1. Plasmin and α2-plasmin inhibitor

The proteolytic enzyme plasmin is the main mechanism through which intravascular fibrin thrombi are degraded. It circulates as its inactive form, plasminogen, at a plasma concentration of approximately 2 μmol/L and is activated intravascularly by tissue plasminogen activator (tPA) [13, 14]. The localization to intravascular thrombi and formation of the active protease occurs more readily after both plasminogen and tPA are bound to fibrin. Any free plasmin is bound by its primary physiological inhibitor, α2-plasmin inhibitor. This circulates at levels of approximately 1 μmol/L in normal plasma (table 1), and neutralizes plasmin so rapidly that the active enzyme is undetectable in plasma. Assays have therefore been aimed at measuring plasminogen, α2-plasmin inhibitor or the plasmin-α2-plasmin inhibitor (PAP) complex.

Plasminogen activity has been most frequently measured using a functional chromogenic assay, but antigenic assays are also available. In the functional assay, an extrinsic activator, streptokinase, which acts on free as well as bound plasminogen, is added to a patient's plasma to convert all of the plasminogen to plasmin, which then acts on a chromogenic substrate [14, 15]. Several commercial kits are available. Where low activity levels are found, plasminogen antigen concentrations can be measured by enzyme-linked immunosorbent assays (ELISA) or nephelometry to distinguish between lack of plasminogen (type 1 deficiency) and dysplasminogenaemia (type 2 defects) [15, 16]. PAP complexes have been assayed by ELISA kits [17, 18], and chromogenic assays have also been used to detect unbound α2-plasmin inhibitor activity [19].

	Plasma concentration		Site of Synthesis	Plasma half life (approximate)
	(µg/ml)	(mol)		
Plasminogen	200	2 µmol/L	Liver	1.8 – 2.7 days
Plasmin	Undetectable	-	-	Very Brief
α2-plasmin inhibitor	70	1 µmol/L	Liver	12 hours
tPA	0.005	70 ρmol/L	Vascular endothelium	5 minutes
PAI-1	0.02	400 ρmol/L	Vascular endothelium, Liver, Adipocytes	2 hours
TAFI	5	75 nmol/L	Liver, Megakaryocytes	10 minutes

Table 1. Synthesis, plasma concentration and half life of fibrinolytic factors [13, 20, 21]

Congenital deficiency and venous thrombosis

The clinical consequences of low plasminogen levels have been studied in patients with congenital deficiency. The prevalence of plasminogen deficiency in the general population has been estimated at 0.3% in a large Scottish cohort of blood donors [22], and 4.3% in a Japanese study [23]. The higher prevalence in the latter population is due the high frequency of a specific plasminogen gene mutation (Ala6012Thr) in East Asian populations causing type 2 deficiency, with similar rates of type 1 disease in each study. Surprisingly, no definite relationship between either type of deficiency and arterial or venous thrombosis has been found [15, 16, 22, 23]. A modestly increased risk suggested by the combined findings of family studies was not statistically significant [15], and has not been confirmed in larger population-based research [22, 23]. Even in severe homozygous plasminogen deficiency there is no excess of thrombotic events; instead the main clinical phenotype is an accumulation of 'ligneous' fibrin-rich, pseudomembranous lesions in the conjunctiva and less commonly in other mucosal membranes [16]. The reason for a lack of thrombotic phenotype is unclear. It may be that residual plasminogen activity in these homozygous patients (the majority display between 4% and 51% activity) is enough to prevent the small vessel thrombosis seen in mouse gene knock-out models where there is no detectable plasminogen [24, 25], or that alternative fibrinolytic proteases released from neutrophils degrade fibrin [26].

Despite the evidence from congenital deficiency states, a small number of studies have investigated plasminogen or α2-plasmin inhibitor levels as a risk factor for venous thrombosis in non-deficient patients. A large case-control study of 770 patients and 743 controls (the MEGA study) found that modest correlations between thrombosis and plasminogen or α2-plasmin inhibitor were lost after adjustment for markers of inflammation and Body Mass Index [27], and the prospective cohort LITE study found no relationship with PAP complexes [18]. A small series of patients with Budd-Chiari syndrome were found to have a slight but statistically significant decrease in plasmin inhibitor levels [28].

Arterial thrombosis

Some large cohort and case-control studies have investigated an association between fibrinolytic proteins and myocardial infarction (MI). High plasminogen levels have surprisingly been consistently associated with a modest elevated risk of myocardial infarction [29-31]. However only one of these studies adjusted for inflammation or smoking [31], which along with elevated cholesterol are potential confounding factors, and the association with MI was lost. An alternative explanation may be that plasmin is known to contribute to the instability of atherosclerotic plaques by activating matrix metalloproteinases [32]. Alpha-2-plasmin inhibitor was also investigated, no association with MI being found in the prospective cohort ECAT study [29], and a slight positive correlation in the retrospective case-control SMILE study [31].

Hyperfibrinolytic states

Raised levels of PAP complexes and decreased levels of α2-plasmin inhibitor have been described in hyperfibrinolytic states, such as acute coagulopathy of trauma [reviewed in 17, 33], disseminated intravascular coagulation (DIC) [34] and the coagulopathy of acute promyelocytic leukaemia [reviewed in 35]. However, no clinical applications have been established, for example as a risk factor of severity.

Rare congenital α2-plasmin inhibitor deficiency has been described [reviewed in 36]. Homozygous deficiency results in a severe bleeding disorder due to increased fibrinolysis with a similar phenotype to congenital haemophilia or Factor XIII deficiency. Conventional haemostasis screening tests are normal, and a functional α2-plasmin inhibitor assay is required to make the diagnosis.

Summary

In summary, research has not resulted in any clinical applications of assays of plasminogen, α2-plasmin inhibitor or PAP complexes in the investigation of fibrinolytic activity despite their central role, perhaps because they circulate at relatively high concentrations and are generally not rate-limiting factors [13]. In rare cases of congenital deficiency of these proteins, functional assays can be used to make the diagnosis.

2.2. Tissue Plasminogen Activator (tPA) and Plasminogen Activator Inhibitor-1 (PAI-1)

Both tPA and PAI-1 have been investigated as markers of fibrinolytic activity. After stimulation, tPA is released locally from endothelial cells and activated platelets, and binds to the fibrin surface of the developing thrombus where it catalyses the formation of plasmin. Once bound, it is protected from its principle inhibitor PAI-1, which circulates in plasma and is also secreted by platelets [13, 37]. Free tPA has a plasma half life of approximately 5 minutes due to the action of PAI-1 and simultaneous clearance by the liver [13]. Therefore resting levels of unbound active tPA in plasma are very low and may be measured by ELISAs that detect both the active form and the tPA – PAI-1 complex. PAI-1 levels have been investigated using functional assays and various ELISAs, which utilise a range of monoclonal antibodies with varying sensitivities for unbound PAI-1 and the tPA-PAI-1 complex [38].

There are several issues that complicate the results of these assays. The first is that measuring resting plasma levels of tPA detects mainly inactive complexes with PAI-1, and so raised levels of tPA antigen may indicate inhibited fibrinolysis rather than increased fibrinolytic potential [2]. An inverse relationship between antigen and fibrinolytic activity has even been found [39, 40]. To overcome this, some investigators have measured acute tPA release following stimulation such as prolonged venous occlusion by a tourniquet. However, it is not clear whether this is a better reflection of the physiological situation [7]. In addition, plasma levels of PAI-1 do not reflect its true contribution in inhibiting fibrinolysis as the majority of PAI-1 is released at the site of thrombus by activated platelets [37, 41] and plasma and platelet pools of PAI-1 vary independently of each other [42].

Levels of PAI-1 and tPA are affected by other factors. PAI-1 in particular has many non-fibrinolytic functions, and may be raised in diabetes mellitus and insulin resistance [reviewed in 2]. Both tPA and PAI-1 are acute phase reactants and elevated with raised lipids and pregnancy [29, 31]. Furthermore, there is marked diurnal variation in their levels, being higher in the morning [43].

Arterial and venous thrombosis

The association between tPA and PAI-1 antigen levels with arterial disease and thrombosis has been investigated in multiple large studies with conflicting results, described in two recent reviews [2, 7]. Although some studies have found increased tPA and PAI-1 levels to be associated with an increased risk of arterial disease or recurrent events [reviewed in 44, 45], some major publications including the Framingham study have reported no association [30, 46], and in two studies even a trend to decreased risk was found in subjects with elevated PAI-1 [47, 48]. The use of assays measuring tPA release has not resulted in any clarity, increased levels being associated with major atherothrombotic events in one study [49] and the inverse in another [29]. These confusing results may be partly accounted for by confounding factors demonstrated by studies that have adjusted for a range other risk factors such as diabetes, cholesterol, obesity, and inflammation. In the ECAT, SMILE and Young Finn studies, apparent associations between PAI-1 or tPA and arterial risk were lost when other these other factors were included in the analyses [29, 31, 50].

The data on tPA and PAI-1 as risk factors for venous thrombosis has similarly failed to find any clinically useful associations [reviewed in 1, 2]. Some prospective studies have found no differences in antigen levels between patients who suffered thrombosis and controls [18, 51, 52], whereas a recent large retrospective study has found PAI-1 to be a risk factor for first venous thrombosis and to be the most important determinant in Clot Lysis Time (CLT), a global test for hypofibrinolysis described later in this chapter [27].

Hyperfibrinolytic states

PAI-1 and tPA levels have been investigated in various hyperfibrinolytic states. PAI-1 has been suggested as a potential therapeutic target in DIC since raised levels correlate with multi-organ failure and outcome [53], whereas in acute traumatic coagulopathy, no association between PAI-1 and severity of injury has been found [17]. In liver cirrhosis, raised tPA levels are proportional to the severity of cirrhosis and risk of variceal bleeding, and may be mediated by a relative deficiency of PAI-1 [discussed in 54].

Summary

Despite a large amount of data on tPA and PAI-1 levels in the literature, no current clinical applications have emerged. The methodological problems and confounding factors discussed above have played a major role in the lack of consistent clinical correlations with disease and outcome.

2.3. Thrombin activatable fibrinolysis inhibitor (TAFI)

TAFI circulates in plasma as a proenzyme and is converted into its active form TAFIa by thrombin or the thrombin-thrombomodulin complex. It then removes specific lysine or arginine residues from partially degraded fibrin, thereby preventing tPA and plasminogen binding which is required for efficient activation of fibrinolysis [13]. It is unstable in plasma, spontaneously degrading to a latent form (TAFIai) with a half life of approximately 10 mins (Table 1).

TAFI can be quantified by ELISA or functional assay. The ELISAs have the advantage of being easy to perform. However there are important differences in the specificities of the antibodies used; they variably measure total antigen, be specific to certain TAFI genotypes, or measure activated TAFI only by being specific for the TAFIa-TAFIai complex [2, 7, 21]. The functional assays measure the ability to cleave residues from small synthetic substrates and have the advantage of measuring all active TAFI, although there may be interference by other carboxypeptidases in plasma. A practical disadvantage is that they are affected by the variable thermal instability of TAFIa, so samples have to be placed on ice immediately and centrifuged at 4^0C, and they also must be collected in tubes containing thrombin and plasmin inhibitors to prevent in-vitro activation [21].

Venous and arterial thrombosis

Raised TAFI levels appear to be consistently associated with venous thromboembolism. In a large case-control study, the Leiden Thrombophilia Study (LETS), TAFI antigen levels above the 90th percentile of controls were found to be associated with an almost two-fold increased risk of first deep vein thrombosis [55], a finding replicated in a smaller case control study using an ELISA specifically designed to be insensitive to different polymorphisms of TAFI [56]. There is some evidence that recurrent venous thromboemboli may be predicted by high TAFI levels; a prospective study of 600 patients with unprovoked venous thrombosis found a two-fold risk of recurrence if their TAFI levels were above the 75th percentile [57]. Disappointingly, this association could not be confirmed in a follow-up to the LETS study, although this may be because patients with provoked thrombotic events were included [58].

The association between TAFI levels and arterial disease are unclear. Some studies have found a link between high TAFIa (but not total TAFI antigen) and coronary artery disease or myocardial infarction [59, 60], but others have found no association [61, 62] and some have found low total TAFI antigen levels to be associated with increased risk [63, 64].

Other diseases

Associations have been investigated between TAFI and a variety of other disease states such as renal failure, hepatic disease, endocrine disorders, cancer, DIC and pregnancy complications [reviewed in 21] without useful clinical applications arising. One recent study has shown an interesting correlation that suggests the variable bleeding phenotype seen in severe Haemophilia A may be associated with TAFI activation levels [65].

Summary

Once again, the problems with TAFI assays and the lack of consistent significant associations with disease mean that there are no current clinical applications. However the possible association of raised TAFI with recurrent unprovoked venous thrombosis warrants further study.

2.4. Other factors affecting fibrinolysis

Lipoprotein(a) or Lp(a) is a homologue of plasminogen that circulates in plasma and is able to inhibit t-PA mediated plasminogen activation at the fibrin surface [7]. It has been investigated as a risk factor for arterial thrombosis in several prospective studies, and a consistent but weak association has been seen with cardiovascular events in both young and elderly patients [reviewed in 7]. A meta-analysis of prospective studies over the last 40 years, involving approximately 127 000 subjects, found that Lp(a) concentrations were an independent risk factor for both coronary disease and stroke but not clinical outcome. The effect was weak, with a hazard ratio of just 1.13 [66]. Therefore on an individual patient basis, assays of Lp(a) are unlikely to be useful.

Annexin A2 receptors on the endothelial cell surface bind both plasminogen and tPA, and accelerate plasminogen activation 60-fold [13]. Recent publications have shown that autoantibodies to annexin A2 are associated with thrombosis in patients with antiphospholipid syndrome [67]. Another interesting finding has been that autoantibodies to annexin A2 occur in a subset of patients with cerebral sinus thrombosis with or without antiphospholipid antibodies; testing for anti-annexin antibodies may have a role in establishing aetiology in these patients whose thrombosis is otherwise often thought to be idiopathic [68].

2.5. D-dimers

D-dimers are a specific cross-linked fibrin degradation product. Their formation depends on thrombin converting fibrin to fibrinogen and activating factor XIII (FXIIIa), which then cross-links the D-domains of adjacent fibrin strands prior to cleavage by plasmin. Thus D-dimers can be seen as an indirect marker of both coagulation and fibrinolysis, although low levels can be seen under normal physiological conditions, and raised levels may occur in pregnancy, advancing age and a wide range of inflammatory and malignant conditions as well as thrombosis [reviewed in 69]. For these reasons specific, evaluation of the fibrinolytic system with D-dimer results alone is problematic, and we will only briefly summarise the assays and their established clinical applications below.

D-dimers can be measured using monoclonal antibodies that have variable specificity for an antigen found in the FXIIIa cross-linked fragments of fibrin compared to other fibrin degradation products. Multiple assays have been developed using three techniques: quantitative ELISAs, whole blood agglutination (qualitative), and latex bead agglutination assays that can be performed on routine laboratory coagulation analysers and may be quantitative or qualitative [69]. It is important to note that results are not comparable between different assays, even between those of similar formats. For this reason it is important that clinicians and researchers are aware of the performance characteristics of the individual assay they are using, and the clinical setting for which it has been validated [70]. In addition, many of the commonly used assays may give false positive results due to lipaemia, hyperbilirubinaemia, intravascular haemolysis or high levels of rheumatoid factor [69], and anticoagulation reduces D-dimer levels even within 24 hours of commencement [71].

Venous thromboembolism

D-dimers are typically elevated in acute VTE. However, because they are increased in a variety of other non-thrombotic disorders, raised D-dimers are a sensitive but not specific marker. As mentioned above, D-dimer assays vary; the latex agglutination and ELISA methods are the most sensitive (93-96%) but least specific (43-53%) [72], and consequently a 'negative' or normal range result in these has a high negative predictive value. Multiple studies have shown the D-dimer assay can be successfully combined with clinical probability scoring systems in the diagnosis of suspected lower extremity DVT or PE [reviewed in 69] and their use has been recommended in recent guidelines [73]. In patients with a low or moderate pre-test probability of DVT, a negative D-dimer test of high sensitivity can exclude a DVT without the need for further investigations. Similar strategies can be used in patients with suspected PE [69], but not in upper limb venous thrombosis [73], and the test is less useful in the elderly, hospital inpatients or those with malignancy due to the high prevalence of elevated D-dimers in these groups reducing assay specificity [74].

There is an increased risk of recurrent VTE in patients with evidence of ongoing activation of the coagulation and fibrinolytic systems, as indicated by a raised D-dimer after the cessation of anticoagulant therapy [69, 75]. This may be used to inform treatment decisions regarding the duration of anticoagulation; a major study (PROLONG) randomised patients to restarting anticoagulation or observation if their D-dimer was raised a month after treatment had ceased. The recurrent VTE rate was demonstrated to be significantly less in those who had restarted anticoagulation [76].

http://dx.doi.org/10.5772/57316

Disseminated Intravascular Coagulation

DIC can be characterised as a syndrome with uncontrolled activation of the both coagulation and fibrinolytic systems, and consequently raised D-dimer levels are a sensitive but non-specific marker [69]. As no single test can establish the diagnosis, D-dimers have been used in scoring systems to establish the likelihood of DIC and monitor the effect of interventions, such as the one developed by the International Society on Thrombosis and Haemostasis (ISTH) [12].

3. Global fibrinolytic assays

The difficulties described above in using individual fibrinolytic markers to measure the fibrinolytic potential of a patient's plasma has lead to increasing interest in global tests that provide an overview of the entire process. Below we discuss thromboelastography, and fibrin generation and lysis assays which have current or potential clinical applications.

3.1. Thromboelastography

Thromboelastography uses viscoelastic changes during coagulation to produce a graphical representation of the fibrin polymerisation process and subsequent fibrinolysis, and as such it has the potential to provide a global evaluation of clot initiation, formation and lysis. First described in 1948 in Germany, two commercial analysers are currently available: the Thromboelastograph or 'TEG' (Haemonetics, MA, USA) and the Rotational Thromboelastogram or 'ROTEM' (Tem International GmbH, Munich, Germany). Both of these are suitable for use as 'point of care' (POC) devices, and this setting is where thromboelastography has developed its main clinical applications.

The principle of the thromboelastogram is as follows [8, 9]; whole blood is added to an incubated cup at 37°C, into which a pin is suspended connected to a detector system. As cup and pin are oscillated relative to each other, the increasing viscosity from the developing fibrin polymerisation affects the magnitude of the movement of the pin, which is converted by a mechanical–electrical transducer to a signal which is displayed as a trace (Figure 1a). As fibrinolysis occurs, the viscosity falls and is also recorded on the trace. As well as the graphical output, values are calculated for various parameters which include: time until initial fibrin formation, clot formation time, rate of polymerisation of fibrin, maximum clot firmness, and clot lysis. Table 2 lists these and the haemostatic variables they are proposed to measure.

Although the TEG and ROTEM are similar in their technologies, there are some important differences. Firstly, in the TEG, the movement is initiated in the cup and a torsion wire monitors the changes in the sample, whereas in the ROTEM, the pin moves on a ball bearing and there is an optical detection system. Some authors claim this modification has led to the ROTEM being more robust in busy clinical settings such as emergency departments and operating theatres [78, 79]. The ROTEM system also has an electronic pipette to help standardise the method. Both systems use proprietary initiators or modifiers of haemostasis, and the TEG can run two assays in series, whereas the ROTEM can run four. The TEG initiates coagulation with

TEG Parameter	ROTEM Parameter	Description	Proposed measured variables
R (Reaction)	**CT**	Clot Time – period to 2mm amplitude	Coagulation factors, platelets, anticoagulants
K	**CFT**	Clot Formation Time – period between 2 – 20mm amplitude	Coagulation factors, fibrinogen, platelets
α - angle	**α - angle**	Rate of clot formation – slope of trace	Coagulation factors, fibrinogen, platelets
MA	**MCF**	Maximum amplitude – maximum clot firmness on trace	Fibrinogen, platelets, fibrinolysis
G	**MCE**	Shear elastic modulus strength or clot elasticity – a representation of clot strength	Platelet function, fibrinogen
LY30, LY60	**LI 30**	Percent decrease in amplitude 30 or 60 minutes after MA is reached	Fibrinolytic factors, fibrinogen
EPL	-	Estimated Percentage Lysis - rate of change of amplitude after MA is reached	Fibrinolytic factors, fibrinogen
-	**ML**	Maximum Lysis at the end of ROTEM test (20 - 40 mins)	Fibrinolytic factors, fibrinogen

Table 2. TEG and ROTEM nomenclature for measured parameters [8, 9, 77]

kaolin or a combination of tissue factor and kaolin (± heparinase), and in the ROTEM there are multiple reagent options that may help to distinguish between the causes for abnormal traces, described in table 3 [8, 9]. Relevant to measuring fibrinolysis, one of these (APTEM) contains the fibrinolytic inhibitor aprotinin; correction of an abnormal trace by adding this reagent has been used to suggest the presence of hyperfibrinolysis. It is important to note also that reference ranges vary considerably between the two technologies, and hence results are not directly comparable between the instruments [80].

A major advantage of the thromboelastogram and one that has lead to its principle uses during major surgery, is that it can be used as a bedside measure of global haemostasis, the graphical output appearing as a real-time representation of the patient's clot formation and lysis over a 20-30 minute assay time, avoiding delays inherent in sending samples for laboratory analysis. Furthermore, non-anticoagulated whole blood can be used, and therefore many of the interactions between coagulation, platelets and fibrinolytic factors are preserved. A limitation is that the coagulation is being measured under static (no shear) conditions in a plastic cuvette rather than an endothelialised blood vessel [9], although of course this disadvantage is shared with almost all other *in vitro* assays.

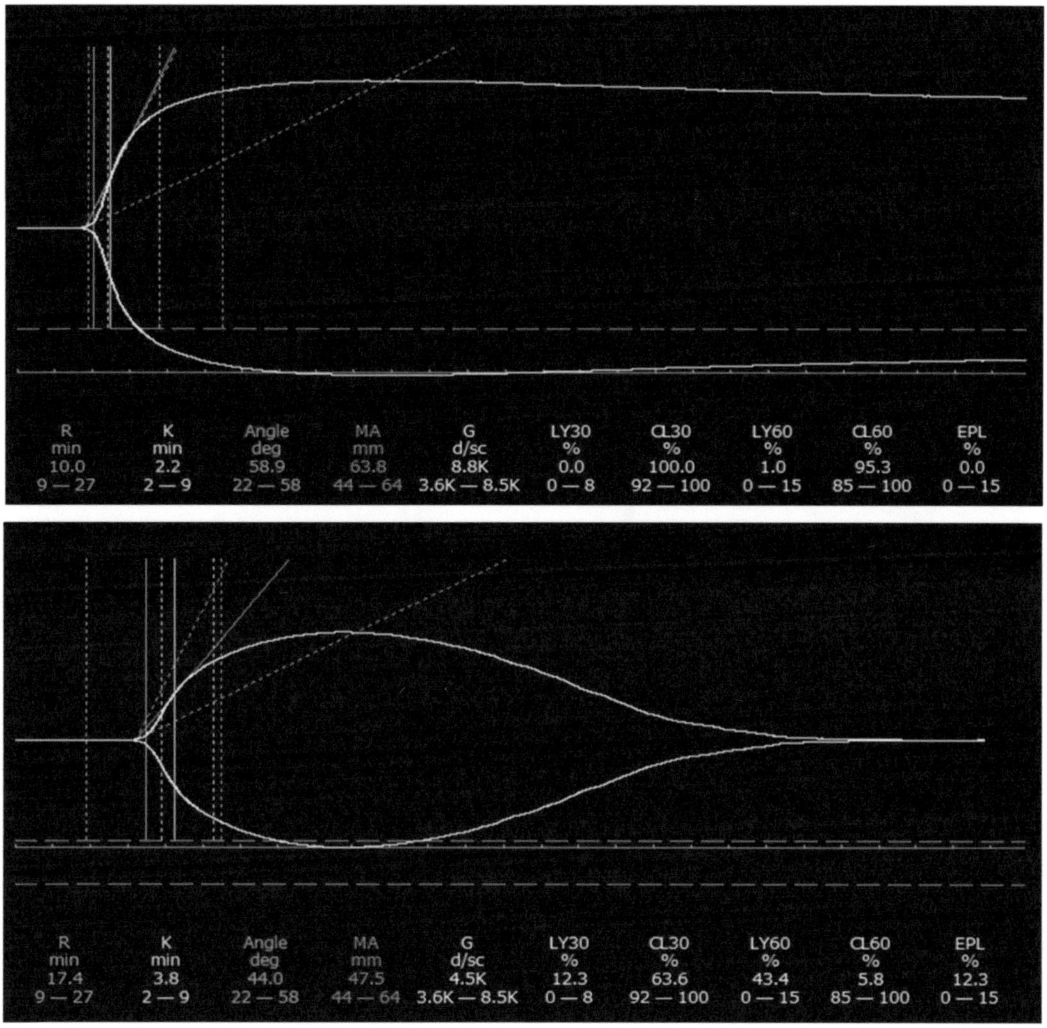

Figure 1. (a) Normal TEG trace. The patient's thromboelastographic trace is shown in white and is produced in real time. The *x-axis* is time; the *y-axis* is millimetres of deviation representing increasing visco-elasticity of the sample as clot forms. Derived parameters are listed below the trace with their proposed normal ranges. R = Clot time; K = Clot formation time; Angle deg = α – angle or Rate of Clot formation; MA = Maximal Amplitude; G = Shear elastic modulus strength; LY30/60 = Percent Lysis at 30/60 minutes; CL30/60 = Inverse of LY30/60 parameter; EPL = Estimated Percentage Lysis; **(b) TEG trace showing hyperfibrinolysis.** The patient's trace in white shows early convergence representing a reduction in visco-elasticity caused by complete fibrinolysis. The key to the derived parameters displayed below the trace is given in Figure 1a above

A concern with thromboelastography has been in the standardisation of methods and reproducibility of results. Pre-analytical variables such as site of blood sampling, time from sampling to analysis, type of reagent and instrument used can alter results significantly [reviewed in 8]. In addition to native whole blood, re-calcified citrate samples may be used when thromboelastography is performed in the haemostasis laboratory, or when a delay

Assay	Reagents	Proposed Use
TEG		
Kaolin	Kaolin	Overall coagulation assessment
Rapid TEG	Kaolin + Tissue Factor	Shorter test time / faster results
Heparinase	Kaolin + Heparinase	Detection of heparin
ROTEM		
In-TEM	Contact activator	Assessment of intrinsic pathway
Ex-TEM	Tissue Factor	Assessment of extrinsic pathway
Hep-TEM	Contact activator + Heparinase	Detection of heparin
Ap-TEM	Tissue Factor + Aprotinin	Detection of fibrinolytic effect when used with EX-TEM
Fib-TEM	Tissue Factor + Platelet antagonist	Qualitative assessment of fibrinogen

Table 3. Selected TEG and ROTEM reagents [9]

between sampling and analysis is expected in a POC setting. However it has been reported that stable results are not produced until after 30 minutes of collection in citrate, which defeats the purpose of the technique as a 'real-time' assessment of haemostasis, and values from citrate samples cannot be correlated to those from non-anticoagulated samples [81].

Operating the TEG or ROTEM in a POC setting means that non-laboratory staff must run these moderately complex tests and hence sufficient numbers need to be properly trained to operate and maintain the equipment to avoid further errors. Quality assessment (QA) must be carried out on a regular basis, the TEG for example requiring quality control (QC) samples to be run each time the machine is switched on, every 8 hours or if the analyser moved [10]. Commercial samples for internal quality control are available and external QA schemes exist, but the results from the latter have been disappointing [82]. Coefficient of variation (CV) results between centres have been reported between 7.6 – 39.9% in the TEG and 3.6 - 83.6% in the ROTEM [82, 83] for coagulation variables on plasma samples, although much better results in both devices can be produced in a single centre using whole blood if the manufacturer's method is followed exactly [9, 84].

No data on the reproducibility on fibrinolytic measures between centres has been published. The effect of fibrinolysis on TEG or ROTEM instruments can be detected using the parameters that are listed in Table 2. However, operators can also use a qualitative difference in the shape of the traces to diagnose hyperfibrinolysis, an example of which is shown in Figure 1b. Although subjective, experienced operators have used this strategy successfully in complex surgery to guide treatment of hyperfibrinolysis as described below, and the effect of giving an anti-fibrinolytic agent *in vivo* or adding aprotinin *in vitro* in the APTEM is clearly demonstrated in the traces of these patients [77, 78, 85-87]. However, the validity and sensitivity of this approach is unclear and in some reviews it has been suggested that only marked hyperfibrinolysis can be identified this way [33, 88]. Some investigators using the TEG have attempted to standardise the definition of hypofibrinolysis as an 'Estimated Percent Lysis' (EPL) of greater than 15% [88]; this is calculated by the TEG software comparing the area under the curve at the MA amplitude and 30 minutes later. Validation of this definition as a measure of hyperfibrinolysis is lacking, but a recent publication has shown that increasing concentrations of tPA at pathophysiological levels added *in vitro* lead to higher EPL levels in a dose dependent way (but not in the less sensitive RapidTEG) [89]. Also, important clinical correlations with outcome have been found with this EPL threshold (see the studies reviewed below). In the ROTEM there is some data to suggest the maximum lysis measure at 1 hour correlates with tPA, PAPs and PAI-1 [79], and the clot lysis index at 30 mins has 71% sensitivity for hyperfibrinolysis when compared to the less quantitative euglobulin clot lysis test (described in a later section) [78].

In discussing the literature regarding the use of thromboelastography as an assay of fibrinolysis, first the established uses as a POC device in surgery and trauma will be summarised, although detection of hyperfibrinolysis in these situations is only a component of the data utilised. Following this, the research concerning the use of the technique in pregnancy, haemophilia and hypercoagulable states will be discussed.

Hepatic surgery

One of the first clinical applications described was in orthotopic liver transplantation where the TEG can be used to monitor coagulation and guide blood component and anti-fibrinolytic therapy [90]. The haemostatic defect in these patients is complex; they often start with a thrombocytopenia and depletion of clotting factors due to end stage liver disease, but also have low levels of the natural anticoagulant proteins C, S and antithrombin. During surgery they may have a rapidly changing picture due to consumption of factors and dilution. Patients may also develop hyperfibrinolysis caused by tPA build up during the anhepatic stage, followed by a surge of tPA release from the reperfused transplant liver [91, 92]. However, unnecessary use of anti-fibrinolytics should be avoided due to the risk of hepatic artery thrombosis. POC thromboelastography can produce timely information at intervals throughout the surgery on the nature of the defect and requirements for coagulation factor replacement or anti-fibrinolytic therapy, and has been shown to decrease the need for red cell transfusion and plasma products [90, 93-95].

Cardiac surgery

Cardiac surgery requiring cardiopulmonary bypass is a complex balance between anticoagulation with heparin, the effect of anti-platelet agents and the need for haemostasis at the end of surgery [10]. Hyperfibrinolysis may also be seen, particularly post-bypass. There is good evidence from randomised controlled trials and retrospective analysis that the use of thromboelastography-guided algorithms for heparin reversal, blood component and anti-fibrinolytic support reduce the need for blood product transfusion and the rates of surgical re-exploration due to post-operative bleeding [96-100]. For example, a randomised prospective trial of 105 patients undergoing complex cardiac surgery compared TEG-guided transfusion therapy with standard care and found significantly fewer transfusions in the TEG group due to less postoperative requirements [97]. This trial also showed a 75% drop in the number of patients having FFP infusion and a 50% fall in platelet transfusion. Because the use of TEG and ROTEM has been shown to reduce the potential risk to the patient and to reduce costs [96, 101], their use has been recommended in both US and European guidelines [102, 103].

Trauma

Increased understanding of trauma associated coagulopathy has shown that fibrinolysis is a key component which is associated with increased mortality and can be reliably detected by thromboelastography in the emergency department, combat settings and operating theatres [for recent reviews see 10, 33]. Interest in this area has grown further since the publication of the large multi-centre CRASH-2 study which showed decreased mortality if trauma patients were given tranexamic acid to inhibit fibrinolysis within three hours [11]. However the inclusion criteria were very broad in this study, and POC testing with TEG may be able to target anti-fibrinolytic therapy to those who would benefit most. For example, a recently published prospective study used TEG to evaluate a severely injured cohort of patients for hyperfibrinolysis, defined as an EPL of 15% or more [104]. The incidence was 11% overall, but these patients had 25 times the risk of early mortality. The TEG assay was reported to rapidly identify hyperfibrinolysis within the first hour in all patients, allowing potential early use of anti-fibrinolytics. The results replicate a smaller study using the ROTEM [105]. These developments warrant further prospective randomised trials to demonstrate a reduced morbidity or survival benefit in trauma patients monitored by thromboelastography and treated accordingly.

Haemophilia

Little has been published on the use of thromboelastography in inherited bleeding disorders. However, the TEG has been used to demonstrate hyperfibrinolysis in Haemophilia A, and this was correctable with either recombinant FVIIa or an anti-fibrinolytic or both [86, 106], and the TEG is also able to monitor the effect of rFVIIa used to treat haemophilia patients with acquired inhibitors [107].

Hypercoagulable or hypofibrinolytic states

Thromboelastography has been less successful in demonstrating hypofibrinolysis. This may be because normal subjects only show a minor degree of fibrinolysis in unmodified TEG or ROTEM assays, for example one study showing the normal range of the ROTEM Maximum Lysis at 60 minutes to be 0 – 12% (mean 3%) [84]. Modifications have been suggested to increase the sensitivity to hypofibrinolysis by adding exogenous tPA to the cuvette prior to clot initiation, but there has been little published on the success of this approach; one group described a standard method for measuring tPA induced fibrinolysis using the TEG and subsequently used it to show that children with idiopathic venous thrombosis have significantly reduced fibrinolysis compared to controls [108, 109]. The data concerning the use of thromboelastography in hypercoagulable states has otherwise concentrated on the ability of the technique to show shortened clotting times, rapid fibrin polymerisation or increased clot strength [e.g. 110], and is outside the scope of this chapter.

http://dx.doi.org/10.5772/57316

Pregnancy

Pregnancy is a hypercoagulable state in which many of the component s of the coagulation and fibrinolytic system are altered, but conventional assays fail to provide an overall picture of the patient's haemostatic potential. Thromboelastography has been used in this regard, and has been successful in guiding therapeutic anticoagulation with LMWH and assessing the risk of neuraxial anaesthesia [reviewed in 8, 10]. A minor degree of hypofibrinolysis can be detected by TEG at the end of the third trimester compared to 8 weeks post partum [111], and an algorithm for TEG-guided treatment of post partum haemorrhage has been suggested, similar to those used in trauma [112].

Conclusion

Thromboelastography has an established clinical role in the detection of hyperfibrinolysis in major hepatic and cardiac surgery, and its use in the management of trauma victims is growing. As further awareness and understanding of the assay occurs, further applications in bleeding patients [112], haemophilia and pregnancy are likely [113]. However, an expansion of its role into detection of hypofibrinolysis is unlikely given the insensitivity of current methodologies.

4. Fibrin generation and lysis assays

Attempts had been made to time the dissolution of plasma clots as an overall measure of fibrinolysis even before the development of molecular markers and their immunoassays. However, spontaneous fibrinolysis of plasma clots is an extremely slow process, for example taking as long as 20 hours to achieve just 10% lysis [114]. Laboratory assays were subsequently developed that could measure fibrinolysis over a shorter period, principally the euglobulin clot lysis time (ECLT) [115] and the dilute whole blood clot lysis time (DWBCLT) [116]. However they have not been widely adopted because of several drawbacks. The ECLT measures lysis in only a fraction of plasma precipitated by utilising a low pH and ionic strength; the main determinants are fibrinogen, tPA and plasminogen only, the natural inhibitors being absent. DWBCLT is performed in the absence of calcium and hence excludes the interplay of the coagulation and fibrinolytic systems, and both of these tests were also labour intensive and unsuited to modern clinical laboratories.

4.1. Clot lysis time (CLT)

More recently an automated assay called the clot lysis time (CLT) has been developed to assess the dissolution of a tissue factor induced fibrin clot by exogenous tPA [117]. Citrated platelet-poor plasma (PPP) is added to a microtitre plate at 37°C with tissue factor, calcium, phospholipid to initiate clot formation and exogenous tPA to trigger fibrinolysis. The turbidity at 405nm is measured over time. The CLT is defined as the time from the midpoint of clot formation (between clear and maximum turbidity) to the midpoint of clot lysis (between maximum turbidity and clear). It has a mean (± SD) in normal individuals of 83.8 (± 11.1) minutes [118].

The CLT has several advantages. Firstly, it is relatively simple and easy to run. It can be done on previously frozen samples and is insensitive to method of PPP preparation [118]. It provides an assessment of the overall fibrinolytic capacity of the plasma, being affected by most of the individual factors. Plasminogen, α2-plasmin inhibitor, PAI-1 and TAFI all have been shown to be important variables in the CLT, whilst prothrombin, fibrinogen and factors VII, X and XI have a progressively more minor effect [27]. However, the concentration of the exogenous tPA is above physiological levels, and important interactions with platelets are not accounted for.

The CLT has been poorly standardised between groups, but a recent publication has sought to address this and investigate the biological variation within healthy individuals [118]. It was identified that the assay has a total analytical CV of 13.4%, and there is substantial biological variance over time within normal individuals. Sequential samples are therefore required to establish the true fibrinolytic potential of an individual; the authors suggest a single result may differentiate up to 20% from the true value. These should be done at the same time of day because the assay is affected by the diurnal variation in fibrinolysis that was previously noted in plasma levels of tPA and PAI-1, but no seasonal variation was detected. As it is a turbidometric assay, results may also be affected by marked lipaemia or paraproteinaemia.

Venous thromboembolism

There is definitive evidence that reduced fibrinolytic potential as shown by prolonged CLT is a risk factor for first venous thromboembolism (VTE). The LETS case control study determined the CLTs for 421 patients following their first DVT selected consecutively from anticoagulation clinics and excluded only if aged over 70 or if they had a malignancy [117]. Samples were taken at least 6 months after the diagnosis and at least 3 months after the cessation of anticoagulant and were matched with 469 control samples from patient's partners. A dose-dependent correlation was seen between increased CLT and DVT, with those with CLTs above the 90th percentile having twice the risk of controls, even when corrected for age, sex, clotting factors, antithrombin and TAFI levels. A second smaller study investigated lysis times in a group of 100 patients with a first idiopathic VTE using a similar turbidometric assay [119]. Patients were excluded if they had any known congenital or acquired risk factors for thrombosis or evidence of an underlying inflammatory state; the included VTE patients showed mean clot lysis times that were a 31.9% longer than controls. Findings were replicated in the Multiple Environmental and Genetic Assessment (MEGA) study of 2090 patients with first DVT or PE and 2564 controls [120]. Patients were between 18-70 years and were excluded if death or end-stage disease prevented follow-up samples being taken, whilst the control group was comprised of the patient's partners and random healthy individuals. Again, a dose dependent increase in risk of DVT was seen for increasing CLTs. The authors defined hypofibrinolysis as those with a CLT above the 75th percentile, and these patients had a two-fold risk compared to those in the first quartile. Interestingly, a synergistic effect was seen when CLT was combined with other known risk factors. Immobilisation increased the risk of VTE 4.3-fold in this study, but combined with hypofibrinolysis the risk was over 10 times that of controls. The overall risk with Factor V Leiden heterozygosity increased from 3.5 to 8.1-fold but the combination with prothrombin 20210A mutation did not show the same effect. Most markedly, for women under 50 years on the oral contraceptive, the risk of first VTE went up from 2.6-fold to over 20-times the risk if they also had hypofibrinolysis. Previously it had been shown that OCP use had either a minor [121] or no effect [122, 123] on prolonging the clot lysis time by itself.

Recurrent VTE

The establishment of hypofibrinolysis defined by CLT as a risk factor for first VTE has led to interest in whether it could predict recurrent events, and therefore be used in clinical decision-making on the duration of anti-coagulation in patients. The LETS population was prospectively studied to see if prolonged CLTs detected after the first DVT predicted recurrent VTE [58]. In a group of 447 patients with a mean follow-up of 7.3 years, no significant association was seen in the 90 patients with recurrence. In a second study, 704 patients with a first unprovoked VTE and no genetic risk factor, malignancy, lupus anticoagulant or other requirement for long-term anti-coagulation, were studied [124]. In the female population (n=378), there was a 3.28-fold risk of recurrence for those with a CLT in the fourth quartile, but no association with recurrence was found in men or the overall population. Whilst these results are disappointing, there may be reasons why some effect was not detected; it should be noted that in the LETS study, patients with temporary risk factors such as immobility were included in the study although they had a low risk of recurrence, and in both studies patients who remained on anti-coagulation for any reason were excluded, including those continuing because they were thought to be high risk for recurrence. In neither of these studies were CLTs combined with other known predictors of recurrence, such as elevated D-dimer or Factor VIII levels, to see if their predictive power could be increased.

Uncommon thrombotic disorders

Some recent interesting research suggests using global methods such as the CLT may provide insight into the pathogenesis of some poorly understood hypercoagulable diseases. For example, CLTs were significantly longer (p=0.001) in 81 patients with retinal vein occlusion compared to a matched control group, even when multivariate analysis adjusted for cardiovascular risk factors [125]. Another study showed CLTs above the 95th percentile gave a 3.4-fold increase risk of Budd-Chiari syndrome [28], and 92 patients with pre-eclampsia were found to have significantly prolonged clot lysis times compared to controls, independent of the presence of antiphospholipid antibodies [126].

Arterial thrombosis

Clot lysis times have also been studied as a risk factor for arterial disease in 3 recent studies. The first used samples from the large case control study population from the Study of Myocardial Infarction Leiden (SMILE) to test CLT in 421 men and 642 controls [127]. Samples in the study group were taken a median 2.6 years after first MI. In men under 50 years the overall risk of MI was 3.2 times (95% CI 1.5-6.7) increased for CLTs in the highest quartile; however, once cardiovascular risk factors were adjusted for the risk was attenuated to just 1.8 (95% CI 0.7-4.8), and no relationship was seen in the over 50s. Another case-control study (from the 'ATTAC' study) examined the association between CLTs and ischaemic stroke, peripheral vascular disease as well as MI in both sexes [123]. Even after adjusting for cardiovascular risk factors there was an approximately 2-fold increase in risk of arterial event associated with CLTs above the 80th percentile (compared to the risk associated with diabetes which was 2.5), and the association was similar in the 3 categories of disease. Finally, a third case-control group (the RATIO study) found a significant association between CLT and arterial thrombosis in young women aged 18-50 [128]. The risk of MI was increased for those with CLT in the third tertile, but surprisingly the risk of ischaemic stroke was only increased by shortened CLTs, i.e. with hyperfibrinolysis, a finding which is yet to be validated or explained.

Anticoagulants and hypocoagulable states

Given the evidence that some patients with thrombosis have impaired fibrinolysis, one interesting area of investigation concerns the effect of different anticoagulants on fibrinolysis measured by the CLT. Data on their effect could help to interpret CLT studies on patients with VTE without the need to take them off their anticoagulation, which was a methodological problem in the studies on recurrent VTE risk described above. Another possible benefit might be the ability to individualise anticoagulant choices for patients with hypofibrinolysis. Three studies have addressed the effect of anticoagulants. CLTs were measured in an in-vitro study where varying concentrations of anticoagulants including a low molecular weight heparin (LMWH), a selective anti-Xa drug (fondaparinux) and thrombin inhibitors (hirudin and PPACK) [129]. The LMWH and fondaparinux both had a significant effect in shortening CLTs, whereas no effect was seen with the thrombin inhibitors. A second study looked at the in-vivo use of unfractionated heparin (UFH) and LMWH in the treatment of acute PE, and found that fibrinolysis was enhanced significantly in the UFH group versus those on LMWH [130]. A third study showed that fondaparinux shortened CLTs in vitro and in healthy subjects, and this could be partially reversed with rFVIIa [131].

There has been comparatively little research on the utility of CLT in measuring hypocoagulable or hyperfibrinolytic conditions. In haemophilia A, hyperfibrinolysis has been demonstrated by shortened CLTs, and can be abolished by adding FVIII, TAFI or recombinant activated Factor VII (rFVIIa) [132, 133]. Another study used shortened CLTs to demonstrate hyperfibrinolysis in liver cirrhosis [134].

4.2. Overall Haemostatic Potential (OHP)

A limitation of the CLT is that only a single timed variable representing fibrin degradation is produced from the process of fibrin generation and subsequent lysis. A more comprehensive method for investigating this process is provided by the *Overall Haemostatic Potential* assay which was first developed in Sweden by Blombäck and colleagues [135] and modified in subsequent publications [136-138]. The principle of the OHP is the generation of fibrin formation and lysis curves to represent the shifting balance between fibrin generation and lysis using serial spectrophotometric measurements plotted against time. Two other assays with very similar methods have been described and will be also considered in this section. These are the *Clot Formation and Lysis* (CloFAL) assay [139] and the *Coagulation Inhibitor Potential* (CIP) assay [140, 141].

The modified OHP [136, 138] uses a small amount of thrombin to trigger coagulation. Fresh or thawed citrated PPP is added to a microtitre plate well at 37°C containing buffer with calcium chloride and thrombin at a final concentration of 0.03 – 0.04 IU/ml. Light absorbance at 390 or

405nm is recorded every minute for 40-60 mins. As the fibrinogen is gradually converted to fibrin by generated thrombin, the absorbance increases and is recorded at each time point, with the area under the curve (AUC) reflecting the total fibrin generated. The measurements from this well are termed the Overall Coagulation Potential (*OCP*). Each sample is run in parallel with another well containing the same reagents but with added tPA at 330 – 350ng/mL. In this analysis, called the Overall Haemostatic Potential (*OHP*), complete fibrinolysis occurs after initial fibrin generation, recorded by a fall in absorbance over time. The difference between the AUCs of the *OCP* (without tPA) and the *OHP* (with tPA) represents the overall fibrinolytic potential (*OFP*) and is expressed as a percentage of the *OCP*. Examples of these curves are shown in Figures 2a and b. Other derived measures include the *Delay*, which is the time from start of the analysis to onset of fibrin generation and correlates with the APTT, the maximum optical density (*Max OD*) representing the maximal amount of fibrin generated (correlating to plasma fibrinogen levels), and the velocity (*Max Slope*) to describe the rate of fibrin generation [138]. In addition, the OFP may be corrected for variations in *Delay* by standardising the time period over which it is calculated to the 45 minutes starting from the onset of fibrin generation (OFP 45).

Tests are performed in duplicates in a microtitre plate. In a single laboratory the intra-assay CVs were approximately 3.1 – 8.7% and the inter-assay CVs 4.2 – 5.1% for the OCP and OHP values respectively [136]. Experiments in our laboratory have shown that standard precautions may be applied regarding pre-analytical variables; fresh samples are stable if processed within 2 hours or may be frozen and analysed later, and different methods of PPP preparation did not alter assay results either (unpublished data).

The OHP has demonstrated sensitivity to changes in both coagulation and fibrinolytic factors. In vitro experiments using factor deficient plasma have demonstrated significant correlations between OHP parameters and concentrations of factors II, V, VII, VIII, IX and X and XI [142]. These results were replicated in our laboratory, and we also have shown using in-vitro experiments that the OFP parameter is sensitive to varying concentrations of plasminogen, α2-plasmin inhibitor, PAI-1, TAFI and the fibrinolytic inhibitor tranexamic acid [unpublished data and 143]. In vitro spiking experiments have shown fibrinogen concentration outside the normal range also has a negative correlation with fibrinolysis parameters; however, whereas fibrinogen levels can have a marked effect on the CLT assay because of the increase in the clot's peak light absorbance, the nature of the OFP parameter as a ratio of the OCP-OHP:OCP controls for the maximum OD and is a reasonable expression of clot lysis.

The OHP can also be used as a screening assay for heritable thrombophilias; previously unpublished evidence from our laboratory shows sensitivity to antithrombin deficiency with both hypercoagulable and hypofibrinolytic changes (figure 3), the latter defect likely related to increased TAFIa levels. The *Coagulation Inhibitor Potential* (CIP) assay is a newer modification of the OHP specifically designed for thrombophilia screening which uses heparin pentasaccharide to potentiate antithrombin and the snake venom Protac to activate Protein C [140, 141]. It has shown excellent sensitivity of 100% and reasonable specificity of 70-80% in two small series of patients with FV Leiden, or Protein C, S or antithrombin deficiency [140, 144].

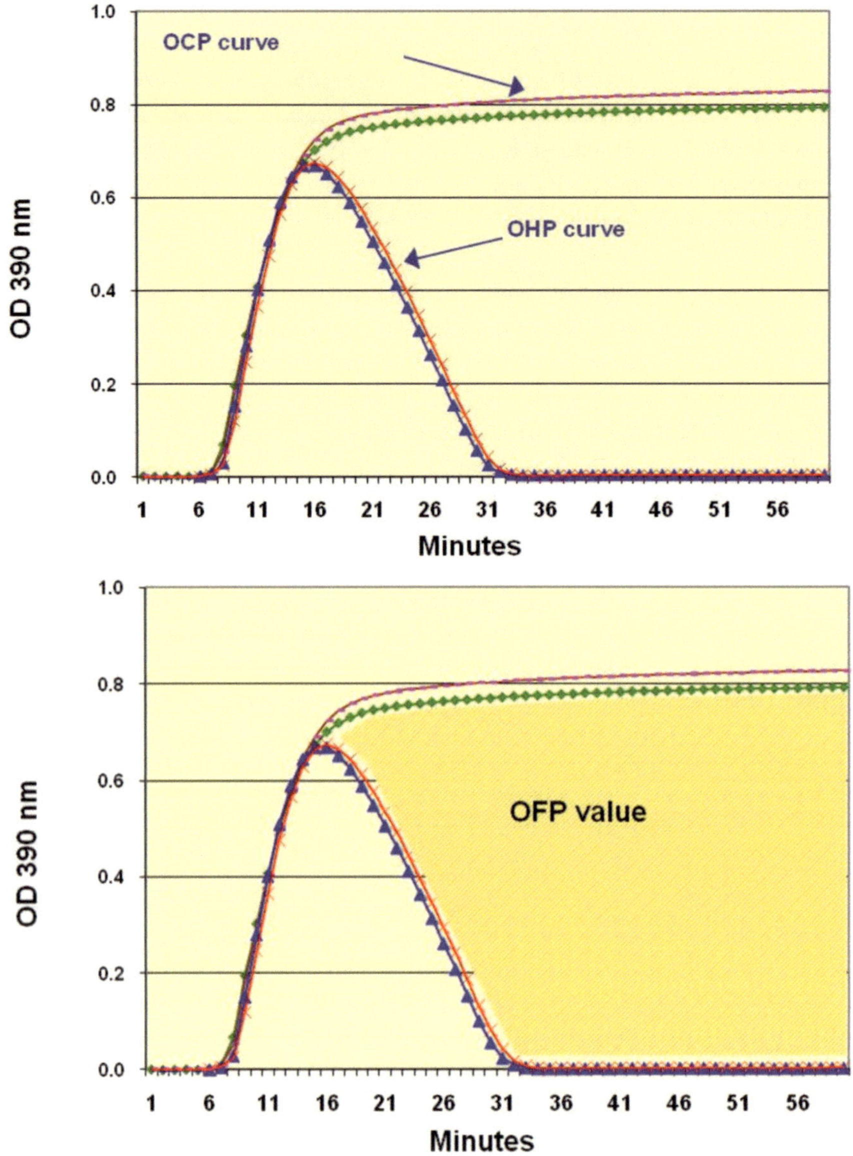

Figure 2. (a) Examples of Overall Coagulation Potential (OCP) and Overall Haemostatic Potential (OHP) curves. **(b)** The Overall Fibrinolytic Potential (OFP) is the difference of the area under the curves of the Overall Coagulation Potential (OCP) and Overall Haemostatic Potential (OHP)

Whilst there are clear advantages of the OHP as an assay for fibrinolysis, such as its simplicity, inexpensiveness and reproducibility, there have been several criticisms of the method [145]. The first is that thrombin is used to initiate coagulation. In earlier versions of the assay, higher thrombin concentrations were used and there was evidence of direct fibrinogen activation

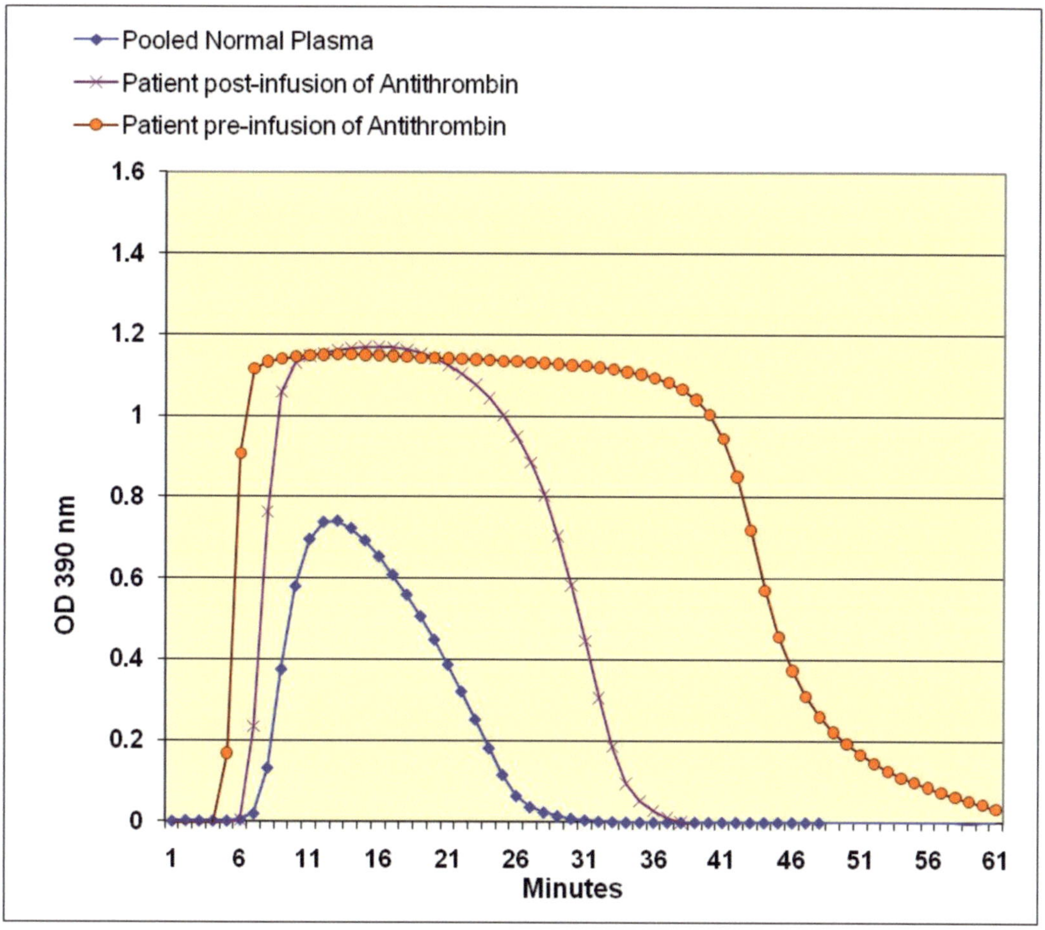

Figure 3. Overall Haemostatic Potential (OHP) curves of a patient with congenital antithrombin deficiency before and after antithrombin concentrate infusion compared to a pooled normal plasma control. The pre-infusion OHP curves show decreased *Delay*, increased *Max Slope* and *Max OD*, and impaired fibrinolysis. *Delay*, *Max Slope* and fibrinolysis are partially corrected by antithrombin infusion.

occurring from the exogenous thrombin. However the very low concentrations used in the modified version produce no detectable clot in thrombin deficient plasma, suggesting the exogenous thrombin is only enough to trigger coagulation via a feedback reaction and not directly converting fibrinogen [145]. Even so, a further refinement of the method has been published which replaces the thrombin with a low concentration of tissue factor and phospholipid to more accurately mirror in-vivo coagulation and this method has also been shown to be sensitive to changes in coagulation factor and PAI-1 concentrations [137]. The *CloFAL* assay has also been independently developed with a very similar method to the OHP using tissue factor as an initiator, and a different algorithm to evaluate fibrinolysis [139].

A second criticism of the OHP is that plasminogen activation depends almost exclusively on the exogenous tPA, a modification of the method which is essential to produce measurable fibrinolysis within a reasonable time frame but which makes the assay insensitive to changes in endogenous plasminogen activators [145]. Thirdly, the effects of the cellular components are excluded by the use of PPP, unlike in the TEG for example. Finally, the OHP and related assays currently lack standardisation and are not available commercially, and variations in type of initiator, concentrations of reagents and derived parameters making results between groups difficult to compare. As yet, no inter-laboratory CVs have been published. OFP results are also likely to show a diurnal variation due to their sensitivity to higher PAI-1 levels in the morning, and this has been demonstrated in patients with obstructive sleep apnoea [146].

Arterial thrombosis

Impaired fibrinolysis demonstrated by the OHP assay has been found in patients with coronary heart disease. A large retrospective study compared 800 patients three months after their first MI with 1123 normal controls from the local population [147]. Fibrinolytic parameters below the 10th percentile of the control group's values conferred an odds ratio of first MI of 1.66 (95% CI 1.22-2.27) after correction for cardiovascular risk factors in multivariate analysis. In another study, serial samples from patients admitted to hospital with acute coronary syndrome showed decreased fibrinolysis that improved on treatment with LMWH [148]. Patients with stable coronary artery disease also have reduced fibrinolysis; 56 patients with angiography proven coronary atherosclerosis had significantly reduced OFP values compared to controls [149]. The lowest tertile of OFP results conferred an odds ratio of 16.1 for coronary artery disease compared to the highest tertile. This major increase in risk was partly accounted for by higher PAI-1 levels although the global OFP measure remained an independent risk factor when adjusted for this.

The OHP has also demonstrated hypofibrinolysis in patients with cerebrovascular events. In one study, samples were taken from a group of 44 young patients a median of 5 years after they had experienced an episode of acute cerebral ischaemia and compared to healthy age matched controls. Little difference in the incidence of traditional thrombophilic measures was seen between the groups, but increased OCP parameters and decreased OFP results were demonstrated [150]. Another study examined TAFI levels and the OHP in patients at the time of acute ischaemic stroke and 60 days later [151]. Patients had impaired global fibrinolysis compared to controls which was partly, but not fully, explained by raised TAFI levels.

Venous thrombosis

Currently there is less published evidence regarding the use of the OHP to detect hypofibrinolysis in patients with venous thrombosis, although the assay does show promise in this area. The Swedish group first published data on a group of 88 women who had had a pregnancy related VTE, with the majority having evidence of activated protein C resistance with or without the Factor V Leiden mutation [152]. Blood samples were taken for OHP analysis from the patients 8 months to 13 years after the last VTE and compared to samples from a control group of healthy women. They were able to demonstrate a significant persisting hypercoagulability and hypofibrinolysis in the group which was most marked in those who had Factor V Leiden. Subsequently another publication studied 161 patients referred to haematology clinic with clinically defined hypercoagulable states [138]. The study group was heterogenous and included patients with VTE (n=73), arterial thrombi, antiphospholipid antibodies or lupus anticoagulant, and pregnancy complications. Despite this, significant differences in fibrin generation and lysis were found in the study population compared to a control group of blood donors, giving the OHP assay an estimated sensitivity of 96% for detection of clinically defined hypercoagulable states. The results of this study complement the excellent sensitivity the OHP has demonstrated in detecting inherited thrombophilic states that was described previously [140], and data showing that the OHP can discriminate factor XII deficient patients with a prothrombotic phenotype [153].

These promising results merit further prospective study to investigate whether the OHP assay can predict first or recurrent VTE. It may be particularly useful in identifying hypercoagulability in patients with otherwise unprovoked idiopathic VTE; in our laboratory we have noted impaired fibrinolysis in this group (unpublished), and similar results have been published using the CloFAL assay in paediatric VTE [154].

Pregnancy

The OHP assay demonstrates both significantly increased fibrin generation and decreased hypofibrinolysis in normal pregnancy [J Curnow et al, personal communication, 136]. In high risk pregnancy, these changes have also been described [155] and unpublished data from our laboratory shows a significant worsening in these parameters compared to patients with uncomplicated pregnancy, which may indicate a role for the OHP in prospective studies of thrombosis risk.

Anticoagulation monitoring

The OHP shows potential applications in the monitoring of overall coagulation and fibrinolytic changes with anticoagulation. As described above, improvement of fibrinolysis was seen in acute coronary syndrome patients once LMWH was started [148], and similar improvement may be seen with warfarin and the new oral anticoagulants (unpublished data). However, the response appears to be variable even when conventional assays show anticoagulation to be within the therapeutic window; for example, in a study of pregnant women with previous thromboembolism, dalteparin prophylaxis was shown to improve hypercoagulable OHP variables in the majority, but some patients were seen to remain hypercoagulable even with therapeutic anti-Xa results [155]. Further study is required to investigate if this translates to an increased thrombosis risk and whether changing treatment based on OHP results can result in improved patient care.

Hypocoagulable states

As mentioned previously, the OHP is sensitive to factor deficiencies in vitro. Results from Haemophilia A patients indicate the OHP may even be a better predictor of clinical phenotype than APTT levels or FVIII assays [145], and in patients with inhibitors, the OHP may be used to monitor the fibrin generation response to recombinant FVIIa treatment [143]. Studies evaluating the OHP's ability to monitor FVIII dosing are ongoing [145].

Summary

Fibrin generation and lysis assays show sensitivity to both hypo- and hyperfibrinolytic states, unlike the thromboelastography. Although they have not entered clinical practice currently, they show great promise in identifying global changes in coagulation and fibrinolytic tendency. In this regard, the OHP has an advantage over the CLT because both aspects of haemostasis are derived. Clearly, further study is required, but the OHP and related assays have the potential to better characterise global coagulation responses than conventional assays, possibly leading to individualised treatment for patients with thrombotic and bleeding conditions.

5. Conclusions

Currently, fibrinolysis is rarely measured in clinical practice. This has been mainly due to the failure of assays of the specific factors to show consistent relationships with disease. In part, this failure has been related to methodological flaws in the assays, for example in the variable specificities of the antibodies used to detect TAFI or PAI-1. However, the principle problem is that the validity of one-off sampling of individual factors as a representation of the complex fibrinolytic pathway is questionable, especially when the sampling has occurred at a time distant to the pathological event being investigated.

D-dimer assays have been one notable success in clinical practice where they have established applications in the diagnosis of VTE and DIC. However, as a non-specific marker of thrombosis and fibrinolysis, they provide little information of the fibrinolytic potential of an individual. Global assays have the ability to improve clinical fibrinolytic testing in this regard. Thromboelastography is increasingly establishing itself as a tool to detect hyperfibrinolysis, particular in point-of-care settings such as cardiothoracic and liver transplant surgery. Fibrin generation and lysis assays such as the CLT and OHP have the disadvantage of requiring platelet poor plasma, but in contrast to thromboelastography, appear to be sensitive to both hyper- and hypofibrinolysis. Results in studies of arterial and venous thrombosis have been encouraging, but further research needs to be undertaken to find out whether the data has clinical applications, for example in predicting an individual patient's risk of recurrent thrombosis. In the meantime, the development of new whole blood tests is ongoing [156, 157], with the hope of achieving a better simulation of in-vivo fibrinolytic conditions.

Author details

Dominic Pepperell, Marie-Christine Morel-Kopp and Chris Ward*

*Address all correspondence to: cward@med.usyd.edu.au

Northern Blood Research Centre, Kolling Institute of Medical Research, The University of Sydney and Department of Haematology and Transfusion Medicine, Royal North Shore Hospital, Sydney, NSW, Australia

References

[1] Prins MH, Hirsh J. A critical review of the evidence supporting a relationship between impaired fibrinolytic activity and venous thromboembolism. Arch Intern Med. 1991 Sep;151(9):1721-31.

[2] Meltzer ME, Doggen CJ, de Groot PG, Rosendaal FR, Lisman T. The impact of the fibrinolytic system on the risk of venous and arterial thrombosis. Semin Thromb Hemost. 2009 Jul;35(5):468-77.

[3] Spencer FA, Emery C, Joffe SW, Pacifico L, Lessard D, Reed G, et al. Incidence rates, clinical profile, and outcomes of patients with venous thromboembolism. The Worcester VTE study. J Thromb Thrombolysis. 2009 Nov;28(4):401-9.

[4] Prandoni P, Noventa F, Ghirarduzzi A, Pengo V, Bernardi E, Pesavento R, et al. The risk of recurrent venous thromboembolism after discontinuing anticoagulation in patients with acute proximal deep vein thrombosis or pulmonary embolism. A prospective cohort study in 1,626 patients. Haematologica. 2007 Feb;92(2):199-205.

[5] Baglin T, Luddington R, Brown K, Baglin C. Incidence of recurrent venous thromboembolism in relation to clinical and thrombophilic risk factors: prospective cohort study. Lancet. 2003 Aug 16;362(9383):523-6.

[6] Hansson PO, Sorbo J, Eriksson H. Recurrent venous thromboembolism after deep vein thrombosis: incidence and risk factors. Arch Intern Med. 2000 Mar 27;160(6): 769-74.

[7] Gorog DA. Prognostic value of plasma fibrinolysis activation markers in cardiovascular disease. J Am Coll Cardiol. 2010 Jun 15;55(24):2701-9.

[8] Luddington RJ. Thrombelastography/thromboelastometry. Clin Lab Haematol. 2005 Apr;27(2):81-90.

[9] Ganter MT, Hofer CK. Coagulation monitoring: current techniques and clinical use of viscoelastic point-of-care coagulation devices. Anesth Analg. 2008 May;106(5): 1366-75.

[10] MacIvor D, Rebel A, Hassan ZU. How do we integrate thromboelastography with perioperative transfusion management? Transfusion. 2013 Jul;53(7):1386-92.

[11] Shakur H, Roberts I, Bautista R, Caballero J, Coats T, et al. Effects of tranexamic acid on death, vascular occlusive events, and blood transfusion in trauma patients with significant haemorrhage (CRASH-2): a randomised, placebo-controlled trial. Lancet. 2010 Jul 3;376(9734):23-32.

[12] Taylor FB, Jr., Toh CH, Hoots WK, Wada H, Levi M, Scientific Subcommittee on Disseminated Intravascular Coagulation of the International Society on T, et al. Towards

definition, clinical and laboratory criteria, and a scoring system for disseminated intravascular coagulation. Thromb Haemost. 2001 Nov;86(5):1327-30.

[13] Rijken DC, Lijnen HR. New insights into the molecular mechanisms of the fibrinolytic system. J Thromb Haemost. 2009 Jan;7(1):4-13.

[14] Bachmann F. Plasminogen-Plasmin Enzyme Systems. In: Colman R, Hirsh J, Marder V, Clowes A, George J, editors. Haemostasis and Thrombosis, Basic Principles and Clinical Practice. Fourth ed. Philadelphia, PA: Lippincott, Williams and Wilkins; 2001.

[15] Brandt JT. Plasminogen and tissue-type plasminogen activator deficiency as risk factors for thromboembolic disease. Arch Pathol Lab Med. 2002 Nov;126(11):1376-81.

[16] Tefs K, Gueorguieva M, Klammt J, Allen CM, Aktas D, Anlar FY, et al. Molecular and clinical spectrum of type I plasminogen deficiency: A series of 50 patients. Blood. 2006 Nov 1;108(9):3021-6.

[17] Ostrowski SR, Sorensen AM, Larsen CF, Johansson PI. Thrombelastography and biomarker profiles in acute coagulopathy of trauma: a prospective study. Scand J Trauma Resusc Emerg Med. 2011;19:64.

[18] Folsom AR, Cushman M, Heckbert SR, Rosamond WD, Aleksic N. Prospective study of fibrinolytic markers and venous thromboembolism. J Clin Epidemiol. 2003 Jun; 56(6):598-603.

[19] Clason SB, Meijer P, Kluft C, Ersdal E. Specific determination of plasmin inhibitor activity in plasma: documentation of specificity of manual and automated procedures. Blood Coagul Fibrinolysis. 1999 Dec;10(8):487-94

[20] Wiman B. The fibrinolytic enzyme system. Basic principles and links to venous and arterial thrombosis. Hematol Oncol Clin North Am. 2000 Apr;14(2):325-38, vii.

[21] Heylen E, Willemse J, Hendriks D. An update on the role of carboxypeptidase U (TAFIa) in fibrinolysis. Front Biosci (Landmark Ed). 2011;16:2427-50.

[22] Tait RC, Walker ID, Conkie JA, Islam SIAM, McCall F. Isolated familial plasminogen deficiency may not be a risk factor for thrombosis. Thrombosis and Haemostasis. 1996 December;76(6):1004-8.

[23] Okamoto A, Sakata T, Mannami T, Baba S, Katayama Y, Matsuo H, et al. Population-based distribution of plasminogen activity and estimated prevalence and relevance to thrombotic diseases of plasminogen deficiency in the Japanese: the Suita Study. J Thromb Haemost. 2003 Nov;1(11):2397-403.

[24] Bugge TH, Flick MJ, Daugherty CC, Degen JL. Plasminogen deficiency causes severe thrombosis but is compatible with development and reproduction. Genes and Development. 1995 01 Apr;9(7):794-807.

[25] Bugge TH, Kombrinck KW, Flick MJ, Daugherty CC, Danton MJS, Degen JL. Loss of fibrinogen rescues mice from the pleiotropic effects of plasminogen deficiency. Cell. 1996 15 Jan;87(4):709-19.

[26] Zeng B, Bruce D, Kril J, Ploplis V, Freedman B, Brieger D. Influence of plasminogen deficiency on the contribution of polymorphonuclear leucocytes to fibrin/ogenolysis: studies in plasminogen knock-out mice. Thrombosis and Haemostasis. 2002 Nov; 88(5):805-10.

[27] Meltzer ME, Lisman T, de Groot PG, Meijers JC, le Cessie S, Doggen CJ, et al. Venous thrombosis risk associated with plasma hypofibrinolysis is explained by elevated plasma levels of TAFI and PAI-1. Blood. 2010 Jul 8;116(1):113-21.

[28] Hoekstra J, Guimaraes AH, Leebeek FW, Darwish Murad S, Malfliet JJ, Plessier A, et al. Impaired fibrinolysis as a risk factor for Budd-Chiari syndrome. Blood. 2010 Jan 14;115(2):388-95.

[29] Juhan-Vague I, Pyke SD, Alessi MC, Jespersen J, Haverkate F, Thompson SG. Fibrinolytic factors and the risk of myocardial infarction or sudden death in patients with angina pectoris. ECAT Study Group. European Concerted Action on Thrombosis and Disabilities. Circulation. 1996 Nov 1;94(9):2057-63.

[30] Folsom AR, Aleksic N, Park E, Salomaa V, Juneja H, Wu KK. Prospective study of fibrinolytic factors and incident coronary heart disease: the Atherosclerosis Risk in Communities (ARIC) Study. Arterioscler Thromb Vasc Biol. 2001 Apr;21(4):611-7.

[31] Meltzer ME, Doggen CJ, de Groot PG, Rosendaal FR, Lisman T. Plasma levels of fibrinolytic proteins and the risk of myocardial infarction in men. Blood. 2010 Jul 29;116(4):529-36.

[32] Lijnen HR. Plasmin and matrix metalloproteinases in vascular remodeling. Thromb Haemost. 2001 Jul;86(1):324-33.

[33] Davenport R. Pathogenesis of acute traumatic coagulopathy. Transfusion. 2013 Jan;53 Suppl 1:23S-7S.

[34] Favaloro EJ. Laboratory testing in disseminated intravascular coagulation. Semin Thromb Hemost. 2010 Jun;36(4):458-67.

[35] Breen KA, Grimwade D, Hunt BJ. The pathogenesis and management of the coagulopathy of acute promyelocytic leukaemia. Br J Haematol. 2012 Jan;156(1):24-36.

[36] Carpenter SL, Mathew P. Alpha2-antiplasmin and its deficiency: fibrinolysis out of balance. Haemophilia. 2008 Nov;14(6):1250-4.

[37] Torr-Brown SR, Sobel BE. Attenuation of thrombolysis by release of plasminogen activator inhibitor type-1 from platelets. Thromb Res. 1993 Dec 1;72(5):413-21.

[38] Declerck PJ, Collen D. Measurement of plasminogen activator inhibitor 1 (PAI-1) in plasma with various monoclonal antibody-based enzyme-linked immunosorbent assays. Thromb Res Suppl. 1990;10:3-9.

[39] MacCallum PK, Cooper JA, Howarth DJ, Meade TW, Miller GJ. Sex differences in the determinants of fibrinolytic activity. Thromb Haemost. 1998 Mar;79(3):587-90.

[40] van der Bom JG, de Knijff P, Haverkate F, Bots ML, Meijer P, de Jong PT, et al. Tissue plasminogen activator and risk of myocardial infarction. The Rotterdam Study. Circulation. 1997 Jun 17;95(12):2623-7.

[41] Katsaros KM, Kastl SP, Huber K, Zorn G, Maurer G, Glogar D, et al. Clopidogrel pretreatment abolishes increase of PAI-1 after coronary stent implantation. Thromb Res. 2008;123(1):79-84.

[42] Simpson AJ, Booth NA, Moore NR, Bennett B. The platelet and plasma pools of plasminogen activator inhibitor (PAI-1) vary independently in disease. Br J Haematol. 1990 Aug;75(4):543-8.

[43] Grimaudo V, Hauert J, Bachmann F, Kruithof EK. Diurnal variation of the fibrinolytic system. Thromb Haemost. 1988 Jun 16;59(3):495-9.

[44] Smith A, Patterson C, Yarnell J, Rumley A, Ben-Shlomo Y, Lowe G. Which hemostatic markers add to the predictive value of conventional risk factors for coronary heart disease and ischemic stroke? The Caerphilly Study. Circulation. 2005 Nov 15;112(20):3080-7.

[45] Kinlay S, Schwartz GG, Olsson AG, Rifai N, Bao W, Libby P, et al. Endogenous tissue plasminogen activator and risk of recurrent cardiac events after an acute coronary syndrome in the MIRACL study. Atherosclerosis. 2009 Oct;206(2):551-5.

[46] Wang TJ, Gona P, Larson MG, Tofler GH, Levy D, Newton-Cheh C, et al. Multiple biomarkers for the prediction of first major cardiovascular events and death. N Engl J Med. 2006 Dec 21;355(25):2631-9.

[47] Cushman M, Lemaitre RN, Kuller LH, Psaty BM, Macy EM, Sharrett AR, et al. Fibrinolytic activation markers predict myocardial infarction in the elderly. The Cardiovascular Health Study. Arterioscler Thromb Vasc Biol. 1999 Mar;19(3):493-8.

[48] Itakura H, Sobel BE, Boothroyd D, Leung LL, Iribarren C, Go AS, et al. Do plasma biomarkers of coagulation and fibrinolysis differ between patients who have experienced an acute myocardial infarction versus stable exertional angina? Am Heart J. 2007 Dec;154(6):1059-64.

[49] Cortellaro M, Cofrancesco E, Boschetti C, Mussoni L, Donati MB, Cardillo M, et al. Increased fibrin turnover and high PAI-1 activity as predictors of ischemic events in atherosclerotic patients. A case-control study. The PLAT Group. Arterioscler Thromb. 1993 Oct;13(10):1412-7.

[50] Raiko JR, Oikonen M, Wendelin-Saarenhovi M, Siitonen N, Kahonen M, Lehtimaki T, et al. Plasminogen activator inhitor-1 associates with cardiovascular risk factors in healthy young adults in the Cardiovascular Risk in Young Finns Study. Atherosclerosis. 2012 Sep;224(1):208-12.

[51] Crowther MA, Roberts J, Roberts R, Johnston M, Stevens P, Skingley P, et al. Fibrinolytic Variables in Patients with Recurrent Venous Thrombosis: a Prospective Cohort Study. Thromb Haemost. 2001;85:390-4.

[52] Ridker PM, Vaughan DE, Stampfer MJ, Manson JE, Shen C, Newcomer LM, et al. Baseline fibrinolytic state and the risk of future venous thrombosis. A prospective study of endogenous tissue-type plasminogen activator and plasminogen activator inhibitor. Circulation. 1992 May;85(5):1822-7.

[53] Hack CE. Fibrinolysis in disseminated intravascular coagulation. Semin Thromb Hemost. 2001 Dec;27(6):633-8.

[54] Ferguson JW, Helmy A, Ludlam C, Webb DJ, Hayes PC, Newby DC. Hyperfibrinolysis in alcoholic cirrhosis: relative plasminogen activator inhibitor type 1 deficiency. Thromb Res. 2008;121(5):675-80.

[55] van Tilburg NH, Rosendaal FR, Bertina RM. Thrombin activatable fibrinolysis inhibitor and the risk for deep vein thrombosis. Blood. 2000 May 1;95(9):2855-9.

[56] Verdu J, Marco P, Benlloch S, Sanchez J, Lucas J. Thrombin activatable fibrinolysis inhibitor (TAFI) polymorphisms and plasma TAFI levels measured with an ELISA insensitive to isoforms in patients with venous thromboembolic disease (VTD). Thromb Haemost. 2006 Mar;95(3):585-6.

[57] Eichinger S, Schonauer V, Weltermann A, Minar E, Bialonczyk C, Hirschl M, et al. Thrombin-activatable fibrinolysis inhibitor and the risk for recurrent venous thromboembolism. Blood. 2004 May 15;103(10):3773-6.

[58] Meltzer ME, Bol L, Rosendaal FR, Lisman T, Cannegieter SC. Hypofibrinolysis as a risk factor for recurrent venous thrombosis; results of the LETS follow-up study. J Thromb Haemost. 2010 Mar;8(3):605-7.

[59] Zorio E, Castello R, Falco C, Espana F, Osa A, Almenar L, et al. Thrombin-activatable fibrinolysis inhibitor in young patients with myocardial infarction and its relationship with the fibrinolytic function and the protein C system. Br J Haematol. 2003 Sep; 122(6):958-65.

[60] Tregouet DA, Schnabel R, Alessi MC, Godefroy T, Declerck PJ, Nicaud V, et al. Activated thrombin activatable fibrinolysis inhibitor levels are associated with the risk of cardiovascular death in patients with coronary artery disease: the AtheroGene study. J Thromb Haemost. 2009 Jan;7(1):49-57.

[61] Folkeringa N, Coppens M, Veeger NJ, Bom VJ, Middeldorp S, Hamulyak K, et al. Absolute risk of venous and arterial thromboembolism in thrombophilic families is not

increased by high thrombin-activatable fibrinolysis inhibitor (TAFI) levels. Thromb Haemost. 2008 Jul;100(1):38-44.

[62] Morange PE, Tregouet DA, Frere C, Luc G, Arveiler D, Ferrieres J, et al. TAFI gene haplotypes, TAFI plasma levels and future risk of coronary heart disease: the PRIME Study. J Thromb Haemost. 2005 Jul;3(7):1503-10

[63] de Bruijne EL, Gils A, Guimaraes AH, Dippel DW, Deckers JW, van den Meiracker AH, et al. The role of thrombin activatable fibrinolysis inhibitor in arterial thrombosis at a young age: the ATTAC study. J Thromb Haemost. 2009 Jun;7(6):919-27.

[64] Meltzer ME, Doggen CJ, de Groot PG, Meijers JC, Rosendaal FR, Lisman T. Low thrombin activatable fibrinolysis inhibitor activity levels are associated with an increased risk of a first myocardial infarction in men. Haematologica. 2009 Jun;94(6): 811-8.

[65] Foley JH, Nesheim ME, Rivard GE, Brummel-Ziedins KE. Thrombin activatable fibrinolysis inhibitor activation and bleeding in haemophilia A. Haemophilia. 2012 May; 18(3):e316-22.

[66] Emerging Risk Factors C, Erqou S, Kaptoge S, Perry PL, Di Angelantonio E, Thompson A, et al. Lipoprotein(a) concentration and the risk of coronary heart disease, stroke, and nonvascular mortality. Jama. 2009 Jul 22;302(4):412-23.

[67] Cesarman-Maus G, Rios-Luna NP, Deora AB, Huang B, Villa R, Cravioto Mdel C, et al. Autoantibodies against the fibrinolytic receptor, annexin 2, in antiphospholipid syndrome. Blood. 2006 Jun 1;107(11):4375-82.

[68] Cesarman-Maus G, Cantu-Brito C, Barinagarrementeria F, Villa R, Reyes E, Sanchez-Guerrero J, et al. Autoantibodies against the fibrinolytic receptor, annexin A2, in cerebral venous thrombosis. Stroke. 2011 Feb;42(2):501-3.

[69] Bates SM. D-dimer assays in diagnosis and management of thrombotic and bleeding disorders. Semin Thromb Hemost. 2012 Oct;38(7):673-82.

[70] Dempfle CE. Validation, calibration, and specificity of quantitative D-dimer assays. Semin. 2005 Nov;5(4):315-20.

[71] Couturaud F, Kearon C, Bates SM, Ginsberg JS. Decrease in sensitivity of D-dimer for acute venous thromboembolism after starting anticoagulant therapy. Blood Coagul Fibrinolysis. 2002 Apr;13(3):241-6.

[72] Di Nisio M, Squizzato A, Rutjes AW, Buller HR, Zwinderman AH, Bossuyt PM. Diagnostic accuracy of D-dimer test for exclusion of venous thromboembolism: a systematic review. J Thromb Haemost. 2007 Feb;5(2):296-304.

[73] Bates SM, Jaeschke R, Stevens SM, Goodacre S, Wells PS, Stevenson MD, et al. Diagnosis of DVT: Antithrombotic Therapy and Prevention of Thrombosis, 9th ed: Ameri-

can College of Chest Physicians Evidence-Based Clinical Practice Guidelines. Chest. 2012 Feb;141(2 Suppl):e351S-418S.

[74] Schouten HJ, Geersing GJ, Koek HL, Zuithoff NP, Janssen KJ, Douma RA, et al. Diagnostic accuracy of conventional or age adjusted D-dimer cut-off values in older patients with suspected venous thromboembolism: systematic review and meta-analysis. Br Med J. 2013;346:f2492.

[75] Heit JA. Predicting the risk of venous thromboembolism recurrence. Am J Hematol. 2012 May;87 Suppl 1:S63-7.

[76] Palareti G, Cosmi B, Legnani C, Tosetto A, Brusi C, Iorio A, et al. D-dimer testing to determine the duration of anticoagulation therapy.[Erratum appears in N Engl J Med. 2006 Dec 28;355(26):2797], [Reprint in J Vasc Nurs. 2007 Jun;25(2):39; PMID: 17531938]. N Engl J Med. 2006 Oct 26;355(17):1780-9.

[77] De Souza RL, Short T, Warman GR, Maclennan N, Young Y. Anaphylaxis with associated fibrinolysis, reversed with tranexamic acid and demonstrated by thrombelastography. Anaesth Intensive Care. 2004 Aug;32(4):580-7.

[78] Levrat A, Gros A, Rugeri L, Inaba K, Floccard B, Negrier C, et al. Evaluation of rotation thrombelastography for the diagnosis of hyperfibrinolysis in trauma patients. Br J Anaesth. 2008 Jun;100(6):792-7.

[79] Spiel AO, Mayr FB, Firbas C, Quehenberger P, Jilma B. Validation of rotation thrombelastography in a model of systemic activation of fibrinolysis and coagulation in humans. J Thromb Haemost. 2006 Feb;4(2):411-6.

[80] Nielsen VG. A comparison of the Thrombelastograph and the ROTEM. Blood Coagul Fibrinolysis. 2007 Apr;18(3):247-52.

[81] Zambruni A, Thalheimer U, Leandro G, Perry D, Burroughs AK. Thromboelastography with citrated blood: comparability with native blood, stability of citrate storage and effect of repeated sampling. Blood Coagul Fibrinolysis. 2004 Jan;15(1):103-7.

[82] Kitchen DP, Kitchen S, Jennings I, Woods T, Walker I. Quality assurance and quality control of thrombelastography and rotational Thromboelastometry: the UK NEQAS for blood coagulation experience. Semin Thromb Hemost. 2010 Oct;36(7):757-63.

[83] Chitlur M, Sorensen B, Rivard GE, Young G, Ingerslev J, Othman M, et al. Standardization of thromboelastography: a report from the TEG-ROTEM working group. Haemophilia. 2011 May;17(3):532-7.

[84] Lang T, Bauters A, Braun SL, Potzsch B, von Pape KW, Kolde HJ, et al. Multi-centre investigation on reference ranges for ROTEM thromboelastometry. Blood Coagul Fibrinolysis. 2005 Jun;16(4):301-10.

[85] Brenni M, Worn M, Bruesch M, Spahn DR, Ganter MT. Successful rotational thromboelastometry-guided treatment of traumatic haemorrhage, hyperfibrinolysis and coagulopathy. Acta Anaesthesiol Scand. 2010 Jan;54(1):111-7.

[86] Ghosh K, Shetty S, Kulkarni B. Correlation of thromboelastographic patterns with clinical presentation and rationale for use of antifibrinolytics in severe haemophilia patients. Haemophilia. 2007 Nov;13(6):734-9.

[87] Dirkmann D, Radu-Berlemann J, Gorlinger K, Peters J. Recombinant tissue-type plasminogen activator-evoked hyperfibrinolysis is enhanced by acidosis and inhibited by hypothermia but still can be blocked by tranexamic acid. J Trauma Acute Care Surg. 2013 Feb;74(2):482-8.

[88] Kashuk JL, Moore EE, Sawyer M, Wohlauer M, Pezold M, Barnett C, et al. Primary fibrinolysis is integral in the pathogenesis of the acute coagulopathy of trauma. Ann Surg. 2010 Sep;252(3):434-42; discussion 43-4.

[89] Genet GF, Ostrowski SR, Sorensen AM, Johansson PI. Detection of tPA-induced hyperfibrinolysis in whole blood by RapidTEG, KaolinTEG, and functional fibrinogen-TEG in healthy individuals. Clin Appl Thromb Hemost. 2012 Nov;18(6):638-44.

[90] Kang YG, Martin DJ, Marquez J, Lewis JH, Bontempo FA, Shaw BW, Jr., et al. Intraoperative changes in blood coagulation and thrombelastographic monitoring in liver transplantation. Anesth Analg. 1985 Sep;64(9):888-96.

[91] Porte RJ, Bontempo FA, Knot EA, Lewis JH, Kang YG, Starzl TE. Systemic effects of tissue plasminogen activator-associated fibrinolysis and its relation to thrombin generation in orthotopic liver transplantation. Transplantation. 1989 Jun;47(6):978-84.

[92] Steib A, Gengenwin N, Freys G, Boudjema K, Levy S, Otteni JC. Predictive factors of hyperfibrinolytic activity during liver transplantation in cirrhotic patients. Br J Anaesth. 1994 Nov;73(5):645-8.

[93] Coakley M, Reddy K, Mackie I, Mallett S. Transfusion triggers in orthotopic liver transplantation: a comparison of the thromboelastometry analyzer, the thromboelastogram, and conventional coagulation tests. J Cardiothorac Vasc Anesth. 2006 Aug; 20(4):548-53.

[94] Trzebicki J, Flakiewicz E, Kosieradzki M, Blaszczyk B, Kolacz M, Jureczko L, et al. The use of thromboelastometry in the assessment of hemostasis during orthotopic liver transplantation reduces the demand for blood products. Ann Transplant. 2010 Jul-Sep;15(3):19-24.

[95] Wang SC, Shieh JF, Chang KY, Chu YC, Liu CS, Loong CC, et al. Thromboelastography-Guided Transfusion Decreases Intraoperative Blood Transfusion During Orthotopic Liver Transplantation: Randomized Clinical Trial. Transplantation proceedings. 2010;42(7):2590-3.

[96] Spiess BD, Gillies BSA, Chandler W, Verrier E. Changes in transfusion therapy and reexploration rate after institution of a blood management program in cardiac surgical patients. Journal of Cardiothoracic and Vascular Anesthesia. 1995;9(2):168-73.

[97] Shore-Lesserson L, Manspeizer HE, DePerio M, Francis S, Vela-Cantos F, Ergin MA. Thromboelastography-guided transfusion algorithm reduces transfusions in complex cardiac surgery. Anesthesia and Analgesia. 1999 February;88(2):312-9.

[98] Royston D, von Kier S. Reduced haemostatic factor transfusion using heparinase-modified thromboelastography during cardiopulmonary bypass. Br J Anaesth. 2001;86(4):575-8.

[99] Anderson L, Quasim I, Soutar R, Steven M, Macfie A, Korte W. An audit of red cell and blood product use after the institution of thromboelastometry in a cardiac intensive care unit. Transfusion Medicine. 2006 February;16(1):31-9.

[100] Avidan MS, Alcock EL, Da Fonseca J, Ponte J, Desai JB, Despotis GJ, et al. Comparison of structured use of routine laboratory tests or near-patient asessment with clinical judgement in the management of bleeding after cardiac surgery. Br J Anaesth. 2004 February;92(2):178-86.

[101] Spalding GJ, Hartrumpf M, Sierig T, Oesberg N, Kirschke CG, Albes JM. Cost reduction of perioperative coagulation management in cardiac surgery: value of 'bedside' thromboelastography (ROTEM). European Journal of Cardio-thoracic Surgery. 2007 June;31(6):1052-7.

[102] Ferraris VA, Ferraris SP, Saha SP, Hessel IEA, Haan CK, Royston BD, et al. Perioperative Blood Transfusion and Blood Conservation in Cardiac Surgery: The Society of Thoracic Surgeons and The Society of Cardiovascular Anesthesiologists Clinical Practice Guideline. Annals of Thoracic Surgery. 2007 May;83(5 SUPPL.):S27-S86.

[103] Dunning J, Versteegh M, Fabbri A, Pavie A, Kolh P, Lockowandt U, et al. Guideline on antiplatelet and anticoagulation management in cardiac surgery. European Journal of Cardio-thoracic Surgery. 2008 July;34(1):73-92.

[104] Ives C, Inaba K, Branco BC, Okoye O, Schochl H, Talving P, et al. Hyperfibrinolysis elicited via thromboelastography predicts mortality in trauma. J Am Coll Surg. 2012 Oct;215(4):496-502.

[105] Theusinger OM, Wanner GA, Emmert MY, Billeter A, Eismon J, Seifert B, et al. Hyperfibrinolysis diagnosed by rotational thromboelastometry (ROTEM) is associated with higher mortality in patients with severe trauma. Anesth Analg. 2011 Nov;113(5): 1003-12.

[106] Hvas AM, Sorensen HT, Norengaard L, Christiansen K, Ingerslev J, Sorensen B. Tranexamic acid combined with recombinant factor VIII increases clot resistance to accelerated fibrinolysis in severe hemophilia A. J Thromb Haemost. 2007 Dec;5(12): 2408-14.

[107] Sorensen B, Ingerslev J. Whole blood clot formation phenotypes in hemophilia A and rare coagulation disorders. Patterns of response to recombinant factor VIIa. J Thromb Haemost. 2004 Jan;2(1):102-10.

[108] Kupesiz A, Rajpurkar M, Warrier I, Hollon W, Tosun O, Lusher J, et al. Tissue plasminogen activator induced fibrinolysis: standardization of method using thromboelastography. Blood Coagul Fibrinolysis. 2010 Jun;21(4):320-4.

[109] Kupesiz OA, Chitlur MB, Hollon W, Tosun O, Thomas R, Warrier I, et al. Fibrinolytic parameters in children with noncatheter thrombosis: a pilot study. Blood Coagul Fibrinolysis. 2010 Jun;21(4):313-9.

[110] O'Donnell J, Riddell A, Owens D, Handa A, Pasi J, Hamilton G, et al. Role of the Thrombelastograph as an adjunctive test in thrombophilia screening. Blood Coagul Fibrinolysis. 2004 Apr;15(3):207-11.

[111] Karlsson O, Sporrong T, Hillarp A, Jeppsson A, Hellgren M. Prospective longitudinal study of thromboelastography and standard hemostatic laboratory tests in healthy women during normal pregnancy. Anesth Analg. 2012 Oct;115(4):890-8.

[112] Hill JS, Devenie G, Powell M. Point-of-care testing of coagulation and fibrinolytic status during postpartum haemorrhage: developing a thrombelastography-guided transfusion algorithm. Anaesth Intensive Care. 2012 Nov;40(6):1007-15.

[113] Othman M, Falcon BJ, Kadir R. Global hemostasis in pregnancy: are we using thromboelastography to its full potential? Semin Thromb Hemost. 2010 Oct;36(7):738-46.

[114] Taylor FB, Jr., Lockhart MS. Whole blood clot lysis: in vitro modulation by activated protein C. Thromb Res. 1985 Mar 15;37(6):639-49.

[115] Comp PC, Jacocks RM, Rubenstein C, Radcliffe R. A lysine-absorbable plasminogen activator is elevated in conditions associated with increased fibrinolytic activity. J Lab Clin Med. 1981 May;97(5):637-45.

[116] Hersch SL, Kunelis T, Francis RB, Jr. The pathogenesis of accelerated fibrinolysis in liver cirrhosis: a critical role for tissue plasminogen activator inhibitor. Blood. 1987 May;69(5):1315-9.

[117] Lisman T, de Groot PG, Meijers JC, Rosendaal FR. Reduced plasma fibrinolytic potential is a risk factor for venous thrombosis. Blood. 2005 Feb 1;105(3):1102-5.

[118] Talens S, Malfliet JJ, Rudez G, Spronk HM, Janssen NA, Meijer P, et al. Biological variation in tPA-induced plasma clot lysis time. Thromb Haemost. 2012 Oct;108(4): 640-6.

[119] Undas A, Zawilska K, Ciesla-Dul M, Lehmann-Kopydlowska A, Skubiszak A, Ciepluch K, et al. Altered fibrin clot structure/function in patients with idiopathic venous thromboembolism and in their relatives. Blood. 2009 Nov 5;114(19):4272-8.

[120] Meltzer ME, Lisman T, Doggen CJ, de Groot PG, Rosendaal FR. Synergistic effects of hypofibrinolysis and genetic and acquired risk factors on the risk of a first venous thrombosis. PLoS Med. 2008 May 6;5(5):e97.

[121] Krzek M, Ciesla-Dul M, Zabczyk M, Undas A. Fibrin clot properties in women heterozygous for factor V Leiden mutation: effects of oral contraceptives. Thromb Res. 2012 Oct;130(4):e216-21.

[122] Meijers JC, Middeldorp S, Tekelenburg W, van den Ende AE, Tans G, Prins MH, et al. Increased fibrinolytic activity during use of oral contraceptives is counteracted by an enhanced factor XI-independent down regulation of fibrinolysis: a randomized cross-over study of two low-dose oral contraceptives. Thromb Haemost. 2000 Jul; 84(1):9-14.

[123] Guimaraes AH, de Bruijne EL, Lisman T, Dippel DW, Deckers JW, Poldermans D, et al. Hypofibrinolysis is a risk factor for arterial thrombosis at young age. Br J Haematol. 2009 Apr;145(1):115-20.

[124] Traby L, Kollars M, Eischer L, Eichinger S, Kyrle PA. Prediction of recurrent venous thromboembolism by clot lysis time: a prospective cohort study. PLoS ONE. 2012;7(12):e51447.

[125] Cellai AP, Lami D, Fedi S, Marcucci R, Mannini L, Cenci C, et al. A hypercoagulable and hypofibrinolytic state is detectable by global methods in patients with retinal vein occlusion. Atherosclerosis. 2012 Sep;224(1):97-101.

[126] Martinez-Zamora MA, Tassies D, Carmona F, Espinosa G, Cervera R, Reverter JC, et al. Clot lysis time and thrombin activatable fibrinolysis inhibitor in severe preeclampsia with or without associated antiphospholipid antibodies. J Reprod Immunol. 2010 Nov;86(2):133-40.

[127] Meltzer ME, Doggen CJ, de Groot PG, Rosendaal FR, Lisman T. Reduced plasma fibrinolytic capacity as a potential risk factor for a first myocardial infarction in young men. Br J Haematol. 2009 Apr;145(1):121-7.

[128] Siegerink B, Meltzer ME, de Groot PG, Algra A, Lisman T, Rosendaal FR. Clot lysis time and the risk of myocardial infarction and ischaemic stroke in young women; results from the RATIO case-control study. Br J Haematol. 2012 Jan;156(2):252-8.

[129] Lisman T, Adelmeijer J, Nieuwenhuis HK, de Groot PG. Enhancement of fibrinolytic potential in vitro by anticoagulant drugs targeting activated factor X, but not by those inhibiting thrombin or tissue factor. Blood Coagul Fibrinolysis. 2003 Sep;14(6): 557-62.

[130] Schutgens RE, Esseboom EU, Snijder RJ, Haas FJ, Verzijlbergen F, Nieuwenhuis HK, et al. Low molecular weight heparin (dalteparin) is equally effective as unfractionated heparin in reducing coagulation activity and perfusion abnormalities during the early treatment of pulmonary embolism. J Lab Clin Med. 2004 Aug;144(2):100-7.

[131] Lisman T, Bijsterveld NR, Adelmeijer J, Meijers JC, Levi M, Nieuwenhuis HK, et al. Recombinant factor VIIa reverses the in vitro and ex vivo anticoagulant and profibrinolytic effects of fondaparinux. J Thromb Haemost. 2003 Nov;1(11):2368-73.

[132] Mosnier LO, Lisman T, van den Berg HM, Nieuwenhuis HK, Meijers JC, Bouma BN. The defective down regulation of fibrinolysis in haemophilia A can be restored by increasing the TAFI plasma concentration. Thromb Haemost. 2001 Oct;86(4):1035-9.

[133] Lisman T, Mosnier LO, Lambert T, Mauser-Bunschoten EP, Meijers JC, Nieuwenhuis HK, et al. Inhibition of fibrinolysis by recombinant factor VIIa in plasma from patients with severe hemophilia A. Blood. 2002 Jan 1;99(1):175-9.

[134] Rijken DC, Kock EL, Guimaraes AH, Talens S, Darwish Murad S, Janssen HL, et al. Evidence for an enhanced fibrinolytic capacity in cirrhosis as measured with two different global fibrinolysis tests. J Thromb Haemost. 2012 Oct;10(10):2116-22.

[135] He S, Bremme K, Blomback M. A laboratory method for determination of overall haemostatic potential in plasma. I. Method design and preliminary results. Thromb Res. 1999 Oct 15;96(2):145-56.

[136] He S, Antovic A, Blomback M. A simple and rapid laboratory method for determination of haemostasis potential in plasma. II. Modifications for use in routine laboratories and research work. Thromb Res. 2001 Sep 1;103(5):355-61.

[137] He S, Zhu K, Skeppholm M, Vedin J, Svensson J, Egberg N, et al. A global assay of haemostasis which uses recombinant tissue factor and tissue-type plasminogen activator to measure the rate of fibrin formation and fibrin degradation in plasma. Thromb Haemost. 2007 Oct;98(4):871-82.

[138] Curnow JL, Morel-Kopp MC, Roddie C, Aboud M, Ward CM. Reduced fibrinolysis and increased fibrin generation can be detected in hypercoagulable patients using the overall hemostatic potential assay. J Thromb Haemost. 2007 Mar;5(3):528-34.

[139] Goldenberg NA, Hathaway WE, Jacobson L, Manco-Johnson MJ. A new global assay of coagulation and fibrinolysis.[Erratum appears in Thromb Res. 2006;118(6):771]. Thromb Res. 2005;116(4):345-56.

[140] Andresen MS, Abildgaard U. Coagulation Inhibitor Potential: a study of assay variables. Thromb Res. 2005;115(6):519-26.

[141] Andresen MS, Iversen N, Abildgaard U. Overall haemostasis potential assays performed in thrombophilic plasma: the effect of preactivating protein C and antithrombin. Thromb Res. 2002 Dec 15;108(5-6):323-8.

[142] Antovic A, Blomback M, Sten-Linder M, Petrini P, Holmstrom M, He S. Identifying hypocoagulable states with a modified global assay of overall haemostasis potential in plasma. Blood Coagul Fibrinolysis. 2005 Nov;16(8):585-96.

[143] Antovic JP, Antovic A, He S, Tengborn L, Blomback M. Overall haemostatic potential can be used for estimation of thrombin-activatable fibrinolysis inhibitor-dependent

fibrinolysis in vivo and for possible follow-up of recombinant factor VIIa treatment in patients with inhibitors to factor VIII. Haemophilia. 2002 Nov;8(6):781-6.

[144] Andresen MS, Abildgaard U, Liestol S, Sandset PM, Mowinckel MC, Odegaard OR, et al. The ability of three global plasma assays to recognize thrombophilia. Thromb Res. 2004;113(6):411-7.

[145] Antovic A. The overall hemostasis potential: a laboratory tool for the investigation of global hemostasis. Semin Thromb Hemost. 2010 Oct;36(7):772-9.

[146] McEwen B, Morel-Kopp MC, Phillips C, Sullivan D, Ward CM, Grunstein R, et al. Circadian changes in thrombotic potential in obstructive sleep apnea (OSA): A randomized, placebo-controlled crossover study. Journal of Thrombosis and Haemostasis. 2011 July;9:841.

[147] Leander K, Blomback M, Wallen H, He S. Impaired fibrinolytic capacity and increased fibrin formation associate with myocardial infarction. Thromb Haemost. 2012 Jun;107(6):1092-9.

[148] Skeppholm M, Kallner A, Malmqvist K, Blomback M, Wallen H. Is fibrin formation and thrombin generation increased during and after an acute coronary syndrome? Thromb Res. 2011 Nov;128(5):483-9.

[149] Reddel CJ, Curnow JL, Voitl J, Rosenov A, Pennings GJ, Morel-Kopp MC, et al. Detection of hypofibrinolysis in stable coronary artery disease using the overall haemostatic potential assay. Thromb Res. 2013 May;131(5):457-62.

[150] Anzej S, Bozic M, Antovic A, Peternel P, Gaspersic N, Rot U, et al. Evidence of hypercoagulability and inflammation in young patients long after acute cerebral ischaemia. Thromb Res. 2007;120(1):39-46.

[151] Rooth E, Wallen H, Antovic A, Von Arbin M, Kaponides G, Wahlgren N, et al. Thrombin activatable fibrinolysis inhibitor and its relationship to fibrinolysis and inflammation during the acute and convalescent phase of ischemic stroke. Blood Coagulation and Fibrinolysis. 2007 June;18(4):365-70.

[152] Antovic A, Blomback M, Bremme K, Van Rooijen M, He S. Increased hemostasis potential persists in women with previous thromboembolism with or without APC resistance. J Thromb Haemost. 2003 Dec;1(12):2531-5.

[153] Antovic JP, Antovic A, Sten-Linder M, Wramsby M, Blomback M. Overall hemostatic potential (OHP) assay-a possible tool for determination of prothrombotic pattern in FXII deficiency. J Thromb Haemost. 2004 Nov;2(11):2058-60.

[154] Bombardier C, Villalobos-Menuey E, Ruegg K, Hathaway WE, Manco-Johnson MJ, Goldenberg NA. Monitoring hypercoagulability and hypofibrinolysis following acute venous Thromboembolism in children: application of the CloFAL assay in a prospective inception cohort study. Thromb Res. 2012 Sep;130(3):343-9.

[155] Antovic A, Blomback M, Bremme K, He S. The assay of overall haemostasis potential used to monitor the low molecular mass (weight) heparin, dalteparin, treatment in pregnant women with previous thromboembolism. Blood Coagul Fibrinolysis. 2002 Apr;13(3):181-6.

[156] Yamamoto J, Yamashita T, Ikarugi H, et al. Gorog Thrombosis Test: a global in-vitro test of platelet function and thrombolysis. Blood Coagul Fibrinolysis. 2003;14:31–9.

[157] Rijken DC, Hoegee-de NE, Jie AF, Atsma DE, Schalij MJ, Nieuwenhuizen W. Development of a new test for the global fibrinolytic capacity in whole blood. J Thromb Haemost. 2008;6:151–7.

Chapter 7

Coagulation and Fibrinolysis Markers and Their Use for the Prediction of High Risk Patients with Venous Thromboembolism Following Total Hip Arthroplasty

Yutaka Inaba, Yohei Yukizawa and
Tomoyuki Saito

Additional information is available at the end of the chapter

http://dx.doi.org/10.5772/57248

1. Introduction

Patients undergoing elective total joint arthroplasty of the lower extremities are at particularly high risk for venous thromboembolism (VTE). Randomized clinical trials have demonstrated the rates of deep vein thrombosis (DVT) following total hip or knee arthroplasty in patients not given thromboprophylaxis to be 42-57 % and 41-85%, respectively [1]. Therefore, perioperative thromboprophylaxis has been a crucial part of the management of these patients for more than 20 years. The administration of anticoagulant drugs, such as vitamin K antagonists, unfractionated heparins, low-molecular weight heparins and a pentasaccharide, is the most effective method of reducing the risk of VTE after major orthopedic surgical procedures. In contrast, although the appropriate uses of these agents are assumed to only minimally increase the bleeding tendency, higher prophylactic efficacy is naturally associated with a higher risk of bleeding complications. The American College of Chest Physicians (ACCP) Guidelines recently downgraded the strength of most pharmaco-prophylactic recommendations in order to achieve a more balanced trade-off between the reduction of thrombotic events and the increase in bleeding events. [2] However, a strong recommendation for routine use of anticoagulants after surgery was included in the previous edition. The American Academy of Orthopaedic Surgeons (AAOS) Guidelines also recommend that orthopedic surgeons evaluate patients' risks for pulmonary embolism (PE) and serious bleeding complications and individualize pharmacologic prophylaxis based on a risk-benefit ratio [3,4]. However, the best way to manage patients depending on their risk for VTE remains controversial because several forms of thromboprophylaxis following surgery are now available.

Approaches to assessing individual risks of hospitalized patients for VTE can be applied to determine whether anticoagulant drugs are indicated for thromboprophylaxis [5-7]. These assessments, however, are usually complex and difficult to use in everyday practice [8]. Also, alternative indications limited to patients undergoing surgery are lacking, and the associations between postoperative VTE and reported risk factors such as obesity, age or varicose veins have not yet been adequately investigated. Only one risk factor, previous history of VTE, has sufficient evidence indicating that some of these patients may be at even higher risk [9, 10].

Measurements of blood coagulation parameters, such as prothrombin time (PT), activated partial thromboplastin time (aPTT), plasma levels of D-dimer, and so on, are frequently used to assess clotting function and the coagulation state in patients. Although previous considerations of these global screening tests did not facilitate the diagnosis of thrombotic events [11, 12], recent biochemical studies of the coagulation and fibrinolysis systems have expanded the availability of specific and sensitive tests which can detect coagulation state abnormalities. Several different markers have been found to be elevated in clinical disorders, in which the coagulation and fibrinolysis states are out of balance (e.g. disseminated intravascular coagulation, acute myocardial infarction, cerebral infarction, and VTE).

Some of these coagulation markers are sensitive to coagulation state changes in patients undergoing invasive procedures. We previously examined changes in the profiles of some coagulation markers in patients undergoing primary total hip arthroplasty (THA). According to our results, the plasma levels of soluble fibrin (SF) and plasminogen-activator inhibitor-1 (PAI-1) sensitively represented hypercoagulable states which might be associated with postoperative VTE, and we suggested a screening method for evaluating VTE risk in patients undergoing THA using these two markers [13]. Although further investigation is needed, this screening test may be useful for grouping postoperative patients into risk categories. This chapter first provides general information about coagulation markers, which we investigated for diagnosing VTE, and then gives a brief overview of our suggestions pertaining to the screening test for evaluating individual postoperative VTE risk.

2. Coagulation markers associated with thrombosis

2.1. D-dimer

D-dimer is a specific fragment of a cross-linked fibrin clot that is released into the blood when a clot is lysed by plasmin. The utility of measuring D-dimer for the diagnosis of VTE has been extensively studied. D-dimer is detectable at levels greater than 500 ng/mL of fibrinogen equivalent units in nearly all patients with VTE. In general, it is a sensitive test but lacks specificity for the diagnosis of DVT and is, therefore, only useful when negative [14, 15] because plasma levels of D-dimer are increased in a variety of inflammatory and prothrombotic conditions associated with activation of coagulation, such as surgery, trauma, and infection.

2.2. Thrombin-antithrombin Complex (TAT)

The activation of coagulation leads to thrombin products in plasma, but this is regulated in part through interactions with protease inhibitors, such as antithrombin III (AT III). TAT complexes are formed following the neutralization of thrombin by ATIII. TAT is a sensitive marker for thrombin formation, and its elevation in plasma is suggested to alter hemostatic activation. However, TAT formation represents only an indirect measurement of an activated coagulation system [16], and is frequently influenced by peripheral blood sampling techniques under venous occlusion. Thus, measurement of TAT has a low diagnostic accuracy for thrombotic events [17], though marked and persistent TAT level increases may deserve further investigation.

2.3. Soluble Fibrin (SF)

Activated thrombin produces fibrinogen, forming a fibrin monomer that rapidly polymerizes to form a clot. Small amounts can dissolve and circulate in plasma as "soluble fibrin". SF molecules have a strong tendency to polymerize and thus have a short half-life and are present physiologically only at very low concentrations. This is why SF is regarded as a very sensitive marker showing a hypercoagulable state when significantly elevated in plasma. The hypercoagulable state is often caused by various invasive procedures, such as surgery, and plasma levels of SF are recognized to rise rapidly during and after surgery [18, 19].

2.4. Plasminogen-activator inhibitor-1 (PAI-1)

PAI-1 is an important component of the coagulation system that down-regulates fibrinolysis in the circulation. PAI-1 is synthesized by the endothelium and smooth muscle cells in arteries. Elevated plasma PAI-1 in non-surgical patients has been documented in subjects who subsequently developed vascular ischemic events [20-22]. Also, plasma levels of PAI-1 are associated with surgical invasion, and the resultant increase in levels of the fibrinolytic inhibitor is regarded as being a major contributor to fibrinolytic shut-down [18, 23].

2.5. Preoperative VTE risk assessment

There are numerous risk factors for VTE in surgical patients, including the type and extent of surgery or trauma, duration of hospitalization, a history of previous VTE or malignancy, and inherited hypercoagulable states [24-27]. To prevent the development of postoperative VTE, surgical patients should be assessed for risk factors and given thromboprophylaxis as indicated. According to the ACCP Guidelines, surgical patients, excluding those undergoing orthopedic surgical procedures, can be divided into 4 risk groups (very low, low, moderate, or high) depending on the operations being performed. Patients undergoing major orthopedic surgery, such as THA, total knee arthroplasty or hip fracture surgery, are always regarded as being at high risk, and the ACCP Guidelines recommend postoperative anticoagulation (Grade 1B) or portable intermittent pneumatic compression (IPC) (Grade 1C) for thromboprophylaxis.

2.6. Postoperative VTE risk assessment according to SF and PAI-1

According to preoperative risk assessment, most patients undergoing major orthopedic surgery will be in the "high risk" group. However, the state of hypercoagulation following surgery may vary depending on many factors (e.g. patient responsiveness to invasive procedures, types of surgery, duration of surgery, and anesthetic technique). To assess how severe the hypercoagulable state is in patients, acute and sensitive coagulation markers are needed. As mentioned above, we investigated coagulation markers to evaluate their utilities for VTE risk screening following primary THA.

We investigated 170 consecutive patients who were scheduled to undergo primary THA. Patients were excluded if they had any of the following conditions: (a) body weight <40kg; (b) cerebral or gastrointestinal bleeding within the previous 6 months; (c) preoperative intake of anticoagulant or antiplatelet agents; (d) severe renal insufficiency (estimated glomerular filtration rate (eGFR) <30 mL/min-1/1.73 m-^{2})[28]; (e) hepatic failure; (f) allergic to contrast agents; or (g) coagulation or fibrinolysis disorder. All patients were operated on under general anesthesia, and THA was performed through a minimally-invasive anterolateral approach with the patient in the lateral decubitus position. Postoperative mobilization followed a set protocol supervised by experienced physiotherapists. Early walking with a tolerable weight load with crutches or a walker was performed from the day after surgery.

Blood samples were obtained from peripheral veins preoperatively, after a brief fast, and on postoperative days 1, 3, 7, and 14. Plasma SF levels were measured with a latex photometric immunoassay (IATRO SF II; Mitsubishi Chemical Medience Corporation, Tokyo, Japan) using IF-43 monoclonal antibody raised against a urea-solubilized fibrin monomer. PAI-1 was measured using a latex photometric immunoassay (LPIA-tPAI Test; Mitsubishi Chemical Medience Corporation, Tokyo, Japan). Plasma D-dimer levels were also assayed employing a latex photometric immunoassay (LPIA-ACE D-dimer; Mitsubishi Chemical Medience Corporation, Tokyo, Japan). The normal limit was <0.7 μg/mL. TAT was measured by enzyme-linked immunosorbent assay (ELISA) with a reference range of 0.1–5.0 ng/mL (Enzygnost TATmicro; Siemens Healthcare Diagnostics Inc., Tokyo, Japan).

There were two patient groups: IPC group (67 patients) and fondaparinux (FPX) group (103 patients). During surgery, IPC was concurrently performed on all patients in both groups under general anesthesia, and the patients were intravenously administered unfractionated heparin (UFH) in a single dose of 20 IU/kg of body weight. IPC was postoperatively maintained until the day patients started walking, usually 1-2 days after surgery, and this was the only thromboprophylaxis for the IPC group. In addition to IPC, the patients in the FPX group were also subcutaneously administered 2.5 mg of FPX daily for 14 days starting on postoperative day 1. For the detection of postoperative VTE including PE and DVT, angiography of the pulmonary artery and deep vein of the pelvis and the lower limbs was performed for all patients on postoperative day 7 by 64-slice multidetector row computed tomography using a nonionic contrast agent.

Postoperative VTE was detected in 17 (25%) of the IPC patients, and 8 (7%) of the FPX patients. The difference in the frequency of VTE occurrence between the IPC and FPX groups was statistically significant ($p < 0.01$). All DVT presented in calf veins, and there were no cases with symptomatic DVT or PE.

In the IPC group, plasma levels of SF on postoperative day 1 were significantly higher in patients with VTE than in those without VTE (Figure 1, p< 0.01). Similar to SF, plasma levels of PAI-1 on day 1 were also significantly higher in the patients with VTE in the IPC group (Figure 1, p< 0.01). On the other hand, SF and PAI-1 levels showed similar tendencies in patients with and without VTE in the FPX group (Figure 2). In both the IPC and the FPX group, plasma D-dimer levels showed bimodal peaks that were evident on postoperative days 1 and 7. In the IPC group, significant differences were found on postoperative day 7 (p< 0.01, Figures 1 and 2). IPC patients with VTE also had higher TAT levels on postoperative day 1 (p< 0.05).

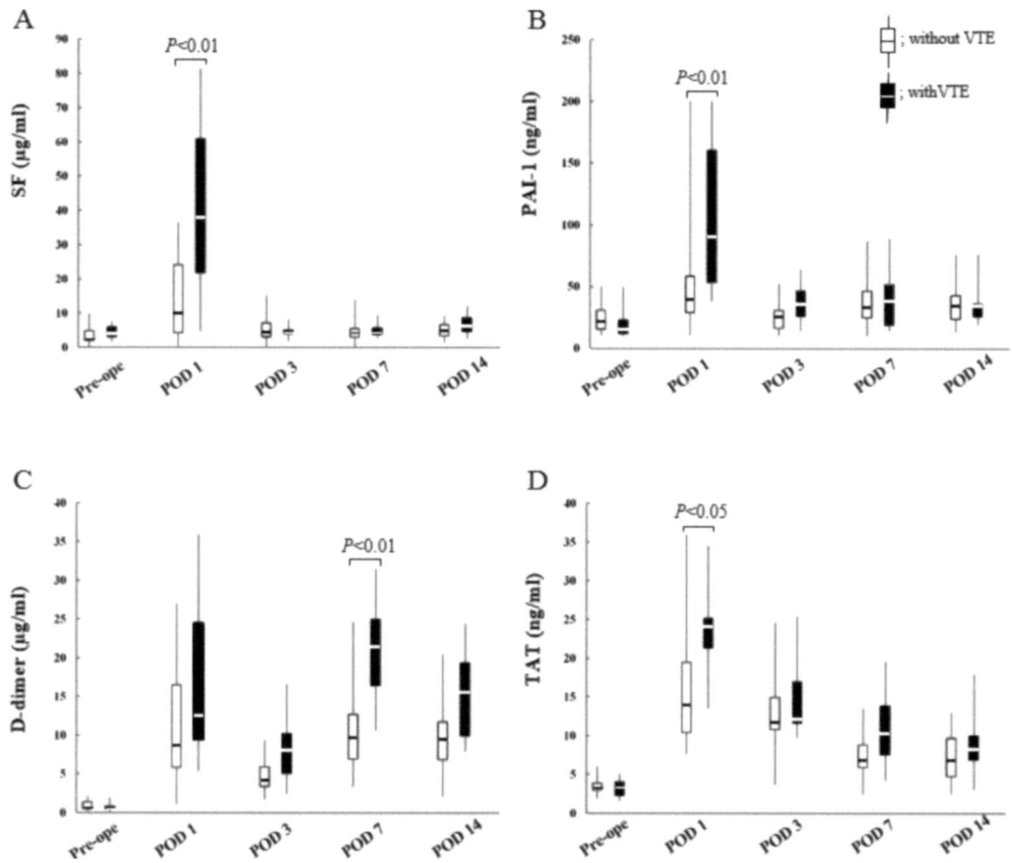

Plasma levels of soluble fibrin (SF) (A), plasminogen activator inhibitor type 1 (PAI-1) (B), D-dimer (C), and thrombin-antithrombin complex (TAT) (D) in patients who received only intermittent pneumatic compression were measured preoperatively (pre-op) and on postoperative days 1 (POD1), 3 (POD3), 7 (POD7), and 14 (POD14). The boxes represent the interquartile ranges. The perpendicular lines (whiskers) represent the 5th and 95th percentiles and the horizontal bars in the boxes indicate the median values. On the day after surgery, the plasma levels of SF, PAI-1, and TAT were found to be significantly increased in the venous thromboembolism (VTE) group as compared with the non-VTE group ($p < 0.01$, $p < 0.01$, $p < 0.05$, respectively). The changes in D-dimer levels showed bimodal peaks on postoperative days 1 and 7 in both groups. Significant differences were observed in the D-dimer levels measured on postoperative day 7 ($p < 0.01$).

Figure 1. Changes in coagulation and fibrinolysis markers in patients who received only intermittent pneumatic compression after total hip arthroplasty

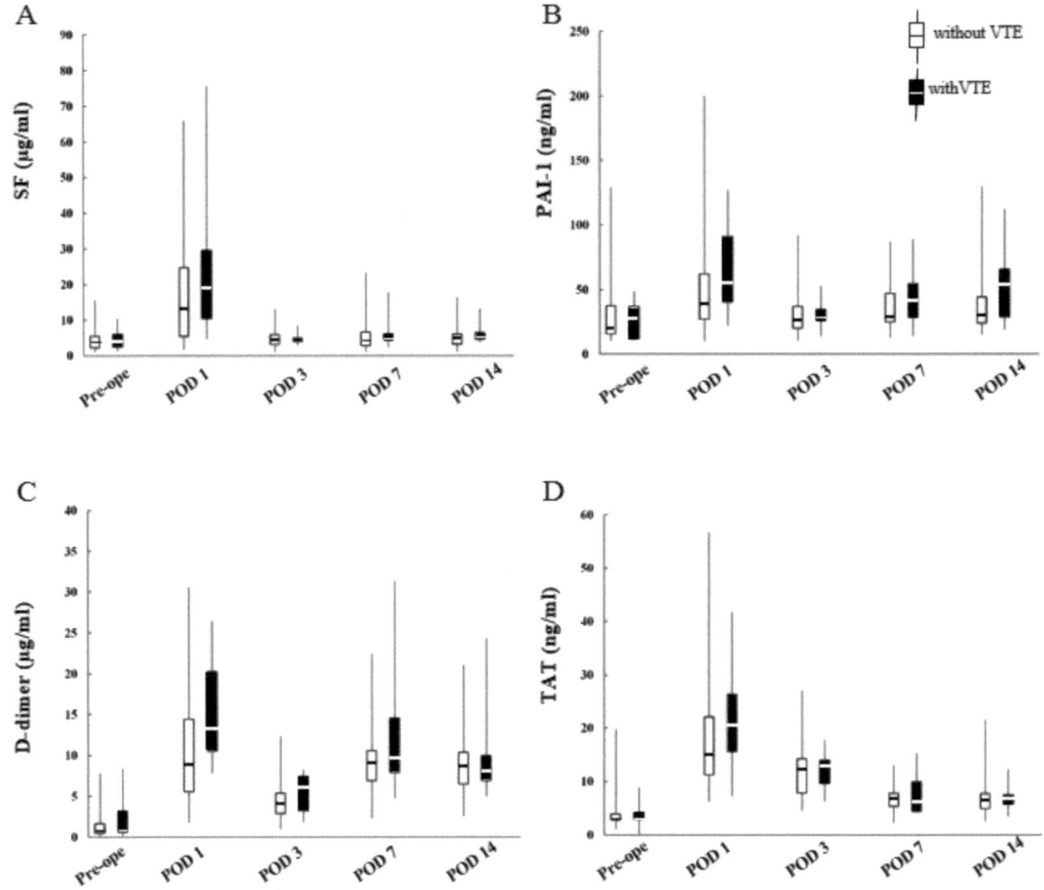

Plasma levels of soluble fibrin (SF) (A), plasminogen activator inhibitor type 1 (PAI-1) (B), D-dimer (C), and thrombin-antithrombin complex (TAT) (D) in patients who received subcutaneous injections of fondaparinux sodium were measured preoperatively (pre-op) and on postoperative days 1 (POD1), 3 (POD3), 7 (POD7), and 14 (POD14). The boxes represent the interquartile ranges. The perpendicular lines represent the 5th and 95th percentiles and the horizontal bars in the boxes indicate the median values. There were no statistically significant differences in the levels of SF, PAI-1, D-dimer, and TAT between the patients with and without VTE in the fondaparinux group.

Figure 2. Changes in coagulation and fibrinolysis markers in patients who received subcutaneous injections of fondaparinux sodium after total hip arthroplasty

Figure 3 shows the receiver operating characteristic (ROC) curve for each marker on postoperative day 1 (for SF, PAI-1, and TAT) and day 7 (for D-dimer). The ROC curves provided the cut-off levels for these markers, and the SF cut-off level was determined to be 19.8 μg/mL with a sensitivity of 88% and a specificity of 62%. The cut-off level of PAI-1 was 53.5 ng/mL with a sensitivity of 78% and a specificity of 72%, and that of TAT was determined to be 18.1 ng/mL with a sensitivity of 85% and a specificity of 66%. Of these markers, multivariate logistic regression analysis revealed SF and PAI-1 to have the strongest associations, statistically, with a thrombotic tendency.

http://dx.doi.org/10.5772/57248

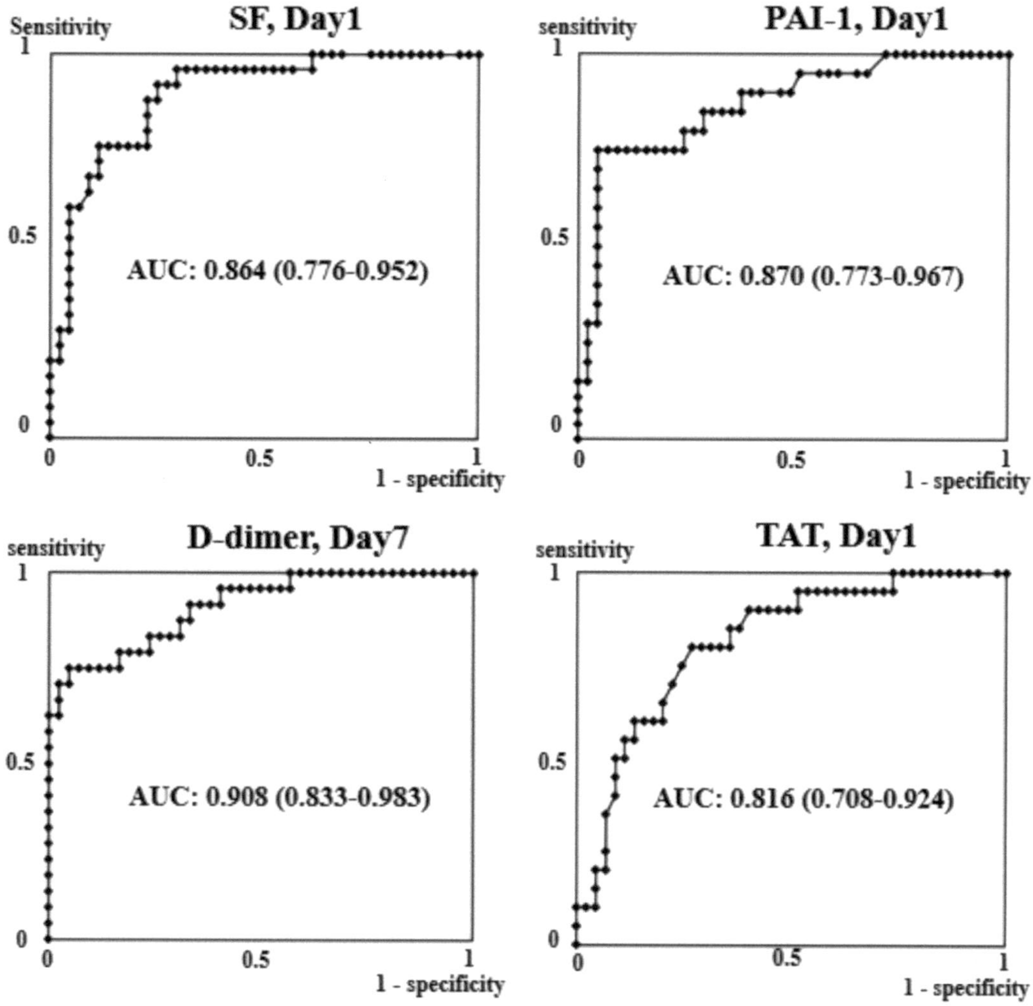

In each diagram, the area under the ROC curve is shown, as well as the 95% confidence interval in parentheses.

Figure 3. Receiver operating characteristic curve analyses of the accuracies of quantitative soluble fibrin (SF), plasminogen activator inhibitor type 1 (PAI-1), and thrombin-antithrombin complex (TAT) levels on postoperative day 1 and D-dimer levels on day 7

Figure 4 shows the scatter graph of SF and PAI-1 levels, with 2 lines at each cut-off level. These lines divide patients into 2 groups, with higher and lower levels, and these divisions provided a sensitivity of 100%, a specificity of 67%, and a positive predictive value of 50% for postoperative VTE. In addition, when this criterion was applied to patients of the FPX group, 7 of the 8 with VTE met the criterion, yielding a negative agreement rate of 98.0% (48/49).

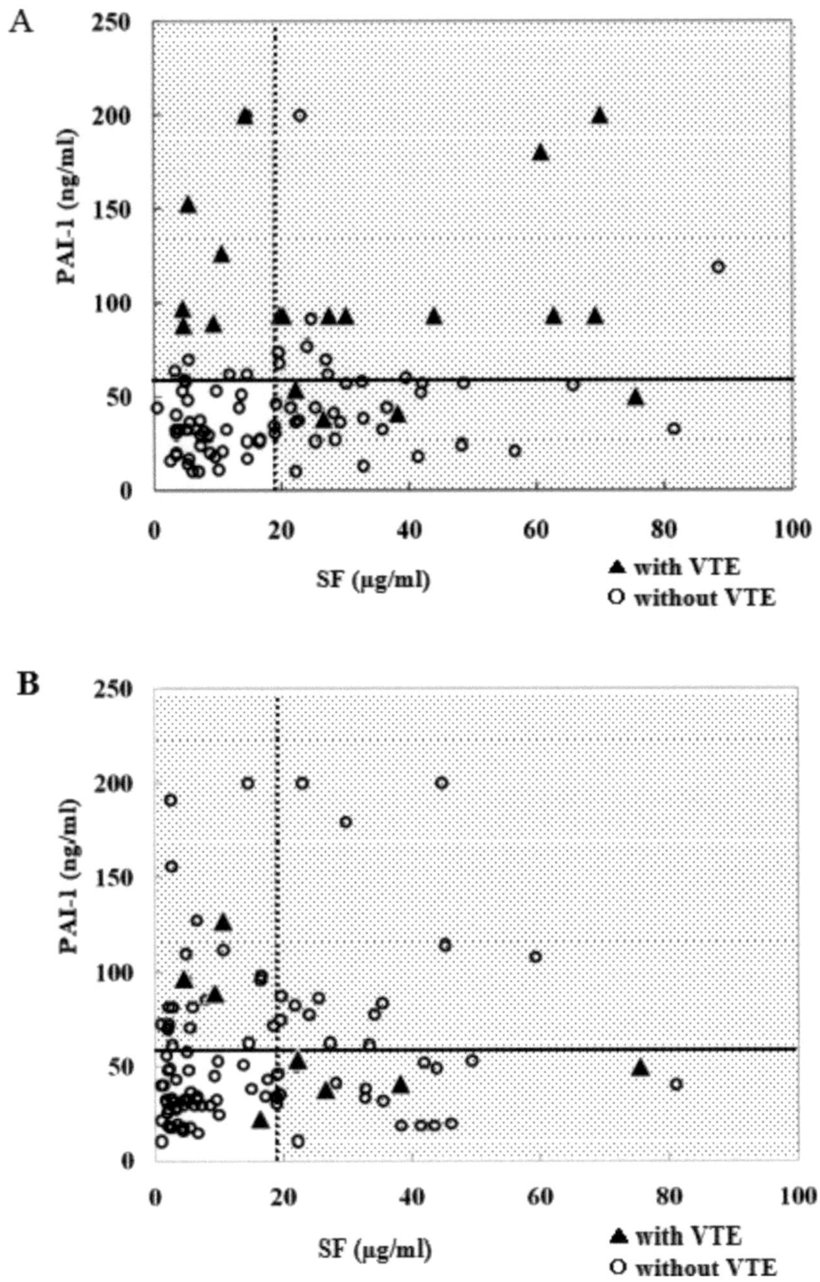

Increases in either SF or PAI-1 on postoperative day 1 above their cut-off levels provided 100% sensitivity and 67% specificity for predicting VTE when patients were not administered fondaparinux sodium postoperatively (A). In addition, when this criterion was applied to patients who received subcutaneous injections of fondaparinux following surgery, 7 of 8 patients with VTE met the criterion, yielding a 98.0% (48/49) negative agreement rate (B).

Figure 4. Discriminating postoperative venous thromboembolism (VTE) using levels of soluble fibrin (SF) and plasminogen activator inhibitor type 1 (PAI-1)

As shown in the scatter graphs, pharmaco-prophylaxis reduced the incidence of VTE especially in the high-risk group. In addition, the incidence of VTE in the low-risk group was not different from those obtained with other methods of thromboprophylaxis. The blood analysis on the day after surgery indicated almost half of patients to be in the low-risk group. It was suggested that patients with low plasma levels of SF and PAI-1 might not need pharmaco-prophylaxis following surgery. The blood analysis, which we have suggested as a means of risk assessment, was very simple to use and would likely be acceptable to many institutions. However, further investigation is necessary due to the small sample size in this study.

Highly invasive surgery has been shown to commonly result in a hypercoagulable state [16, 29], resulting in elevated plasma SF. SF reflects acute intravascular fibrin formation as well because SF is one of the circulating materials contributing to fibrin clots [30]. PAI-1 is also produced at the site of inflammation following tissue injury [18, 23]. It was suggested that plasma levels of SF and PAI-1 in the early phase after surgery reflect an imbalance between coagulation and fibrinolysis which contributes to excessive fibrin deposition in the vascular wall [31]. We believe that the combined measurement of SF and PAI-1 on postoperative day 1 is a useful screening method for patients at high risk for postoperative VTE and for determining whether pharmaco-prophylaxis after THA is indicated.

Because the results of SF and PAI-1 assays can be obtained within several hours on the day after surgery, whether pharmaco-prophylaxis is indicated can be determined on postoperative day 1. However, the optimal timing for the initiation of pharmaco-prophylaxis is one of the issues raised by thromboprophylaxis, and the administration of anticoagulant agents following this screening test might be regarded as being relatively late. There has been debate in the literature regarding the issue of how to maximize efficacy while minimizing bleeding risk [32] because the peak efficacy of anticoagulant agents depends on the timing of the first injection [33, 34]. According to a systematic review [33], the incidence of DVT was 19% in patients to whom low-molecular-weight heparin (LMWH) was administered 12 hours before surgery, 12% in patients given LMWH during surgery, and 14% in those treated postoperatively. In our study, low-dose UFH was administered once during surgery and postoperative anticoagulation was performed 24 hours after surgery. According to our results, the initiation of anticoagulation, as performed in this study, appears to be both reasonable and appropriate.

The present study has limitations. First, VTE could be initiated during the operation [35, 36], in the postoperative period without mobilization [37], or 1-2 months after surgery [38, 39]. Thus, evaluations of VTE occurrence may vary depending on the timing of imaging tests, duration of follow-up, or the duration of postoperative thromboprophylaxis. Second, our study was limited to a single center, and the sample size was too small to draw conclusions about the efficacy of our alternative prophylaxis regimen.

3. Summary

Individual risk assessment is becoming a widespread method for determining whether prophylaxis, especially in patients undergoing major orthopedic surgery, is indicated. VTE developing after surgery might be induced by a hypercoagulable or regulated fibrinolytic state during the early postoperative phase. Thus, the proposed screening test using SF and PAI-1 on the day after surgery may be of value in providing information about whether the coagulation state is unbalanced, and in predicting VTE following THA. We anticipate that selective pharmacological thromboprophylaxis, based on the plasma levels of SF and PAI-1 on the first postoperative day, will be achieved with an alternative thromboprophylaxis regimen.

Characteristics	IPC group		p value	FPX group		p value
	Patients with VTE N = 17	Patients without VTE N = 50		Patients with VTE N = 6	Patients without VTE N = 97	
Age, years	68 (8)	62 (12)	N.S.	58 (8)	61 (12)	N.S.
Gender: Male/Female, no.	3/14	17/33	N.S.	6/0	21/76	N.S.
Weight, kg	58 (14)	58 (13)	N.S.	59 (14)	58 (13)	N.S.
Body mass index	24 (6)	23 (5)	N.S.	24 (5)	24 (5)	N.S.
Primary hip disease, no.			N.S.			N.S.
OA	15	36		4	79	
RA	0	3		0	7	
ANFH	2	6		2	11	
PVS	0	1		0	0	
Preoperative plasma levels of:						
Triglycerides, mg/dL	92 (35)	108 (40)	N.S.	99 (32)	98 (41)	N.S.
Total cholesterol, mg/dL	228 (44)	199 (31)	N.S.	202 (26)	222 (36)	N.S.

Values are presented as means (SD). IPC, intermittent pneumatic compression; FPX, fondaparinux sodium; VTE, venous thromboembolism; OA, osteoarthritis; RA, rheumatoid arthritis; ANFH, avascular necrosis of femoral head; PVS, pigmented villonodular synovitis; N.S., not significant.

Table 1. Patient characteristics

Author details

Yutaka Inaba*, Yohei Yukizawa and Tomoyuki Saito

*Address all correspondence to: yute0131@med.yokohama-cu.ac.jp

Department of Orthopaedic Surgery, Yokohama City University, Yokohama, Japan

http://dx.doi.org/10.5772/57248

References

[1] Geerts WH, Bergqvist D, Pineo GF, Heit JA, Samama CM, Lassen MR, et al. Prevention of venous thromboembolism: American College of Chest Physicians Evidence-Based Clinical Practice Guidelines (8th Edition). Chest 2008; 133(6 Suppl): 381S-453S.

[2] Falck-Ytter Y, Francis CW, Johanson NA, Curley C, Dahl OE, Schulman S, et al. Prevention of VTE in Orthopedic Surgery Patients: Antithrombotic Therapy and Prevention of Thrombosis, 9th ed: American College of Chest Physicians Evidence-Based Clinical Practice Guidelines. Chest 2012; 141(2 Suppl): e278S-325S.

[3] Johanson NA, Lachiewicz PF, Lieberman JR, Lotke PA, Parvizi J, Pellegrini V, et al. American academy of orthopaedic surgeons clinical practice guideline on. Prevention of symptomatic pulmonary embolism in patients undergoing total hip or knee arthroplasty. J Bone Joint Surg Am 2009; 91(7): 1756-7.

[4] Jacobs JJ, Mont MA, Bozic KJ, Della Valle CJ, Goodman SB, Lewis CG, et al. American Academy of Orthopaedic Surgeons clinical practice guideline on: preventing venous thromboembolic disease in patients undergoing elective hip and knee arthroplasty. J Bone Joint Surg Am 2012; 94(8): 746-7.

[5] Mismetti P, Laporte S, Zufferey P, Epinat M, Decousus H, Cucherat M. Prevention of venous thromboembolism in orthopedic surgery with vitamin K antagonists: a meta-analysis. J Thromb Haemost 2004; 2(7): 1058-70.

[6] Eikelboom JW, Quinlan DJ, Douketis JD. Extended-duration prophylaxis against venous thromboembolism after total hip or knee replacement: a meta-analysis of the randomised trials. Lancet 2001; 358(9275): 9-15.

[7] Dentali F, Douketis JD, Gianni M, Lim W, Crowther MA. Meta-analysis: anticoagulant prophylaxis to prevent symptomatic venous thromboembolism in hospitalized medical patients. Ann Intern Med 2007; 146(4): 278-88.

[8] Laaksonen VO, Arola MK, Hannelin M, Inberg MV, Kivisaari S. Effect of anaesthesia on the incidence of postoperative lower limb thrombosis. Ann Chir Gynaecol Fenn 1973; 62(5): 304-17.

[9] Pedersen AB, Sorensen HT, Mehnert F, Overgaard S, Johnsen SP. Risk factors for venous thromboembolism in patients undergoing total hip replacement and receiving routine thromboprophylaxis. J Bone Joint Surg Am 2010; 92(12): 2156-64.

[10] Warwick D, Friedman RJ, Agnelli G, Gil-Garay E, Johnson K, FitzGerald G, et al. Insufficient duration of venous thromboembolism prophylaxis after total hip or knee replacement when compared with the time course of thromboembolic events: findings from the Global Orthopaedic Registry. J Bone Joint Surg Br 2007; 89(6): 799-807.

[11] Bauer KA. Activation markers of coagulation. Baillieres Best Pract Res Clin Haematol 1999; 12(3): 387-406.

[12] Fareed J, Bick RL, Hoppensteadt DA, Walenga JM, Messmore HL, Bermes EW, Jr. Molecular markers of hemostatic activation. Implications in the diagnosis of thrombosis, vascular, and cardiovascular disorders. Clin Lab Med 1995; 15(1): 39-61.

[13] Yukizawa Y, Inaba Y, Watanabe S, Yajima S, Kobayashi N, Ishida T, et al. Association between venous thromboembolism and plasma levels of both soluble fibrin and plasminogen-activator inhibitor 1 in 170 patients undergoing total hip arthroplasty. Acta Orthop 2012; 83(1): 14-21.

[14] Bounameaux H, Cirafici P, de Moerloose P, Schneider PA, Slosman D, Reber G, et al. Measurement of D-dimer in plasma as diagnostic aid in suspected pulmonary embolism. Lancet 1991; 337(8735): 196-200.

[15] Wells PS, Anderson DR, Bormanis J, Guy F, Mitchell M, Gray L, et al. Application of a diagnostic clinical model for the management of hospitalized patients with suspected deep-vein thrombosis. Thromb Haemost 1999; 81(4): 493-7.

[16] Brueckner S, Reinke U, Roth-Isigkeit A, Eleftheriadis S, Schmucker P, Siemens HJ. Comparison of general and spinal anesthesia and their influence on hemostatic markers in patients undergoing total hip arthroplasty. J Clin Anesth 2003; 15(6): 433-40.

[17] Pazzagli M, Mazzantini D, Cella G, Rampin E, Palla A. Value of thrombin-antithrombin III complexes in major orthopedic surgery: relation to the onset of venous thromboembolism. Clin Appl Thromb Hemost 1999; 5(4): 228-31.

[18] Misaki T, Kitajima I, Kabata T, Tani M, Kabata C, Tsubokawa T, et al. Changes of the soluble fibrin monomer complex level during the perioperative period of hip replacement surgery. J Orthop Sci 2008; 13(5): 419-24.

[19] Hosaka A, Miyata T, Aramoto H, Shigematsu H, Nakazawa T, Okamoto H, et al. Clinical implication of plasma level of soluble fibrin monomer-fibrinogen complex in patients with abdominal aortic aneurysm. J Vasc Surg 2005; 42(2): 200-5.

[20] Di Minno G, Mancini FP, Margaglione M. Hemostatic variables and ischemic cardiovascular disease: do we need a concerted effort for more profitable future clinical investigations? Cardiovasc Drugs Ther 1997; 10(6): 743-9.

[21] Meade TW, Ruddock V, Stirling Y, Chakrabarti R, Miller GJ. Fibrinolytic activity, clotting factors, and long-term incidence of ischaemic heart disease in the Northwick Park Heart Study. Lancet 1993; 342(8879): 1076-9.

[22] Ridker PM, Hennekens CH, Stampfer MJ, Manson JE, Vaughan DE. Prospective study of endogenous tissue plasminogen activator and risk of stroke. Lancet 1994; 343(8903): 940-3.

[23] Kluft C, Verheijen JH, Jie AF, Rijken DC, Preston FE, Sue-Ling HM, et al. The postoperative fibrinolytic shutdown: a rapidly reverting acute phase pattern for the fast-act-

ing inhibitor of tissue-type plasminogen activator after trauma. Scand J Clin Lab Invest 1985; 45(7): 605-10.

[24] Heit JA, O'Fallon WM, Petterson TM, Lohse CM, Silverstein MD, Mohr DN, et al. Relative impact of risk factors for deep vein thrombosis and pulmonary embolism: a population-based study. Arch Intern Med 2002; 162(11): 1245-8.

[25] Prandoni P, Samama MM. Risk stratification and venous thromboprophylaxis in hospitalized medical and cancer patients. Br J Haematol 2008; 141(5): 587-97.

[26] Gangireddy C, Rectenwald JR, Upchurch GR, Wakefield TW, Khuri S, Henderson WG, et al. Risk factors and clinical impact of postoperative symptomatic venous thromboembolism. J Vasc Surg 2007; 45(2): 335-341; discussion 341-2.

[27] Haas SK, Hach-Wunderle V, Mader FH, Ruster K, Paar WD. An evaluation of venous thromboembolic risk in acutely ill medical patients immobilized at home: the AT-HOME Study. Clin Appl Throm Hemost 2007; 13(1): 7-13.

[28] Matsuo S, Imai E, Horio M, Yasuda Y, Tomita K, Nitta K, et al. Revised equations for estimated GFR from serum creatinine in Japan. Am J Kidney Dis 2009; 53(6): 982-92.

[29] Sudo A, Wada H, Nobori T, Yamada N, Ito M, Niimi R, et al. Cut-off values of D-dimer and soluble fibrin for prediction of deep vein thrombosis after orthopaedic surgery. Int J Hematol 2009; 89(5): 572-6.

[30] Hamano A, Umeda M, Ueno Y, Tanaka S, Mimuro J, Sakata Y. Latex immunoturbidimetric assay for soluble fibrin complex. Clin Chem 2005;,51(1):,183-8.

[31] Aso Y. Plasminogen activator inhibitor (PAI)-1 in vascular inflammation and thrombosis. Front Biosci 2007; 12: 2957-66.

[32] Warwick D, Rosencher N. The "critical thrombosis period" in major orthopedic surgery: when to start and when to stop prophylaxis. Clin Appl Thromb Hemost 2010; 16(4): 394-405.

[33] Strebel N, Prins M, Agnelli G, Buller HR. Preoperative or postoperative start of prophylaxis for venous thromboembolism with low-molecular-weight heparin in elective hip surgery? Arch Intern Med 2002; 162(13): 1451-6.

[34] Hull RD, Pineo GF, Stein PD, Mah AF, MacIsaac SM, Dahl OE, et al. Timing of initial administration of low-molecular-weight heparin prophylaxis against deep vein thrombosis in patients following elective hip arthroplasty: a systematic review. Arch Intern Med 2001; 161(16): 1952-60.

[35] Shine TS, Feinglass NG, Leone BJ, Murray PM. Transesophageal echocardiography for detection of propagating, massive emboli during prosthetic hip fracture surgery. Iowa Orthop J 2010; 30: 211-4.

[36] Church JS, Scadden JE, Gupta RR, Cokis C, Williams KA, Janes GC. Embolic phenomena during computer-assisted and conventional total knee replacement. J Bone Joint Surg Br 2007; 89(4): 481-5.

[37] Turpie AG, Bauer KA, Eriksson BI, Lassen MR. Fondaparinux vs enoxaparin for the prevention of venous thromboembolism in major orthopedic surgery: a meta-analysis of 4 randomized double-blind studies. Arch Intern Med 2002; 162(16): 1833-40.

[38] Bjornara BT, Gudmundsen TE, Dahl OE. Frequency and timing of clinical venous thromboembolism after major joint surgery. J Bone Joint Surg Br 2006; 88(3): 386-91.

[39] Dahl OE, Gudmundsen TE, Bjornara BT, Solheim DM. Risk of clinical pulmonary embolism after joint surgery in patients receiving low-molecular-weight heparin prophylaxis in hospital: a 10-year prospective register of 3,954 patients. Acta Orthop Scand 2003; 74(3): 299-304.

[40] Sharrock NE, Go G, Sculco TP, Salvati EA, Westrich GH, Harpel PC. Dose response of intravenous heparin on markers of thrombosis during primary total hip replacement. Anesthesiology 1999; 90(4): 981-7.

Chapter 8

Thrombolysis or Operation: That is the Question in Prosthetic Valve Thrombosis

Giuseppe Filiberto Serraino, Roberto Lorusso and
Attilio Renzulli

Additional information is available at the end of the chapter

http://dx.doi.org/10.5772/58479

1. Introduction

The structural changes of mechanical prostheses over the last 3 decades have improved their haemodynamic features and prolonged their durability. Nowadays, they are preferable to bioprostheses in most cases (Figure 1). The risk of complications is still very high, among which thrombosis is the most dreaded. Its incidence varies in the literature between 4% [1] and 8.6% [2] within 5 years from implant. Despite various innovations, even today, prosthetic thrombosis is still associated with a high mortality, even if emergency medical or surgical treatment is promptly established [3, 4, 21]. The knowledge of factors that may determine prosthetic thrombosis is still limited. Numerous studies investigated this tragic complication: the most frequent risk factor as reported in the literature is inadequate or discontinued anticoagulant therapy. Other risk factors are related to previous endocarditis and the prosthetic model, since many authors found a major incidence of thrombosis in tilting disc valves [1, 5]. Predisposing factors are atrial fibrillation, atrial thrombosis, previous embolism, difficult left atrial emptying, low output and turbulence related to prosthetic model [6]. The size of the prosthetic valves does not seem significant, while the role of age greater than 60 years [7] and megaatrium [8] is still controversial. It is noteworthy that thrombosis is absent in young patients (under 20 years old) [9] and its incidence is increased during pregnancy [1].

Some authors investigated other interesting aspects such as the interval between implant and thrombosis and the hypothesis of a genetic predisposition to thrombosis [9]. A lower incidence of thrombosis is reported for the aortic prosthesis compared with mitral and tricuspid implants [1], All prosthetic valves are undoubtedly predisposed to thrombogenicity: they activate coagulation factors and platelets a degree dependent on their prosthetic valve type (material and design). Little attention has been given to the periprosthetic fibroblastic proliferation which would be the primary event of thrombosis when it blocks the movement of the poppet [10]. In the past years, our research group analyzed possible statistically significant risk factors in patients who had undergone surgery for a preoperative diagnosis of thrombosis and the most important finding was the very high incidence of thrombosis in which the moving element of the prosthesis was gradually blocked to a complete arrest by an overgrowth of fibrous tissue that invaded the valve orifice. No bioprosthesis showed fibrous tissue ingrowth and therefore the phenomenon was defined as primary thrombosis: anticoagulant therapy would probably have been effective in preventing or limiting the obstruction while fibrinolytic therapy could resolve the acute obstruction. In our view, fibrous tissue cannot be an organized thrombus but more likely is a fibroblastic proliferation which for long periods remains limited to the periprosthetic endothelial connective tissue coating and may expand for unknown reasons and rapidly envelop the valve orifice [14] (Figure 2).

In a recent publication we reported the case of a patient with one blocked leaflet of a mechanical valve prosthesis on mitral position, that persisted for at least three months, without causing any secondary valve thrombosis. Intraoperatively, no thrombus and/or pannus was present. Despite an abnormal blood flow, the new phrostetic valves are resistant to secondary thrombosis [22].

Based on such data, analysis of our records identified risk factors that could affect this phenomenon: the incidence of obstruction was markedly lower for bioprostheses compared to mechanical valves and this is in agreement with the literature [3]. Obstruction of mechanical prostheses had an incidence at intermediate level as reported in the literature[3, 9], while mortality was high, even if immediate treatment was established. The obstruction was determined in most cases by the overgrowth of connective periprosthetic tissue which blocked the valve movement and 70% had adequate anticoagulant treatment. In the rest of cases with primary prosthetic thrombosis, anticoagulant therapy had been discontinued or was inadequate in a high percentage. No obstruction of tricuspid prostheses was observed and the incidence was markedly lower for aortic compared to mitral valves. Sex was not a significant risk factor while age between 40 and 50 turned to be a major risk. The importance of age has already been investigated in the literature [3]. Regarding the prosthetic design, the incidence of obstruction drops from tilting disc to bileaflet and to ball valves.

How this coating may affect fibroblastic proliferation and thrombogenesis in the context of obstruction of mechanical valves is not well established. Our experience confirms reports in the literature as far as the importance of the modality of transprosthetic flow in the origin of obstruction is concerned [5]. So the most important risk factors are large size, slow flow prostheses, tilting disc mitral valves with a small orifice oriented posteriorly where there is slow and turbulent flow, atrial fibrillation and a large left atrium. In addition the increased risk of thrombosis occurs in a period longer than 4 years after the implantation [3, 14] Primary importance has been attributed to the thrombogenic potential of available prosthetic valves and therefore to adequate anticoagulant therapy. No solution has yet been found for patients receiving adequate anticoagulation and for those receiving both coumadin and antiplatelet drugs who develop prosthetic thrombosis. The results of fibrinolytic therapy and prosthetic thrombectomy are not well documented. As far as the former is concerned, there is a high

http://dx.doi.org/10.5772/58479

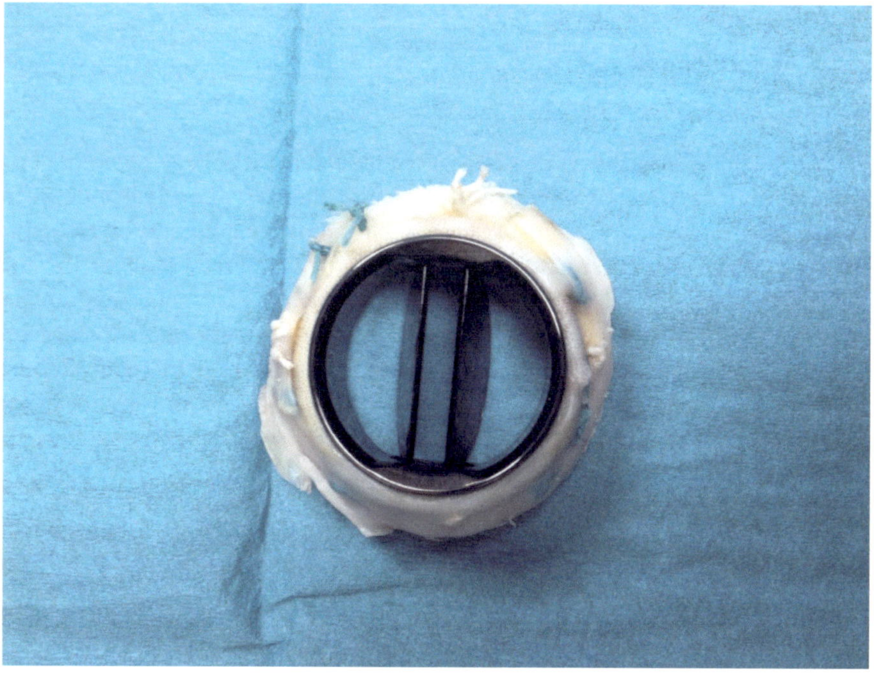

Figure 1. Last generation valve.

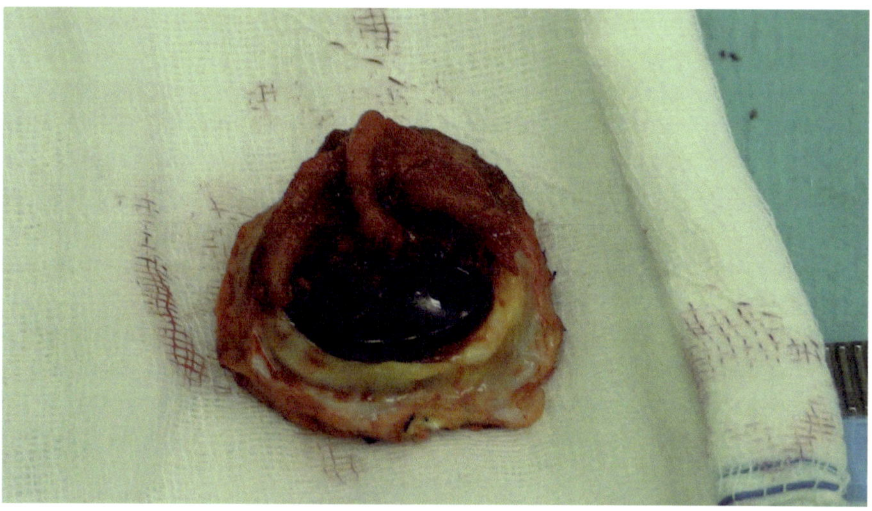

Figure 2. Thrombosis of a mechanical valve.

incidence of cases that do not benefit from this treatment with eventual fatal outcome or require second stage surgery. This incidence may vary from 25% to 38.46% [1]. As far as thrombectomy is concerned, there is a poorly documented high incidence of recurrent thrombosis [12]. A more appropriate subdivision of "biological obstruction" is:

A) primary thrombosis

B) secondary thrombosis

C) absence of thrombosis.

In the first case, thrombosis is determined by a thrombus that is the basic element of prosthetic malfunction; the anticoagulant prophylaxis may play a primary role and fibrinolytic treatment is indicated as confirmed by the almost complete success of this therapy in tricuspid valves where peri-prosthetic fibrous tissue is almost impossible to find. In these cases, thrombectomy may also give good results. In patients in groups B and C, prosthetic malfunction is not primarily determined by thrombosis, but by blockage of the moving element of the prosthesis due to overgrowth of peri-prosthetic fibrous tissue: thrombosis may follow this event (group B) or it may even be absent (group C). Fibrinolysis or thrombectomy may give only temporary and partial results or no result at all. Diagnostic procedures not always document precisely the type of obstruction and therefore the clinical picture and history of the patient, case by case, are more useful. Three different statistical evaluations allowed us to assess those risk factors that are important in determining prosthetic biological obstruction. Such factors are prosthetic design, pyrocarbon coating and valve orientation, time from the implant, local haemodynamic conditions and age. Other important risk factors might be pregnancy, endocarditis, bioprosthetic degeneration, composite conduits and individual predisposition [14]. Therefore, from what has been said before, it is clear that an acute obstruction is a life-threatening complication of mechanical valve prostheses, and is caused by the formation of fresh clot or fibrous tissue overgrowth, or both and the accurate selection of the most appropriate treatment for a particular patient is mandatory. Mechanical valve obstruction is currently the main reason for mechanical valve reoperations. Diagnosis of prosthetic obstruction is based on the presence of certain clinical, echocardiographic, fluoroscopic, and hemodynamic features. Symptoms are various: from palpitation to pulmonary edema or low output syndrome. Fluoroscopy examination can show a reduced or absent excursion of one or both prosthetic leaflets. It is very difficult to determine the morphologic process responsible for thrombosis preoperatively on the basis of the clinical, fluoroscopic, and hemodynamic features. In fact, fluoroscopic and hemodynamic investigations can only confirm the clinical diagnosis of prosthetic obstruction, but cannot give any further information concerning the nature of the obstruction. On the other hand, transesophageal echocardiography (TEE) is a very helpful diagnostic tool, when a prosthetic obstruction is suspected, especially for those obstructions due to primary thrombosis, as its resolution is superior to that of transthoracic echocardiography and it can better visualize thrombi on mechanical prosthetic valves and in cardiac chambers (Figure 3).

TEE has also proved useful for assessing thrombolysis results and for the long-term follow-up of patients after treatment for a thrombosed prosthesis. The TEE evidence of a thrombus seated, on a normal-functioning prosthesis or on the atrial walls is a further indication of thrombotic obstruction, improves the likelihood of successful thrombolysis in this setting (20). Cardiac catheterization may be useful to assess the coronary anatomy and plan the surgical strategy. The greater possibility of a successful treatment is time-dependent, because a thrombolytic agent is more effective on a fresh clot than on an organized one. For this reason, the 15-day

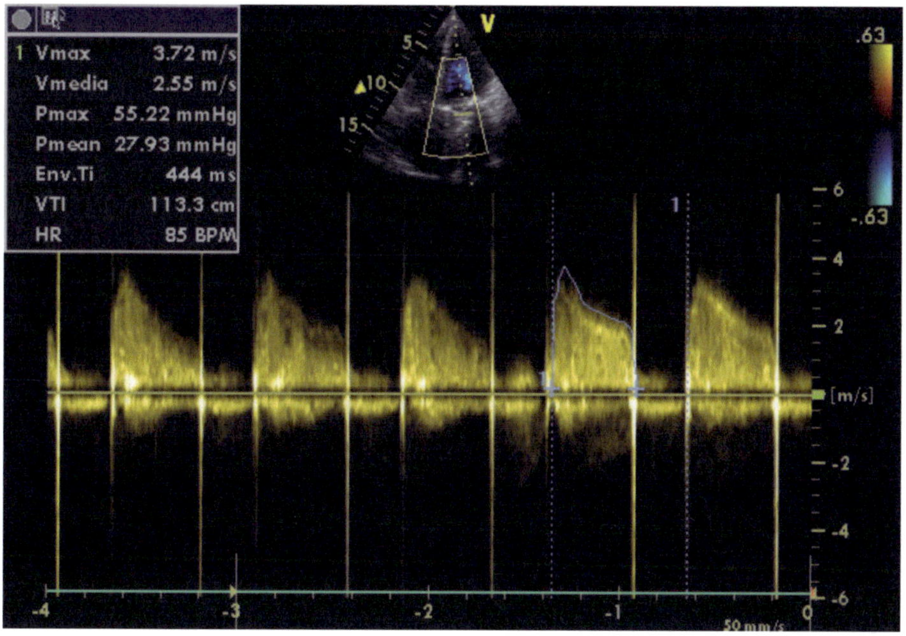

Figure 3. A transesophageal echocardiogram illustrating the presence of a thrombus in a mechanical valve.

cutoff has become the recommended period within which thrombolytic treatment should be initiated for pulmonary embolism [3, 14]. Many studies do not recommend the thrombolytic therapy in patients with left heart prostheses because of the high risk of precipitating cerebral or peripheral embolism. Our previous research found certain incidence of minor embolic complications in our series, and this has been noted by others too. On the other hand, the risk of permanent neurologic deficit or major peripheral embolism is not very high in these patients, as the embolism arises in patients already receiving fibrinolytic treatment. In this situation, if an embolism should occur, this indicates the need for a secondary form of fibrinolysis to reduce the risk of permanent damage. Nevertheless, more patients must be studied to adequately investigate the embolic risk in this setting [3, 14]

Our initial experience demonstrated the utility of thrombolysis in prosthetic valve obstruction. In fact in a previous study we enrolled 20 cases of prosthetic thrombosis treated with thrombolysis using recombinant tissue type plasminogen activator (rt-PA). Indication criteria for thrombolysis were: (i) recent onset of symptoms; (ii) transesophageal echocardiographic (TEE) evidence of clots on the valve or cardiac chambers; and (iii) a partially preserved disc excursion. All patients were fitted with mechanical valves on the left side. Symptoms of obstruction comprised cardiac failure in 11 cases and/or embolism in 10. After rt-PA infusion, normal prosthetic function was restored in all patients, though one underwent successful reoperation five days later. During infusion, five patients had a transient ischemic attack and one a minor transient peripheral embolism. Recurrence of thrombosis occurred in three patients during follow up; subsequent thrombolysis was successful in two, without any complication. A deeper knowledge of mechanism of valve obstruction improved our understanding of the indications, benefits, and limitations of the surgical and fibrinolytic treatment [3, 14].

For this purpose we still consider the following criteria valid indications for thrombolysis: TEE evidence of clots on the valve and chambers, and slightly reduced disc excursion. Thrombolysis in tilting disc valves is reserved only for non-obstructive thrombosis, because obstructive thrombosis in this valve model is generally sustained by pannus [15]. On the other hand, bi-leaflet valves are more prone to primary thrombosis than fibrous tissue overgrowth and sometimes the obstruction affects only one leaflet [15]. Therefore thrombolysis can be considered also when a reduced leaflet excursion is noted [15, 17]. Multi-plane TEE is the best investigative tool for the diagnosis of valve obstruction [18]. It is also useful to monitor thrombolysis outcome [16, 18]. Although some TEE features have been identified to differentiate pannus from thrombus [19], they are not totally reliable and the distinction is still left to the expertise of the echocardiographer. Clinical history and presentation are also helpful. Recombinant tissue-type plasminogen activator was used as it requires only a short course of infusion. A 25% rate of transient embolic complications was observed during treatment. Although no permanent damage resulted because of a secondary fibrinolysis, we acknowledge that the complication rate is high. It can be speculated that while thrombotic material from the mitral valve remains in the left cardiac chambers long enough to be dissolved completely, clot debris from the aortic valve move into the bloodstream immediately after detachment and dissolve only during embolization. As a consequence thrombolysis for aortic valve thrombosis may carry a higher embolic risk. We never had any bleeding complications. No heparin, either in infusion or subcutaneously, was started after thrombolysis and warfarin is restarted the same evening after thrombolysis and dypiridamole is added. We do not agree with the policy of carrying out thrombolysis in patients hemodynamically too unstable to undergo operation [18]. In this subset of patients prosthetic valve replacement is the best option, because thrombolytic drugs take several hours to be effective, and the same refers to heparin (Figure 4); therefore the patient will deteriorate even further, dramatically increasing the risk of redo operation, if fibrinolysis fails. Also, results with replacement have improved over the years, as with any redo procedures. In conclusion, we consider thrombolysis a valid treatment for non-obstructive prosthetic thrombosis only. In the future we may witness an increase in the number of thrombolyses with a decrease of prosthetic valve replacements, as bi-leaflet valves are the most widely implanted valve prostheses. Any time a blocked disc is detected pannus should be suspected, and the patient referred for operation. Patients should also be well informed of the risks of thrombolysis, especially embolism.

Treatment failure is therefore not due to choosing the wrong thrombolytic drug but, instead, to an incorrect perioperative diagnosis. Successful treatment is related to the ability to distinguish patients with primary thrombosis from those with peri-prosthetic fibrous tissue overgrowth. TEE makes this selection possible. In the sub-group of patients with prosthetic fibrotic obstruction, the only effective treatment currently available is prosthetic valve replacement, because, if the patient is in an unstable condition, reoperation is still the best therapeutic option. On the other hand, thrombolysis for the management of primary prosthetic thrombosis has a low incidence of severe complications and the morbidity and mortality related to the surgical procedure are avoided.

Regarding the valve thrombosis during pregnancy, the most suitable treatment seems to be the conservative approach, as confirmed by a single-center, prospective study including a large number of pregnant patients with a prosthetic valve thrombosis which demonstrated that low-dose, slow infusion of tPA is associated with successful thrombus lysis in all episodes, with lower incidence of maternal and fetal adverse events than surgery. So slow infusion of tPA with repeated doses as needed under TEE guidance seems to be effective and relatively safe for both mother and fetus, and the authors suggest that it should be used as first-line therapy for prosthetic valve thrombosis in pregnant women. [13]

2. Conclusions

Treatment failure is therefore not due to choosing the wrong thrombolytic drug but, instead, to an incorrect perioperative diagnosis. Successful treatment is related to the ability to distinguish patients with primary thrombosis from those with peri-prosthetic fibrous tissue overgrowth. TEE is helpful for the diagnosis. For the patients with prosthetic fibrotic obstruction, the only effective treatment currently available is the cardiac surgery with prosthetic valve replacement, because, if the patient is in an unstable condition, reoperation is still the best therapeutic option. On the other hand, thrombolysis for the management of primary prosthetic thrombosis has a low incidence of severe complications and the morbidity and mortality related to the surgical procedure are avoided.

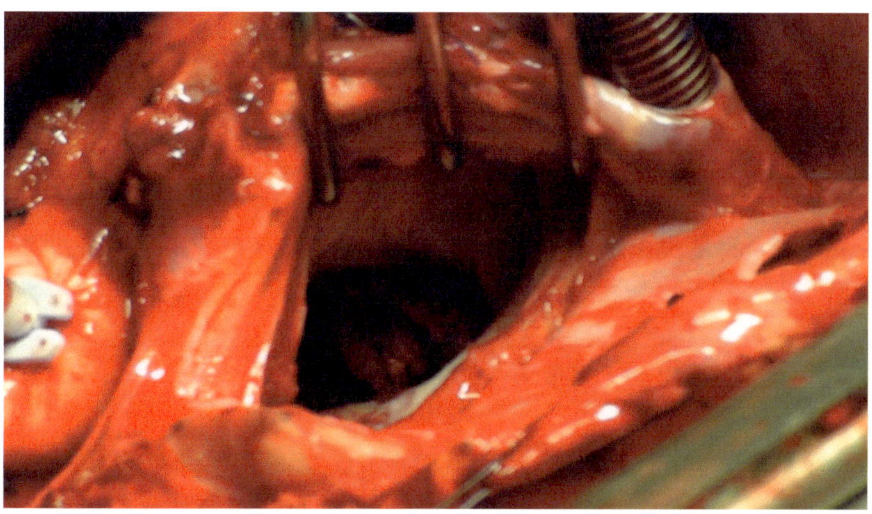

Figure 4. Surgery of mitral valve thrombosis.

Author details

Giuseppe Filiberto Serraino[1], Roberto Lorusso[2] and Attilio Renzulli[1]

1 Department of Cradiac Surgery, University Magna Graecia of Catanzaro, Italy

2 Cardiac Surgery Unit, Spedali Civili Brescia, Italy

References

[1] Edmunds LH Jr (1987) Thrombotic and bleeding complications of prosthetic heart valves. Ann Thorac Surg 44:430-445.

[2] Kontos GJ Jr, Schaff HV, Orszulak TA, Puga FJ, Pluth JR, Danielson GK (1989) Thrombotic obstruction of disc valves: clinical recognition and surgical management. Ann Thorac Surg 48: 60-65

[3] Antunes MJ (1986) Fate of thrombectomized Bjsrk-Shiley valves. J Thorac Cardiovasc Surg 92: 965-966

[4] Ledain LD, Ohayon JP, Colle JP, Lorient-Roudaut FM, Roudaut RP, Besse PM (1986) Acute thrombotic obstruction with disc valve prostheses: diagnostic consideration and ftbrinolytic treatment. J Am Co11 Cardiol 7:743-751

[5] Deville C, Ledain L, Roques X, Fernandez G, Besse P, Baudet E. Fontan F (1987) Traitement thrombolytique chirurgical dans les thromboses valvulaires. Ann Chir: Chir Thorac Cardiovasc 41:135-142

[6] Cabrol C, Cabrol A, Gandjbakhch I, Guiraudon G, Christides C, Mattei MF, Cappe MH (1976) The mitral valve. Publishing Sciences Group, Acton Massachusetts, pp 431-436

[7] Williams JB, Karp RB, Kirklin JW, Kouchoukos NT, Pacifico AD, Zorn GL Jr, Blackstone EH, Brown RN, Piantadosi S, Bradley EL (1980) Considerations in selection and management of patients undergoing valve replacement with glutaraldehydefixed porcine bioprostheses. Ann Thorac Surg 30:247-258

[8] Chaux A, Czer LSC, Matloff JM, De Robertis MA, Stewart ME, Bateman TM, Kass RM, Lee ME, Gray RJ (1984) The St. Jude Medical bileaflet valve prosthesis: a live year experience. J Thorac Cardiovasc Surg 88:706-717

[9] Venugopal P, Kaul U, Iyer KS, Rao IM, Balzam A, Das B, Sampathkumar A, Mukherjee S, Rajani M, Wasiz HS, Bhatia ML, Raghavan V, Reddy KS, Gopinath N (1986) Fate of thrombectomized Bjork-Shiley valves. A long term cinefluoroscopic echocardiographic and haemodynamic evaluation. J Thorac Cardiovasc Surg 91:168-173

[10] Agozzino L, Bellitti R, Schettini S, Cotrufo M (1984) Acute thrombosis of Sorin tilting disc mitral prostheses. Int J Cardiol 5:351-359

[11] Witchitz S, Veyrat C, Moisson P, Scheinman N, Rozens&jn L (1980) Fibrinolytic treatment of thrombus on prosthetic heart valves. Br Heart J 44: 545 – 554

[12] Lebart L, Morineau A, Tabard N (1977) Technique de la description statistique. Dunod, Paris

[13] Mehmet O; Beytullah Ç, Su®leyman K, Ozan MG, Cihan C, Macit K, Ali EO, Sabahattin G, Mehmet AA, Ahmet CA, Zu®beyde B, Murat B, Evren K, Gökhan K, Nilu®fer ED, Mustafa Y Thrombolytic Therapy for the Treatment of Prosthetic Heart Valve Thrombosis in Pregnancy With Low-Dose, Slow Infusion of Tissue-Type Plasminogen Activator. *Circulation.* 2013;128:532-540;

[14] Copans H, Lakier JB, Kinsley RH, Colsen PR, Fritz VU, Barlow JB (1980) Thrombosed Bjerk-Shiley mitral prostheses. Circulation 61:168-174

[15] Vitale N, Renzulli A, Agozzino A, Tedesco N, de Luca Tupputi Schinosa L, Cotrufo M. Obstruction of mechanical mitral prostheses: analysis of pathologic findings Ann Thorac Surg 1997;63:1101– 6.

[16] Renzulli A, Vitale N, Caruso A, Dialetto G, de Luca Tupputi Schinosa L, Cotrufo M. Thrombolysis for prosthetic valve thrombosis: indications and results J Heart Valve Dis 1997;6: 212–8.

[17] Silber H, Khan SS, Matloff JM, Chaux A, DeRobertis M, Gray R. The St Jude valve: thrombolysis as the first line therapy for cardiac valve thrombosis Circulation 1993;87:30–7.

[18] Lengyel M, Fuster V, Keltal M, et al. Guidelines for management of left-sided prosthetic valve thrombosis: a role for thrombolytic therapy J Am Coll Cardiol 1997;30:1521– 6.

[19] Barbetseas J, Naguegh SF, Pitsavos C, Toutouzas PK, Quinones MA, Zoighbi WA. Role of trans-esophageal echocardiography in differentiating pannus from thrombus in obstructed prosthetic valves. J Am Coll Cardiol 1998;31(Suppl 1):463A–4A.

[20] Ozkan M, Gunduz S, Yildiz M et al Diagnosis of the prosthetic heart valve pannus formation with real time three-dimensional transoesophageal echocardiography. Eur J Echocadiogr. 2010; 11: E17.

[21] Cervik C, Izgi C, Dechyapirom W, et al. Treatment of prosthetic valve thrombosis: rationale for a prospective randomized clinical trial. J Heart Valve Dis. 2010;19:161-170.

[22] Jiritano F, Serraino GF, Rossi M, Pisano G, Renzulli A. Resistance to secondary thrombosis of the On-X mitral prosthesis. J Heart Valve Dis. 2013 Sep; 22(5):740-2.

Chapter 9

Coagulation and Fibrinolysis Abnormalities in Patients with Muscular Dystrophy

Toshio Saito

Additional information is available at the end of the chapter

http://dx.doi.org/10.5772/57411

1. Introduction

The cause of the Duchenne muscular dystrophy (DMD) is deficiency of the dystrophin protein leading to dysfunction of many organs. Originally it was thought that the natural history of this disease limits the lifespan of the patients to 20 year. However, positive therapeutic interventions for heart failure, respiratory failure, nutritional management, spinal surgery and the rehabilitation raised the lifespan of patients with DMD in Japan above 30 years of age. (Ishikawa Y, et al. 2011) (Matsumura T, et al. 2011) (Saito T, et al. 2011). Consequently, nowadays complications accompanying the higher survival age of DMD patients should also be considered. This chapter describes a coagulation and fibrinolysis abnormality of muscular dystrophy, and its involvement in the microcirculation disorder accompanying this disease.

2. The old tale of DMD as a microcirculation disorder

Historically before the discovery of dystrophin, a hypothesis was proposed that blood circulation insufficiency due to intravascular obstruction causes muscle necrosis in DMD. This hypothesis was based on muscle histopathology findings similar to necrosis caused by circulation insufficiency. There were some reports that tried to model the pathologic condition of DMD with impaired circulation. However, these trials to reproduce the DMD pathology were unsuccessful. (Bradley WG, et al. 1975) (Gudrun B, et al. 1975) (Leinonen H, et al. 1979)

Meanwhile Miike T, et al. described vascular obstruction and vascular endothelial hyperplasia, namely the blister-like swelling of vascular endothelial cells in the muscle histopathology of non-symptomatic children with DMD, and put forward a hypothesis of the blood flow abnormality that affects the progress of DMD (Miike T, et al. 1987). After the discovery of dystrophin, the mainstream theory for the pathogenesis of DMD became the muscle destruction due to the membranous fragility related to dystrophin defects. Since then the vascular disorders in DMD have been regarded not important.

3. Thrombosis and embolization as complication of DMD

There are some reports related to thrombosis or embolization of patients with DMD.

In 1982, Matsuishi T, et al. reported a basilar artery occlusion in a case of DMD, in which the pathogenesis of infarction was uncertain. (Matsuishi T, et al. 1982) In 1989, Gaffney JF, et al reported left ventricular thrombus and systemic emboli complicating the cardiomyopathy of DMD. (Gaffney JF, et al. 1989) Authors showed anteroseptal mural thrombus and right atrial thrombus as autopsy findings. Riggs T also reported three terminal DMD cases of cardiomyopathy and pulmonary emboli. (Riggs T. 1990) Author showed thrombus formation of ventricle and pulmonary embolus with a ventilation perfusion scan.

The epidemiologic aspects of DMD-related thromboembolism were addressed by Biller J, et al., who reported the frequency of cerebral infarction in patients with inherited neuromuscular diseases including DMD, Becker muscular dystrophy (BMD), myotonic dystrophy, and Freidrich ataxia. According to their data cerebral infarction was seen in 1. 5% of the cases with these diseases and concluded that cerebral infarction is uncommon in neuromuscular diseases.

4. Pioneer studies of coagulation and fibrinolysis abnormalities of DMD in Japan

Among annual reports of clinical research group for muscular dystrophy in Japan, some reports described cases of cerebral infarction and pulmonary embolism in patients with DMD. Ishihara T, et al. reported series of 15 autopsied cases of DMD/BMD with hemorrhagic pulmonary infarction in 1990. He pointed out that this disorder is an important cause of death in DMD. Matsuka Y, et al. reported a DMD case of cerebral infarction and thrombus formation in the left ventricle in 1991, and described elevated levels of thrombin-antithrombin complex (TAT) and platelet factor 4 (PF4) among many DMD cases with CTR>50% in 1993. Hanajima, et al. reported the occurrence of cerebral infarction of DMD in muscular dystrophy wards in Japan to be 5 / 269 DMD patients aged from 16 to 20 years old. Authors concluded that cerebral infarction is not a rare complication of DMD. (Hanajima, et al. 1996)

Based on these findings the clinical research team for the genetic counseling and the clinical research of the pathology and treatment in muscular dystrophy patients (from 1996 to 1998), that was directed by Ishihara T, proposed a research and intervention project to investigate the blood coagulation disorder complicating the muscular dystrophy. In next section, results of the research in this team are described.

http://dx.doi.org/10.5772/57411

5. Abnormal coagulation and fibrinolysis in DMD

Saito Y, et al. reported hypercoagulable state in patients with DMD. (Saito Y, et al. 1997) By the blood coagulation test of patients with DMD and other neuromuscular diseases at rest condition, the authors showed that abnormal findings appear in many coagulation and fibrinolysis parameters such as thrombotest, TAT, and plasmin $-\alpha 2$ Plasmin inhibitor complex (PIC) in DMD. Namely, level of thrombotest, which reflects coagulation activity including effect of PIVKA (used for monitoring warfarin treatment), was low compared to normal range in 78% of DMD, TAT level was elevated in 61% of DMD, and PIC level elevated in 40. 3% of DMD. Abnormality of the coagulation and fibrinolysis was found in most patients with DMD. The frequency of abnormality was high compared with other neuromuscular diseases.

In this report, the ratio of abnormal value of D-dimer and fibrin and fibrinogen degradation products (FDP) was low in DMD, authors described that coagulation cascade is more enhanced than fibrinolysis cascade in patients with DMD. The coagulation and fibrinolysis abnormality was not associated with age, respiratory function, cardiac activity, and activities of daily living. Authors concluded that muscular dystrophy itself is a risk factor for thrombosis.

Based on examination of relation with the muscle destruction Saito T, et al. reported that coagulation and fibrinolysis abnormality is strongly present in younger patients with DMD, BMD, and Fukuyama congenital muscular dystrophy (FCMD). (Saito T, et al. 2001) They showed significant correlation between serum levels of FDP and MM isozyme of creatine kinase (CK-MM), irrespective of type of dystrophy. Figure 1 shows correlation between FDP and CK-MM of patients with DMD, whereas Figure 2 shows correlation between FDP and D-dimer. Levels of FDP were higher at ambulatory young boy with high CK DMD. Authors speculated that enhanced coagulation and fibrinolysis in DMD, BMD, and FCMD is induced by some components that leak from destructed muscle. It is inferred that the disturbances of the coagulation and fibrinolysis result from the muscle destruction. Increase of both plasma levels of D-dimer and serum levels of FDP is an indirect proof of thrombus having been present in vivo. It means that microcirculation disorder is possibly present in DMD, BMD, and FCMD potentially.

In this study advanced DMD patients with low CK showed no abnormal elevation of FDP and D-dimer. However, even DMD patients in advanced stage, whose CK levels were within normal range, showed coagulation abnormalities, if serum CK increased as a consequence of muscle destruction induced by various causative factors. Saito T, et al. reported activated coagulation cascade in a case of advanced DMD that showed transient elevation of serum CK due to convulsion. (Saito T, et al. 2003) These phenomena are possible sources of pulmonary emboli accompanying DMD. Nakayama T, et al. established that CK elevation preceded the development of pulmonary embolism in patients with DMD (Nakayama T, et al. 2000).

6. Abnormal coagulation and fibrinolysis in cases of dystrophinopathy with heart failure

There is evidence for association between cardiac dysfunction and coagulation disorder. Saito T, et al. reported that levels of TAT and prothrombin fragment (F1+2) in DMD patients

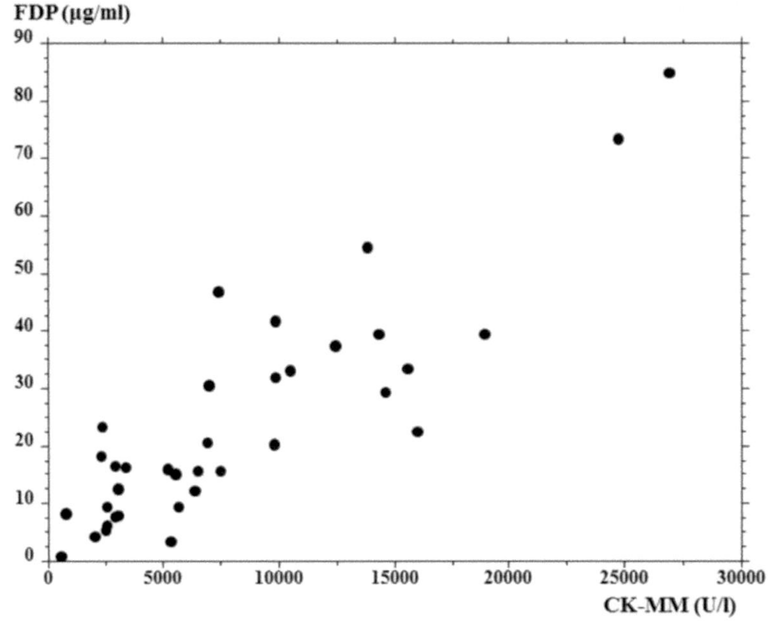

Figure 1. Correlation of serum FDP and CK-MM in patients with DMD, Serum CK-MM level is significantly correlated with FDP. n=36, (modified figure of literature, Saito T, et al. 2001)

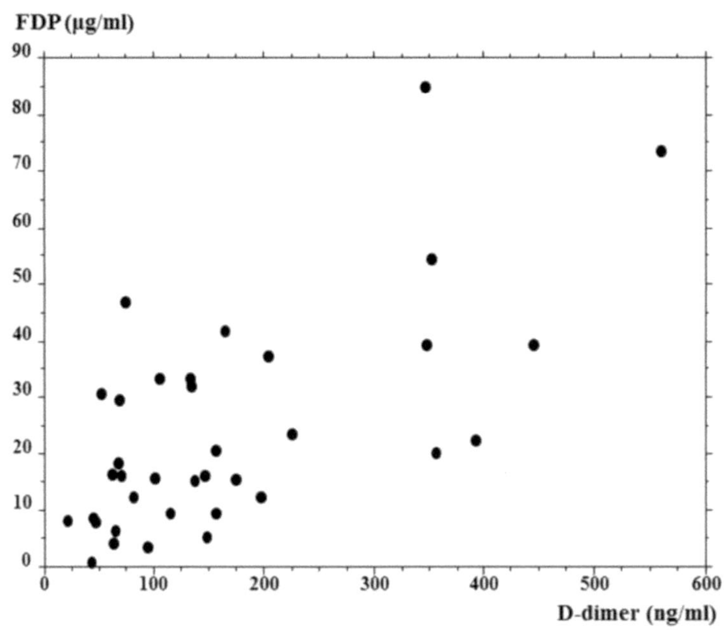

Figure 2. Correlation of serum FDP and plasma D-dimer in patients with DMD, Although correlation between FDP and D-dimer was not significant, both FDP and D-dimer elevated in DMD patients. n=36 (modified figure of literature, Saito T, et al. 2001)

with the markedly depressed cardiac function were significantly elevated compared to DMD patients with preserved cardiac function. Authors concluded that activated coagulation is associated with cardiac dysfunction in patients with DMD. (Saito T, et al. 2005) Porreca E, et al. also reported similar findings in patients with dystrophinopathy including BMD. (Porreca E, et al. 1999) These abnormalities probably induce cerebral infarction through a mechanism similar to the one observed in idiopathic cardiomyopathy. Ikeniwa C, et al. reported two cases of DMD with dilated cardiomyopathy and cerebral infarction. (Ikeni-wa C, et al. 2006)

7. Studies of other factors affecting coagulation and fibrinolysis status

In addition to the cases described above, the clinical research group for muscular dystrophy in Japan reported that infectious diseases activate coagulation cascade by increasing the level of fibrinogen resulting in elevation of D-dimer. However, this acute-phase reaction induced by infection is observed generally in normal subjects too.

An interventional study was also proposed in the form of a clinical trial to administer warfarin for DMD/BMD patients with high risk of thrombosis. Within its framework information regarding the coagulation status of 190 DMD/BMD patients in muscular dystrophy wards in Japan was collected abnormal rate of TAT was 36. 0%, and that of F1+2 was 51. 2% in DMD patients, which demonstrated that enhanced blood coagulation was dominant in DMD patients. However, the number of patients recruited in this clinical trial was too small, so the trial was not started. Instead of clinical trial, they proposed substitute treatment, namely improving congestion in venous return of bedridden patients with DMD, and prevention of dehydration.

8. Platelet abnormalities in DMD

Forst J, et al. reported a significant deficiency of platelet adhesion and ristocetin induced aggregation as well as a marked reduction of expression of glycoprotein IV, although normal plasmatic coagulation and a slight but not significant increase of bleeding time was observed in DMD patients (Forst J, et al. 1998). Authors speculated that the platelet function deficiency occurs because of a decompensation of platelet adhesion as well as aggregation capacity in major spinal surgery, although the deficiency of platelet function in DMD patients does not affect ordinary life or minor surgery.

Further, Matsumura T, et al. reported a case of DMD complicated by thrombotic thrombocy-topenic purpura (TTP). In their report, TTP was confirmed by decreased activity of von Willebrand factor cleaving protease and activity plasma exchange was successful for the patient (Matsumura T, et al. 2003).

9. Pathogenetic aspects of the coagulation abnormalities in Duchenne muscular dystrophy

From the point of view that coagulation disorders induce microcirculation abnormalities, Saito T, et al. speculated that hypoxic and ischemic condition might exist in DMD. They reported that elevated levels of VEGF are observed in dystrophinopathy patients, and supposed that these are induced by relative hypoxic and ischemic condition. (Saito T, et al. 2009) However, these conditions were marked in advanced DMD patients rather than young boy with DMD.

On the other hand, it has been considered that circulation abnormality may participate in disease progression of DMD, which has not been evaluated for a long time since dominance of membrane theory. (Lombard JH. 2011) Functional muscle ischemia has been reported in patients with DMD. (Sander M, et al. 2000) Defect of nNOS due to dystrophin absence induce functional muscle ischemia related muscle exercise, which can induce microcirculation insufficiency of muscle tissue. Asai A, et al. reported effectiveness of Phosphodiesterase-5 Inhibitor to mouse model of muscular dystrophy by improving microcirculation of muscle tissue. (Asai A, et al. 2007)

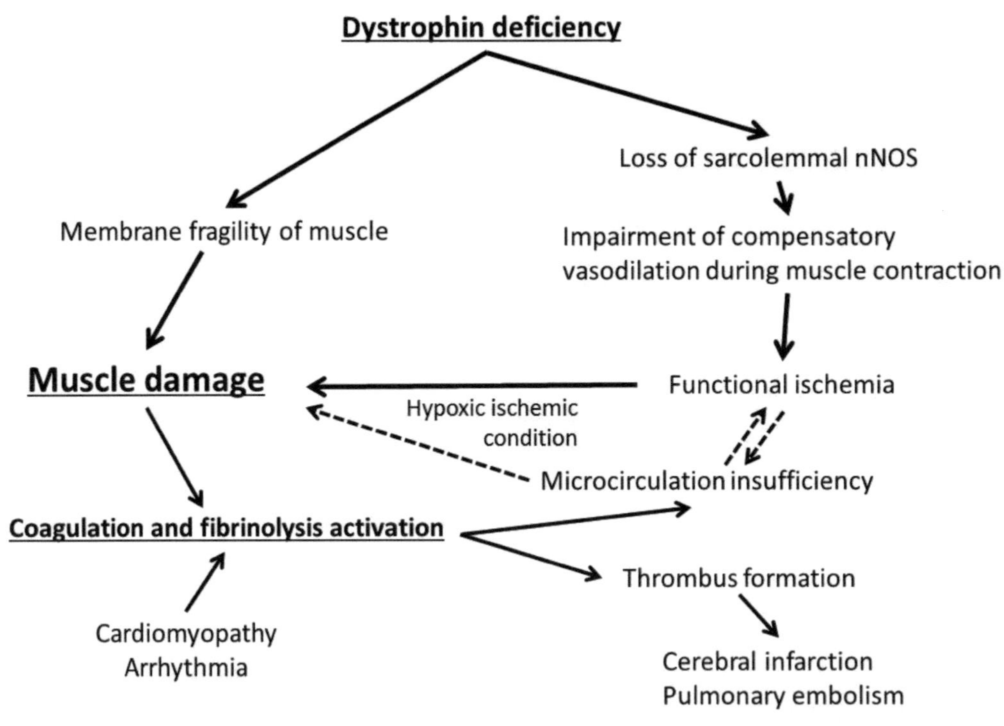

Figure 3. Muscle destruction process and the relation to coagulation and fibrinolysis adnormalities in DMD patients

In Figure 3, I summarize the muscle destruction process and the relation to coagulation and fibrinolysis adnormalities in DMD patients. The origin of DMD is dystrophin deficiency. Dystrophin deficiency induces functional muscle ischemia as well as membrane fragility of muscle, leading to muscle destruction. Muscle destruction activates coagulation and fibrinolysis cascade (, which may be similar to rhabdomyolysis). Activated cascade induces microcirculation insufficiency affecting functional muscle ischemia derive from dystrophin deficiency. On the other hand, cardiomyopathy and arrhythmia cause thrombus formation with mechanism similar to idiopathic dilated cardiomyopathy, which can cause cerebral infarction and pulmonary embolism. Moreover, transient muscle damage even in advanced DMD patients activates coagulation cascade leading to cerebral infarction and pulmonary embolism.

Therefore, improving microcirculation insufficiency, and coagulation and fibrinolysis abnormalities may lead to improving disease progression and prevention of complications in DMD patients. Now, the level of peripheral circulating CD34 positive cells, namely endothelial circulating progenitor cell related with vascular homeostasis, functional maintenance and angiogenesis, is evaluated whether it can be the biomarker reflecting microcirculation abnormality and disease progression of DMD (Saito T, et al. 2013).

Author details

Toshio Saito*

Division of Child Neurology, Department of Neurology, National Hospital Organization Toneyama National Hospital, Japan

References

[1] Asai A, Sahani N, Kaneki M, Ouchi Y, Martyn JAJ, Egusa Yasuhara S. Primary Role of Functional Ischemia, Quantitative Evidence for the Two-Hit Mechanism, and Phosphodiesterase-5 Inhibitor Therapy in Mouse Muscular Dystrophy. PLoS ONE. 2007 2(8) : e806. doi:10. 1371/journal. pone. 0000806.

[2] Bradley WG, O'Brien MD, Walder DN, Murchison D, Johnson M, Newell DJ . Failure to confirm a vascular cause of muscular dystrophy. Arch Neurol. 1975 Jul;32(7) : 466-73.

[3] Biller J, Ionasescu V, Zellweger H, Adams HP Jr, Schultz DT. Frequency of cerebral infarction in patients with inherited neuromuscular diseases. Stroke. 1987 Jul-Aug; 18(4) :805-7.

[4] Forst J, Forst R, Leithe H, Maurin N. Platelet function deficiency in Duchenne muscular dystrophy. NeuromusculDisord. 1998 Feb;8(1) :46-9.

[5] Gaffney JF, Kingston WJ, Metlay LA, Gramiak R. Left ventricular thrombus and systemic emboli complicating the cardiomyopathy of Duchenne's muscular dystrophy. Arch Neurol. 1989 Nov;46(11) :1249-52.

[6] Gudrun B, Andrew GE, Boysen G, Engel AG. Effects of microembolization on the skeletal muscle blood flow. A critique of the microvascular occlusion model ofDuchenne dystrophy. ActaNeurol Scand. 1975 Jul;52(1) :71-80.

[7] Hanajima R, Kawai M. Incidence of cerebral infarction in Duchenne muscular dystrophy. Muscle Nerve. 1996 Jul;19(7) :928.

[8] Ikeniwa C, Sakai M, Kimura S, Wakayama T, Kuru S, Yasuma F, Konagaya M. Two cases of Duchenne muscular dystrophy complicated with dilated cardiomyopathy and cerebral infarction. No To Shinkei. 2006 Mar;58(3) :250-5

[9] Ishikawa Y, Miura T, Ishikawa Y, Aoyagi T, Ogata H, Hamada S, Minami R. Duchenne muscular dystrophy: survival by cardio-respiratory interventions. NeuromusculDisord. 2011 Jan;21(1) :47-51.

[10] Leinonen H, Juntunen J, Somer H, Rapola J. Capillary circulation and morphology in Duchenne muscular dystrophy. Eur Neurol. 1979;18(4) :249-55.

[11] Lombard JH. Microcirculation in a mouse model of Duchenne muscular dystrophy: another blow to the vascular hypothesis? J ApplPhysiol (1985) . 2011 Mar;110(3) : 587-8.

[12] Matsuishi T, Yano E, Terasawa K, Nonaka I, Ishihara O, Yamaguchi Y, Okudera T. Basilar artery occlusion in a case of Duchenne muscular dystrophy. Brain Dev. 1982;4(5) :379-84.

[13] Matsumura T, Saito T, Fujimura H, Shinno S, Sakoda S. A longitudinal cause-of-death analysis of patients with Duchenne muscular dystrophy. RinshoShinkeigaku. 2011 Oct;51(10) :743-50.

[14] Matsumura T, Yokoe M, Saito T, Kunitomi A, Nozaki S, Shinno S. A case of Duchenne muscular dystrophy complicated by thrombotic thrombocytopenic purpura. RinshoShinkeigaku. 2003 Jan-Feb;43(1-2) :31-4.

[15] Miike T, Sugino S, Ohtani Y, Taku K, Yoshioka K. Vascular endothelial cell injury and platelet embolism in Duchenne muscular dystrophy at the preclinical stage. J Neurol Sci. 1987 Dec;82(1-3) :67-80.

[16] Nakayama T, Saito Y, Uchiyama T, Yatabe K, Kawai M. Pathogenesis of pulmonary thrombosis in Duchenne muscular dystrophy; a consideration from changes in serum CK and LDH levels. RinshoShinkeigaku. 2000 Jan;40(1) :55-8.

[17] Porreca E, Guglielmi MD, Uncini A, Di Gregorio P, Angelini A, Di Febbo C, Pierdomenico SD, Baccante G, Cuccurullo F. Haemostatic abnormalities, cardiac involve-

ment and serum tumor necrosis factor levels in X-linked dystrophic patients. ThrombHaemost. 1999 Apr;81(4) :543-6.

[18] Reports of the clinical research team for the genetic counseling and the clinical research of the pathology and treatment in muscular dystrophy patients 1996 – 1998. 1999.

[19] Reports of National Research Group for Establishment of Genetic Counseling and Development of Treatments based on the Pathophysiology in Muscular Dystrophy Patients 1999 – 2001. 2002.

[20] Riggs T. Cardiomyopathy and pulmonary emboli in terminal Duchenne's muscular dystrophy. Am Heart J. 1990 Mar;119(3 Pt 1) :690-3.

[21] Saito T, Kikuchi-Taura A, Tada S, Iyama A, Kimura N, Matsumura T, Fujimura H, Sakoda S. Molecular biomarker of angiogenesis in neuromuscular disorders. Neuromuscul Disord. 2013 23:809.

[22] Saito T, Takenaka M, Miyai I, Yamamoto Y, Matsumura T, Nozaki S, Kang J. Coagulation and fibrinolysis disorder in muscular dystrophy. Muscle Nerve. 2001 Mar; 24(3) :399-402.

[23] Saito T, Matsumura T, Nozaki S, Shinno S. A case of Duchenne muscular dystrophy showing coagulation cascade activation induced by muscle destruction due to convulsion. RinshoShinkeigaku. 2003 May;43(5) :274-6.

[24] Saito T, Yamamoto Y, Matsumura T, Nozaki S, Fujimura H, Shinno S. Coagulation system activated in Duchenne muscular dystrophy patients with cardiac dysfunction. Brain Dev. 2005 Sep;27(6) :415-8.

[25] Saito T, Yamamoto Y, Matsumura T, Fujimura H, Shinno S. Serum levels of vascular endothelial growth factor elevated in patients with muscular dystrophy. Brain Dev. 2009 Sep;31(8) :612-7.

[26] Saito Y, Komiya T, Kawai M. Hypercoagulable state in Duchenne muscular dystrophy. RinshoShinkeigaku. 1997 May;37(5) :374-8.

[27] Sander M, Chavoshan B, Harris SA, Iannaccone ST, Stull JT, Thomas GD, Victor RG. Functional muscle ischemia in neuronal nitric oxide synthase-deficient skeletal muscle of children with Duchenne muscular dystrophy. Proc Natl Acad Sci USA. 2000 97: 13818–23.